Local Health Traditions

Local Health Traditions

Plurality and Marginality in South Asia

Edited by

Arima Mishra

Orient BlackSwan

LOCAL HEALTH TRADITIONS: PLURALITY AND MARGINALITY IN SOUTH ASIA

ORIENT BLACKSWAN PRIVATE LIMITED

Registered Office
3-6-752 Himayatnagar, Hyderabad 500 029, Telangana, India
e-mail: centraloffice@orientblackswan.com

Other Offices
Bengaluru, Bhopal, Chennai, Ernakulam, Guwahati,
Hyderabad, Jaipur, Kolkata, Lucknow, Mumbai,
New Delhi, Noida, Patna, Visakhapatnam

First published by Orient BlackSwan in 2019

ISBN 978-93-5287-661-7

Typeset in
Adobe Jenson Pro 10.5/12.6
by Le Studio Graphique, Gurgaon 122 001

Printed in India at
Glorious Printers, Delhi

Published by
Orient Blackswan Private Limited
3-6-752, Himayatnagar, Hyderabad 500 029, Telangana, India
e-mail: info@orientblackswan.com

Contents

Abbreviations

ABS	Access and benefit sharing
ACPL	Accreditation and Certification of Prior Learning
AICRPE	All India Coordinated Research Project on Ethno-biology
ANANDI	Area Networking and Development Initiatives
ANM	Auxiliary nurse midwife
APU	Azim Premji University
ART	Antiretroviral therapy
ASHA	Accredited Social Health Activist
ATSVS	Akila Thiruvithancore Siddha Vaidhya Sangam
AVP	Arya Vaidya Pharmacy Ltd.
AYUSH	Ayurveda, yoga, naturopathy, unani, siddha and homeopathy
BAMS	Bachelor in Ayurvedic Medicine and Surgery
BHMS	Bachelor of Homeopathic Medicine and Surgery
BMC	Biodiversity Management Committee
BPL	Below poverty line
BSMS	Bachelor in Siddha Medicine and Surgery
CAM	Complementary and alternative medicine
CARe Keralam	Confederation of Ayurvedic Renaissance, Keralam
CBD	Convention on Biological Diversity
CBO	Community-based organisation
C-DIT	Centre for Development of Imaging Technology
CDC	Centre for Disease Control
CTKS	Centre for Traditional Knowledge Systems
DOTS	Directly observed treatment, short course
DRALHT	Documentation and rapid assessment of local health traditions

DMF	Drug master file
FET	Fisher's Exact Tests
FRLHT	Foundation for Revitalisation of Local Health Traditions
GMP	Good Manufacturing Practice
HC	Health Care
ICMR	Indian Council of Medical Research
IGNOU	Indira Gandhi National Open University
ILC	Indigenous and local communities
IPR	Intellectual property rights
ISM&H	Indian Systems of Medicine and Homeopathy
JNTBGRI	Jawaharlal Nehru Tropical Botanical Garden and Research Institute
JSS	Jan Swasthya Sahyog
JSY	Janani Suraksha Yojana
KILA	Kerala Institute for Local Administration
KIRTADS	Kerala Institute of Research, Training and Development Studies of Scheduled Castes and Scheduled Tribes
KSMCS	Kerala Sidha Marma Chikitsa Sangham
KSSP	Kerala Sasthra Sahitya Praishad
LSPSS	Lok Swasthya Parampara Samvardhan Samiti
MATRIKA	Motherhood and Traditional Resources, Information, Knowledge and Action
MBBS	Bachelor of Medicine, Bachelor of Surgery
MCH	Maternal and child health
MDG	Millennium development goals
MGNREGS	Mahatma Gandhi National Rural Employment Guarantee Scheme
MoEF	Ministry of Environment and Forest
MoU	Memorandum of understanding
MSC	Minimum standards of competence
NADRI	National Ayurveda Dietics Research Institute
NBA	National Biodiversity Authority
NCAER	National Council of Applied Economic Research
NEIFM	North Eastern Institute for Folk Medicine

NFHS	National Family Health Survey
NGO	Non-governmental organisation
NIH	National Institute of Health
NK	North Kanara
NRHM	National Rural Health Mission
NSSO	National Sample Survey Organisation
PBR	People's Biodiversity Register
PIC	Prior informed consent
QCI	Quality Council of India
RALHT	Rapid Assessment of Local Health Tradition
RMP	Registered medical practitioner
SAHAJ	Society for Health Alternatives
SARTHI	Social Action for Rural and Tribal Inhabitants of India
SBA	Skilled birth attendant
SEWA (Rural)	Society for Education Welfare and Action
SK	South Kanara
TBA	Traditional birth attendant
TBGRI	Tropical Botanic Garden and Research Institute
TCHP	Traditional community health care providers
TKDL	Traditional Knowledge Digital Library
TK	Traditional knowledge
TKD	Traditional knowledge documentation
TKIK	Traditional Knowledge Innovation, Kerala
UHC	Universal health coverage
UNESCO	United Nations Educational, Scientific and Cultural Organization
USAID	United States Agency for International Development
VCSTCHP	Voluntary Certification Scheme for Traditional Community Healthcare Providers
WHO	World Health Organization
WIPO	World Intellectual Property Organization

Tables, Images, and Appendices

Tables

Images

Appendices

Acknowledgements

This volume on 'local health traditions' has indeed been a collective journey of thinking, reflecting and writing together. Many people have contributed in different ways to this volume. While I may not be able to mention all the names here, I mean to sincerely acknowledge every single person, experience and input that helped in bringing this volume to its fruition.

The idea for this volume emerged from our research study on 'Policy lessons *of* and *for* revitalization of local health traditions in three southern states' (2014–16). The ethnographic research journey for this study has been unusual yet exciting, even as we initially struggled to decipher the category of local health traditions and identify terms of usage in different field sites and people we worked with. It looked familiar, yet not quite so. Thanks to all the traditional healers [we spoke to in Karnataka, Kerala and Tamil Nadu] who have helped us realise the significance of different ways of knowing, learning and practising health and medicine. I am so thankful to all the members of the research team, including Devaki Nambiar, Harilal Madhavan, Pooja Ventakesh, Sarika Kadam, Steffy P., Lakshmi Priya, Praveen Lal, Shrish N., Maya Elias, and Rajeev B. R. as we collectively sailed through this reflective process of learning together.

I am so grateful to the Research Centre at the Azim Premji University for supporting this study. Our study made us realise that we need a space for an enriching conversation around local health traditions in the contemporary context. I thank each of the contributors who agreed to join this conversation. They are from different disciplinary backgrounds, but are bound by a shared commitment to this marginal category of community health knowledge and practice.

I thank the participants in the seminars and conferences where some of the chapters were presented. Their inputs have helped in sharpening the ideas discussed in these chapters. Thanks to Ravi Narayan, Thelma

Narayan [SOCHARA], Ritu Priya [JNU], and Hariramamurthi G. [FRLHT/TDU] for their support and encouragement in engaging with discussions on local health traditions.

I thank my Master's students at the University who have been part of several discussions around local health traditions discussed in the book. I have benefitted from their views and experiences shared in the most creative ways during class discussions.

A very special note of thanks goes to Devaki Nambiar, my friend, colleague and collaborator. I have enjoyed every moment of our discussing and writing together on various aspects of local health traditions. This book owes her a lot for the inputs she has shared at different stages, from conceptualisation to writing.

I thank *Deccan Herald, Siraj Daily,* Shine Vaidyar and Christian Sebastian for allowing us to use the newspaper clippings and other pictures in the book.

Thanks to the team at Orient BlackSwan, including Roopa, Nilanjana and Proteeti, who have taken great care to turn the manuscript into this book.

Lastly but most importantly, the book owes a lot to the good wishes and continuous support of my family members, including my parents, brothers and sister, my husband Umesh and son Abhinav.

Introduction

Arima Mishra

The study of medical pluralism has produced a rich body of knowledge in medical anthropology, beginning with the seminal work of Charles Leslie in the early 1970s. Anthropological scholarship has had several turning points while trying to capture the complexity of pluralism in health and medicine, thus moving from a description of syncretism (Leslie 1976)—'new' medical pluralism (Cant and Sharma 1999), pluralism as part of scientisation, hybridisation and globalisation (Nichter and Lock 2002; Society for Medical Anthropology 2017), to, more recently, an explicit articulation of this field resting on asymmetrical conversations among different bodies of medical knowledge and practices (Naraindas, et al. 2014). Medical pluralism is one of those few thematic areas that continues to intrigue generations of medical anthropologists, either in trying to disentangle epistemological conundrums, explain health-seeking behaviour or map global assemblages of medical and healing ideas and practices. It is an eclectic field that defies binaries of religion/science, tradition/modernity, local/global, folk/classic or ethno-medicine/biomedicine, and is yet paradoxically confronted with the dominant power of biomedicine (and the State), thus continuously drawing and redrawing its own meanings and boundaries. With such a thick body of already-existing scholarship on medical pluralism, where does one locate the present volume?

The idea for a volume on local health traditions was conceived in three related contexts and objectives. The first is the seemingly sharper policy attention to traditional medicine globally, and in India in recent times. The former director general of the World Health Organization (WHO) put it succinctly:

> The time has never been better, and the reasons never greater, for giving traditional medicine its proper place in addressing the many ills that face all our modern—and our traditional—societies ... I believe that the strong calls we are hearing for a renewal of primary health care create an ideal opportunity to revisit the place of traditional medicine, to take a positive look at its many contributions to health care that is equitable, accessible, affordable, and people-centred. (Chan 2008)

The WHO (2002a) defines traditional medicine broadly to include diverse health practices, approaches, knowledge and beliefs, incorporating medicines from plant, animal and/or mineral sources, spiritual therapies, manual techniques and exercises. Several factors, including a rising burden of non-communicable diseases, the failure of the grand narrative of biomedicine, increasing commercial demand for and viability of herbal medicine, the growing complementary and alternative medicine movement, clamour for universal health coverage and strengthening of primary health care bring back the focus on traditional medicine, though each of these factors imposes different sets of demands and directions for traditional medicine (Banerjee 2009; Bode and Unnikrishnan 2013; Bodekar and Kronenberg 2002; Unnikrishnan and Suneetha 2012; WHO 2002a, 2002b, 2003; Wilder 2000). WHO, in its first ever global Traditional Medicine Strategy (2002–05), called for developing national traditional medicine policies in country contexts, specifically where the population depends on such medicine. However, its safety, efficacy and quality has not been adequately evaluated and/or appropriately integrated into national health systems. Bodekar, et al. (2007) note that 31 per cent of WHO member-countries have established some policies on traditional and complementary medicines. While in several countries, specifically in Asia and Africa, traditional medicine policies have followed different paths, either of integration (through medical education and practice, like in China and Vietnam) or of parallel streams (like India, South Korea and select African countries), the role of traditional medicine in the current policy climate has received fresh impetus (Bodekar 2001; Bodekar and Kronenberg 2002; Richter 2003; Unnikrishnan and Suneetha 2012; Wreford 2005). This upsurge is reinforced in related policy frameworks and conventions, including the World Summit on Sustainable Development (United Nations 2002), Convention on Biological Diversity (CBD 1992, 2010) and World Intellectual Property Organisation's (WIPO 2007) Intergovernmental

Committee on Intellectual Property and Genetic Resources, Traditional Knowledge and Folklore, among others.

In the Indian context, this recent turn towards traditional medicine has unfolded in interesting ways. The Indian government came up with its first ever national policy on Indian Systems of Medicine and Homeopathy in 2002 with a clear recognition that 'there is a need for ending the long neglect of these systems in our health care strategy' (Government of India 2002: 3). More significantly, the remorse at the long neglect was extended to folk medicine through the coinage of the term 'local health traditions'. Such traditions are referred to as 'folk traditions related to birth attendants, herbal healers, bone setters, Visha (poison) healers' (ibid.: 14).[1] The policy document adds that 'such knowledge over the years gets eroded causing irreversible damage. Research councils have already documented 10,000 forms of folk medicine but many more remain to be documented. The providers of such knowledge have not been given due acknowledgement, financial benefit and support to patent their knowledge' (ibid.).

Thus, for the first time in the policy document, such a body of knowledge and practices (the erstwhile 'folk medicine') not only found an official space in the State register, but its formal induction was also marked by the coinage of a unified category called 'local health traditions'. This is irrespective of how blurry this taxonomy is in referring to the range of heterogenous forms of knowledge and therapeutic practices, including bone-setting, the dai tradition, *vishavaidyam* (indigenous toxicology), *marmavaidyam* (vital spot massaging and treatment), *siddhavaidyam* (practice of traditional siddha medicine), *ottamoolis* (practised in Kerala, this refers to special single-ingredient medicines used for the treatment of specific diseases), and many others.

From a statist lens, what brings these heterogeneous practices together is their litotic[2] identification as those that are *not* ayurveda, yoga, naturopathy, unani, siddha and homeopathy (AYUSH) and *not* biomedicine (two sets of officially recognised systems of medicine), implying that these are *non*-codified, *non*-institutionalised, *non*-certified and *non*-licensed. This induction, on the one hand, gives these health traditions/community-based health knowledge visibility (worthy of recognition), yet at the same time reinforces the hierarchy of legitimacy by nesting it within AYUSH but keeping it distinct and subservient to these systems of medicine through the litotic terms of reference.

Sharing concern over the possible erosion of such knowledge, the policy calls for its revitalisation through identification, documentation, validation and promotion. The agenda of revitalisation of local health traditions is reinforced in subsequent policy discussions and documents including the National Rural Health Mission (NRHM) (Government of India 2005), the Eleventh (2007–11) and Twelfth (2012–15) Five-Year Plan documents (Government of India 2007, 2012b), recent National Health Policy (2017) and commissioned reports (Chandra 2011; Government of India 2009, 2012a; Karnataka Knowledge Commission 2009). The NRHM (2005) proposed a twin strategy of mainstreaming AYUSH and revitalising local health traditions as part of its overall architectural correction of the public health delivery system. This strategy implies that AYUSH was marginal—needing to be mainstreamed while local health traditions were nearing extinction—needing to be revitalised. The National Health Policy (Government of India 2017: 12) that upholds pluralism as one of the key principles furthers the revitalisation objective through advocating for supporting the documentation and validation of 'local, home and community based practices' as well as research and validation of tribal medicine. It also advocates for certification of the 'prior knowledge' of traditional community health providers.

The act of taxonomy is key to understanding the dynamics of power implicated in practices of medical pluralism. As is well-known, non-allopathic systems of medicine in India have witnessed several nomenclatures, including indigenous medicine, traditional medicine, Indian systems of medicine and, more recently, AYUSH. Each of these categories bears symbolic and political significance in delineating its relationship with the State *vis-à-vis* other systems of medicine (as well as non-systems like folk medicine). The nomenclature of 'local health traditions' seems to have gained prominence in the 1980s through the work of several non-governmental organisations (NGOs)/civil society organisations, networks including the Lok Swasthya Parampara Samvardhan Samiti (LSPSS), People's Health Movement, and others in the context of community ownership and strengthening of primary health care (Balasubramaniam and Radhika 1989; Mukhopadhyay 1992; Shankar and Unnikrishnan 2004; Shodhini Collective 1997). The evolution of this nomenclature of 'local health traditions' is significant in terms of its meaning and legitimacy in the pluralism landscape.

The 'making' of local health traditions in the State register witnessed an eclectic policy history (Mishra, et al. 2018), marked by several years of State neglect to sporadic attention to a recent, seemingly explicit turn towards revitalising these traditions. Studies have shown how the modern, developmentalist State's governance mechanisms of professionalisation, standardisation and institutionalisation have created a hierarchy of legitimacy and established categories of inclusion and exclusion of systems of medicine (Banerjee 2002; Lambert 2012a, 2012b; Priya 2012; Sujatha and Abraham 2009, to cite a few). Thus, forms of medicine and healing that are non-institutionalised and are practised largely based on experiential knowledge, handed over through the apprentice mode of training, fall outside the officially recognised systems of medicine. These became the residua that supposedly, 'in modernist narratives of progress, are always-already disappearing' (Lambert 2012a: 1030). As argued elsewhere,

> Belying the heterogeneity of these therapeutic practices and traditions, in deeming them an 'other' category, the state has been in fact relieved of the obligation to expand, elaborate, or operationalise further. In this one taxonomic act, moreover, these practices are not only de-legitimised by their confirmed distance to the State, but also from the traditional medical systems with which they have had historical and epistemological links (ayurveda, for example) (Mishra, et al. 2018: 43).

While such distance might look complete in the statist frame, in practice, as the existing studies, including select chapters in this volume, demonstrate, the interactions between the official traditional systems of medicine (institutionalised systems like ayurveda, siddha, unani, etc.) and folk medicine (oral/vernacular traditions) are much more complex (Girija 2017; Sax and Bhaskar Nair 2014; Sujatha and Abraham 2012).

With several years of de-recognition, during the 1970s and 1980s, the State did turn to the practitioners of folk medicine and healing as community-based facilitators of development programmes. This was fuelled by several developments, including the Srivastava Committee Report's (Government of India 1975) recommendation on the involvement of indigenous healers as 'local para professionals' for managing everyday illnesses, the 1981 Manual of Community Health Workers as well as the WHO Alma Ata Declaration (1978) seeking to strengthen comprehensive primary health care. This temporary attention has by no means been paradoxical as their inclusion was conceived in a biomedical frame of inclusion, thus requiring a (re)training of folk practitioners. For example, during this period, the traditional midwifery (or dai) training was actively supported by the State as well as several national and international NGOs and networks (Kruske and Barclay 2004; Pigg 1995; Sadgopal 2009). However, this training and the services of dais in maternal and child health (MCH) programmes were soon discontinued as the discourse changed from traditional birth attendant to skilled birth attendant and institutional births.

The formal induction of folk medicine as 'local health traditions' in policy texts since 2000, hence, is an important development and bears significance in the historical and policy context of the State governance mechanisms and processes towards systems of medicine. The upsurge in this interest, however, rests on parallel and potentially contradictory discourses—one that posits the revitalisation as a signifier of economic possibility (drug discovery), while the other approaches it as an opportunity to strengthen primary health care, both of which place very different demands on local health traditions and modes of revitalisation (Mishra, et al. 2018).

It is, hence, pertinent to ask: How does one situate the State's reclaiming of this body of knowledge and practice, which has been outside its frame of recognition by virtue of not conferring on it the governance instruments of professionalisation, licensing, certification and standardisation? How earnestly does the State view the revitalisation agenda? Does revitalisation entail redefining scientific legitimacy or relooking at contours of medical pluralism? What sort of new demands are made of local health traditions to share space in the already-hierarchical medical pluralism landscape? Is revitalisation a means to respond to the consumerist demands for herbal medicine, medical tourism or intellectual property rights? If documentation, validation and promotion are deemed as the way ahead for revitalising these traditions, who, what and how can such knowledge be documented? How do practitioners of local health traditions navigate this in the contemporary scenario? What has revitalisation meant for them? How does the notion of the 'local' evolve and how is it reflected in the knowledge and practices of such traditions? How has it effected different traditions differently, that is, what would revitalisation entail for the indigenous midwifery tradition when the State actively promotes institutional and biomedical practices in childbirth? What has led many of these practices to continue despite the absence of State recognition? The volume critically engages with this recent turn through interrogating the category of the 'local health traditions' through multiple perspectives and practice settings. The apparent visibility of local health traditions in the policy register is an opportune moment to revisit the contours of medical pluralism, and the contributions in the volume speak to this objective.

The second, linked context where the current volume seeks to contribute is the relative invisibility of local health traditions in the literature on medical pluralism. Barring a few, the discussions of local health traditions find a peripheral and derivative space in this literature. A larger space has been devoted to studying 'systems' of medicine, thus leaving out those that fall off the radar of systems, science and the State (Hardiman and Mukharji 2012; Lambert 2012a, 2012b; Pordie 2007). Few studies have explored individual forms of local health traditions including bone-setting, dais, and faith healing (Lambert 2012a, 2012b; Lohokare and Davar 2010; Quack 2009; Raje 2012; Sadgopal 2009; Sax and Nair 2014; Unnikrishnan, et al. 2010). On folk medicine/healing, the role of faith/spiritual healing in mental health practices is extensively discussed, engaging with interesting conversations around religion/science, rituals/medicinal practices, and care and recovery (Basu 2014; Halliburton 2009; Jagadisha, et al. 2016; Quack 2014; Raghuram, et al. 2002; Ranganathan 2014; Sébastia 2009). While some approach local health traditions through a symbiotic lens of *loka/prakriti* (people, nature) and *sastra* (classical texts of ayurveda, siddha, unani, etc.) (Shankar and Unnikrishnan 2004), others underscore the epistemic autonomy of this genre of medical knowledge as 'medical lore', though it may have references to classical/codified forms (Sujatha 2007).

Hardiman and Mukharji (2012), on the other hand, situate local health traditions as the 'subaltern therapeutics'—that which are not recognised by the State. Pointing out the limitations of existing formulations to approach such therapeutics (traditional/Western, folk/modern, oral/textual, etc.), Hardiman and Mukharji caution against limiting the study of medical pluralism to State-regulated sectors alone. They view such an approach as limited, 'since it effaces stratification across and within therapeutic domains, asymmetries in the kinds of treatments and resources available in different localities as well as modes of governance' (Attewell, et al. 2012: 3). They argue that medical pluralism needs to focus upfront on the relationship of power in the field of medicine and its governance. Subaltern therapeutics need to be seen in this context of relationships of power with the State as well as institutionalised systems of medicine. Through a set of historical and anthropological contributions, Hardiman and Mukharji (2012) show how subaltern therapeutics are neither historical nor timeless; instead, they adapt, transform and negotiate to recast themselves in contemporary reality. The present volume takes this conversation further by examining how local health traditions have evolved, are practised across different sites through their interactions/negotiations with the State, NGOs, healers' associations and networks, institutionalised systems of medicine and local communities in contemporary times. The volume turns the lens of pluralism upside down by locating the category of 'local health traditions' at the centrestage of our discussions and engaging with medical pluralism through this marginal space.

Third, the volume turns its attention to the existing literature on ethno-medicine in medical anthropology, which has traditionally engaged with folk medicine in a manner not well-integrated with the literature on medical pluralism. Medical anthropological scholarship has contributed a great deal to trying to explore local conceptions of health and practices among different communities. Largely within the field of indigenous/tribal health or health among specific ethnic groups, there are numerous studies that have sought to document local conceptions of body, health and modes of seeking treatment and healing.[3] While these studies have offered valuable insights into plural conceptions of body, disease, health and healing, these have tended to project such knowledge as rather bounded and also in line with early anthropological work, which is limited to the study of the indigenous/tribal/primitive. For instance, Hughes (1968) defines ethno-medicine as a

> medical system of the primitive which has been evolved in their own cultural milieu and recognized as the methods of diagnosis and treatment which are natural or not. It includes all the body of beliefs, therapeutic practices including pharmacopeia which they use for curing diseases even if they attribute the cause to natural or supernatural (cited in Nair 1994: 136).

Several studies in the field of tribal/indigenous health describe such beliefs and pharmacopeia, resulting in a large body of knowledge on ethno-botany/ethno-medicine/ethno-pharamacology. Advancing the field of the study of ethno-medicine, Nichter (1992) points towards the limitations of the assumed limited scope of ethno-medicine to the study of folk illness, herbal remedies and healing rituals. He argues that ethno-medicine is not the 'study of the spectacular or the quintessential be this in the forms of exotic healing, surgical procedures or cultural bound syndrome' (ibid.: ix). He rightly draws attention to two methodological cautions in the study of ethno-medicine. One is that of theoretical closure that rests on treating ethno-medicine as a discrete domain of empirical enquiry and interpretation of beliefs and practices to a fixed set of values, thus subscribing to an objectified and reified notion of culture. An additional note of caution relates to the construction of the 'other', reflected in 'nostalgic and paternalistic scientific accounts or descriptions of the knowledge and practices of health' (ibid.). Expanding the scope and reorienting the approach of ethno-medicine as a dynamic field, Nichter advocates for greater empirical and methodological rigour in the study of ethno-medicine engaging with newer methods and approaches.

This volume extends this call by joining the growing body of work of anthropologists in 'studying up' as well as 'studying sideways' (as much as 'studying below') in trying to capture different perspectives and sites of power in the study of health policies and practices (Ahlin, et al. 2016; Pfeiffer and Nichter 2008; Storeng and Mishra 2014). Contributions, hence, engage with multiple perspectives, including a range of traditional healers, NGOs and their networks that have been involved in the revitalisation of local health traditions, the users of such traditions as much as that of the State and international agencies. These multiple perspectives are critical to situate the recent upsurge in policy interest in local health traditions and what these have meant for those inhabiting the local health tradition space. Set in contemporary modern India, this volume extends anthropological scholarship in the study of ethno-medicine to critically engage with issues of sites of recognition and legitimacy, practices of documentation of traditional medical knowledge, and gender in healing.

Contributions to the Volume

Section I: Legitimacy and Recognition

Chapters in this section interrogate a set of questions on recognition and legitimacy: What are the boundaries of State recognition? What are the other modes of accruing formal recognition, and strengthening of the knowledge and practice of traditional healers? How does one understand social legitimacy? The chapters address these questions through multiple perspectives, including those of healers, users as well as organisations involved in sustained advocacy on revitalising local health traditions.

Chapter 1, 'Authenticity, Alliance and Results: Notions of Legitimacy Held by Traditional Healers in South India' by Devaki Nambiar, Arima Mishra, Harilal Madhavan, Sarika Kadam, Shrish N. R., Steffy Dhayalan and Pooja Venkatesh, draw attention to the different sources of legitimacy as expounded by traditional healers or *paramparikavaidyas*. They argue how, in the absence of an explicit legal status of their practice and/or knowledge, traditional healers employ several legitimating strategies to garner their place in India's plural therapeutic landscape. Based on data collected from 51 traditional healers in three southern states of India as well as through a two-day dialogue among healers, academics, civil society and government representatives, the authors discuss myriad strategies, reflecting corresponding variation and plurality around notions of legitimacy. For some healers, legitimacy entailed highlighting the *authenticity* of knowledge. The sacred origins of practice and its linkage to nature were the defining features of this knowledge. On the one hand, the rituals and requirements of generational knowledge-transfer differentiated 'traditional' (*paramparik*) healers from potential quacks, while others saw legitimacy as a question of *alliances* with their peers through associations, and with other advocates for local health traditions, including academic partners and civil society organisations. In select cases, legitimacy was established through emphasis on results, through proud narratives of healing diseases like cancer and diabetes. Markers of results and reputation included treating 'reputed' clients (lawyer, minister, film celebrity, etc.); being felicitated by local associations or State actors; extending the client base beyond the immediate 'locale', both in terms of care provided (visiting other places to offer service) and received (healing patients who come to the healers from other states and even countries); and receiving media attention, further extended through a word-of-mouth referral network of loyal clients. Interestingly, all notions of legitimacy were construed in relational terms, reflecting the simultaneity of plurality and asymmetry inherent in their practice.

Can pluralism thrive in the absence of an explicit State recognition of a specific body of knowledge and practice? Naraindas, et al. (2014: 7) rightly remind us that

> a healing system that has the support of the state apparatus and its regulatory function has distinct advantages over one that does not: the latter can hardly generate the comprehensive social-economic-political 'loops' of the former and the inability to do so is a cause and consequence of its weaker position.

In this regard, what sort of official recognition is warranted for local health traditions and to what effect? Unnikrishnan Payyappallimana, Hariramamurthi Govindaswamy, Sarin Sasikumar and Debjani Roy take up this question in Chapter 2, 'Accreditation, Certification and Self-regulation: An Innovative Approach for Strengthening and Reintegrating Traditional Community Health Care Providers'. Based on their own experiences of being involved in a pilot programme on Accreditation and Certification of Prior Learning, a collaborative effort of the Foundation for Revitalisation of Local Health Traditions (FRLHT), Indira Gandhi National Open University (IGNOU) and Quality Council of India, they share the scope of this innovative experiment in accruing recognition and strengthening such traditions. Systematically documenting the steps involved in this programme, the authors show how this is a bottom-up approach to recognition, foregrounding the views and experiences of community members, village panchayat and healers, while allowing conversations with institutionalised knowledge and practitioners (ayurvedic physicians). While such a model holds great promise for the formal recognition of traditional community health practitioners, the authors rightly express caution against the possible AYUSHisation (subsumed under AYUSH) of such tradition.

In this regard, drawing on experiences in other Asian countries, they wonder if strengthening local health traditions in its own right as an independent branch of knowledge (as folk medicine/local health traditions/community health practice) through appropriate nurturing might be a way forward. They strongly argue that traditional community health providers could play an important role in strengthening primary health care by serving as the first site (home/community) of care that is effectively linked to the subsequent tiers in health service delivery. Mechanisms and processes of formal recognition should speak to such a potential role of community health providers. Renu Khanna, in Chapter 11 in the final section of this volume, also expands on this suggestion with specific reference to dais (the chapter is described in detail further on).

Such advocacy also demands a robust and granular understanding of the role of community health/traditional practitioners *vis-à-vis* others in health-care provision in historical and changing contexts through users' perspectives. Emphasising methodological rigour in health-seeking behaviour studies to understand how pluralism is deployed in everyday contexts, Mark Nichter in Chapter 3, 'Whom Do the Rural Poor Consult for Health Care and How Much Do They Spend in India's Pluralistic Health Care Arenas?', revisits data collected in the 1980s from two districts in Karnataka. Though the data are somewhat dated, the chapter's strength is in its methodological robustness and implications for current and future research on therapeutic pluralism. Critiquing the existing health-seeking behaviour studies, Nichter demonstrates the importance of considering interregional as well as intraregional differences when assessing patterns of practitioner consultation and expenditure among the poor in India. The data draw on rural households as a means to better understand practitioner consultation for non-catastrophic health problems and how much these households spend on various types of diagnosis/divination and treatment across a range of practitioners. The study focused on understanding health care-seeking behaviour and expenditure in two different districts (considering the criteria of caste, class and proximity to town) over a period of one year. Health care needs were defined as encompassing the curative, palliative, protective and promotive needs of individual members of households. It also considered a household as a unit of analysis when the illness of one member was interpreted as a sign that the entire household was vulnerable. Such a definition allowed for uncovering a layered analysis of the differences in practitioner consultation and expenditure across and within caste and class groups. Based on an insightful set of findings from this data, Nichter demonstrates how longitudinal data focusing on an expanded notion of health care, across a full range of practitioners and inter and intraregional and cultural consideration, challenges a number of assumptions about from whom, where and why people seek health care. Systematically documenting nine such research observations, Nichter shows how trends in health-care seeking among vulnerable populations also reflect psychosocial needs, perceived risks and social as well as structural insecurities, ways in which distress and concern are expressed and experienced culturally at the site of the body, and actions taken to both reduce harm and secure protection. Such health care-seeking studies could better inform us of the place of different systems and forms of medicine and healing in a pluralism setting.

Taking this further, Sultana Mustafa Khanum in Chapter 4, 'Medical Pluralism and Political Economy of Obstetric Care among Bangladeshi Women in Britain', explores the nuances of social legitimacy for indigenous knowledge and practices through the creative deployment of pluralism in obstetric care among the Bangladeshi migrants in the United Kingdom. Based on intensive fieldwork conducted over a period of 27 years, involving first-, second- and third-generation Bangladeshi migrant/Briton women in Manchester, UK, this chapter explores how perceived/experienced institutional racism and own cultural agencies lead women to blend the use of biomedicine with indigenous medicine (particularly ayurvedic and unani medicine, use of medicinal herbs and practices relating to childbirth) and healing practices. Such blending goes beyond individual bodily practices. For example, both biomedicine and indigenous medicines become items of gift exchange between the women living in England and their relatives back home, thus enabling them to maintain a sense of belongingness. Yet, at the same time, perceived belongingness to two cultures creates ambivalent responses towards the medicalisation of pregnancy and imperatives of technological interventions at childbirth. For these women, while biomedicine was perceived as essential to regain strength or prevent further complications, indigenous medicine was viewed as indispensable to expelling the side effects of such medicine. Finally, while such hybrid medicine is desired, the availability of both biomedicine and indigenous medicine depended on the position of the woman in her family as well as in the wider society, where the power of both family elders and medical personnel are decisive factors. While on the one hand this chapter unravels the complexities of negotiation in the deployment of medical pluralism, it draws attention to the symbolic, political and cultural connotations of indigenous knowledge and practices and how the material 'herbs' travel across borders, healing the individual and social body (the Bangladeshi migrants in the UK), on the other. In such cases, ayurveda/unani (identified through its specific herbal drugs brands) and knowledge of women, including dais, on obstetric care all become part of the same cultural and therapeutic repository.

Section II: Documentation of Traditional Medical Knowledge and Practice

In the broader policy arena, documentation of traditional knowledge has been seen to be the primary mode of promotion and revitalisation, including protection from biopiracy and commercial exploitation. Documentation and other related efforts to protect, preserve and promote traditional knowledge, including genetic resources, agricultural knowledge, cultural expression and other customary practices, in addition to health practices, have been addressed in several international policy frameworks and conventions, including the Convention on Biological Diversity (1992), the World Summit on Sustainable Development declaration (2002) and WIPO.[4] Several organisations and initiatives exist in different parts of the world including India, documenting indigenous/ traditional medical knowledge. This section draws on four contributions that discuss ongoing documentation efforts in different states in India and critically engage with the objectives, processes and outcomes of such efforts.

Brigitte Sébastia, in Chapter 5, 'From Siddha Corpus to Siddha Medicine: Reflection on the Reduction of Siddha Knowledge through Exploration of Manuscripts', discusses how the siddha 'corpus' encompassing the composite body of knowledge where medical matter is inextricably enmeshed with other subjects, namely alchemy, magic, philosophy, spirituality and astrology, gets reduced to 'medicine' through its transmission in institutional settings. Drawing on her collaborative project on digitisation and cataloguing of siddha manuscripts, Sébastia follows the origin, authorship, collection, translations and promotion of siddha medical knowledge through the family manuscripts. These manuscripts, which have originally been kept with families of practitioners or specifically collected by members of traditional siddha practitioners associations, contest the notion that traditional knowledge is necessarily undocumented. The material artifacts like photographs, medicine box and instruments used in the preparations of medicine are an integral part of the manuscripts which have symbolic (many siddha practitioners display it to project the siddha lineage and, thus, authenticity of their practice) as much as healing values. The chapter draws attention to the complexity of translating and making sense of the vast knowledge encrypted in these manuscripts.

This chapter is important as it draws our attention to the need to decipher what is already available in documentation formats (family manuscripts) and how these can be used to contribute to the training and practice of siddha traditional medicine for the generations to come. While there is a growing demand for 'authentic' siddha practice that has its roots in familial tradition of siddha (thus the demand for knowledge encapsulated in family manuscripts), at the same time the institutional mode of instruction (siddha colleges) highlights those aspect of knowledge that are more decipherable and in line with 'scientific' understanding, thus reducing the siddha corpus to siddha medicine.

Harilal Madhavan and Praveen Lal in Chapter 6, 'Family Repositories to Knowledge Commons: The Discourse of Documenting Local Health Traditions in Contemporary Kerala', discuss the myriad documentation efforts in the state of Kerala. The state offers an interesting site for several reasons. It witnesses the existence of vibrant plural medical traditions and practitioners ranging from the local indigenous healer communities, experts in vishavaidyam, *manorogachikitsa* (mental health), the *astavaidya*[5] families to institutionally trained ayurveda physicians, all of them playing a significant role. Traditional medical knowledge and its revitalisation draws the involvement of several stakeholders, including the NGOs, government organisations and a vibrant ayurvedic pharmaceutical market. Ambiguously situated, traditional medical knowledge is projected as an 'indigenous alterity' in the medical and cultural landscape in Kerala. The authors in this chapter closely follow three models of documentation. Each of these has distinct objectives, processes and outcomes of documentation. The Tropical Botanic Garden and Research Institute (TBGRI) follows a community-academia-market linkage model as a viable source of protection and sustenance of traditional knowledge. The Kerala State Biodiversity Board rests on a decentralised model in seeking to empower the communities through the process of documentation. Thus, the People's Biodiversity Register (PBR) seeks to document the knowledge of occurrence, practices of propagation, sustainable harvests and conservation, as well as economic uses of biodiversity resources that reside with India's local communities. The third, Traditional Knowledge Innovation, Kerala, works on the open-source public-domain model of documentation of manuscripts and pamphlets of traditional physician families for wider use, including potential for drug innovations. These models brought to the fore the politics of actors/institutions/ideologies that decide the fate of these documentation efforts. Yet the credit for some of the efforts lies in the fact that the state was a frontrunner in initiating discussions around intellectual property rights and benefit sharing mechanisms much before the international policy frameworks did on these issues.

Moe Nakazora, in Chapter 7, 'Documenting "Folk" Ayurvedic Knowledge in Uttarakhand: Insights from Critical Medical Anthropology', weaves insights from medical anthropology and science and technology studies to reflect on specific documentation exercises and their implications in Uttarakhand, the projected 'herbal state' of India. Following Bruno Latour (1987), she focuses on the socio-material processes of making scientific knowledge (in this case documenting valuable folk medical knowledge) and the politics of inclusion and exclusion embedded in such a process. Through ethnographic fieldwork in 2010–11 and closely observing the work of one NGO, she talks about how the subject-making process of the identification of authentic *vaidyas* (a practitioner of traditional medicine), whose knowledge is to be documented, follows a rather *ad hoc* criteria of those demonstrating active interest in the cultivation of medicinal plants. The documentation in the process of following the CBD guidelines of benefit sharing reinstates a notion that is not in line with the local health tradition. Many such knowledge-holders consider service or duty as a form of exchange of knowledge than benefits in a more materialistic or instrumental sense. The methodological process further reduces notions of benefits to 'help' from the government, thus reorienting the spirit of knowledge exchange (entitlements to recipients). Nakazora's chapter underscores the significance of examining the methodological *processes* of documentation to understand the inclusion and exclusion of knowledge and knowledge-holders. She argues that while the objective of documentation in itself may not be problematic, the larger neoliberal ideology of intellectual property-driven documentation models undermine other modes of protecting and sharing knowledge held by several vaidyas whose knowledge is sought to be documented.

Drawing on fieldwork in the states of Tamil Nadu and Karnataka, Arima Mishra and Devaki Nambiar in Chapter 8, 'Documentation of Traditional Health Knowledge: To What End?', discuss the who, what and why of documentation efforts. They interrogate whether and what forms of documentation indeed revitalise community forms of knowledge and, in the process, understand the role of the State *vis-à-vis* community and other stakeholders involved in the documentation and revitalisation of local health traditions. The authors argue that in the absence of clarity on the objectives of documentation and their alignment with methodological processes, such efforts might marginalise local health traditions rather than strengthening it. Documentation, for example, when it includes only tangible aspects of knowledge, more specifically, knowledge on medicinal plants (name, usage and ailments), would systematically exclude other aspects of the knowledge or the social context in which such knowledge is produced and practised (timing, space of collection of plants, prescriptions and proscriptions regarding diet, other aspects of lifestyle, chanting of hymns that are believed to add effectiveness to the therapeutic process, etc.). Thus, documentation cannot be a mode of revitalisation if this is not linked to its practice, thus drawing attention to the anomaly of promoting knowledge but not the knowledge-holders. Further, a focus only on herbal medicine would exclude the knowledge of other healers (bone setters, dais or faith healers), whose primary mode of healing may not necessarily be herbs alone. The chapter leads to a discussion of emerging documentation efforts that adopt participatory methodologies of cooperative enquiry, active listening and/or a practice-driven mode of documentation that indeed have an important contribution to creating a dynamic space of pluralism drawing on strengths from different bodies of knowledge and practices, thus advancing our understanding of conversations across different bodies of knowledge and their practitioners.

Section III: Gender in Local Health Traditions and Healing

While aspects of caste, ethnicity and religious aspects of medicine and healing have been dealt with, studies on gender in healing (in traditional medical practice) are very few (Flueckiger 1997; McClain 1995; Sujatha and Abraham 2012). The statist frame of approaching local health traditions' marginality, though critical, has rendered many other pertinent issues within local health traditions non-problematic. Within (or in addition to) this broader frame of marginality, the contributions to this section show that women's role in traditional healing are marked by further layers of marginalities, rendering them invisible or selectively visible. Women healers' role tends to be associated with traditional midwives. Though feminists have contributed extensively on traditional midwives (dais in India), these speak more to literature on the maternal health or reproductive policy and practices contexts than traditional medicine. This volume, thus, consciously includes two chapters on dais to integrate them into the discussion on local health traditions. A gender lens to the study of local health traditions and healing has allowed the identifying of the myriad roles women play as herbal healers, bone setters, local homeopathic practitioners and spiritual healers. It also offers rich insights into revisiting some of the existing notions of ritual pollution, public/domestic and natural/cultural binaries, or even the gendered context of healing.

Chapter 9 by Arima Mishra, Maya Annie Elias, Devaki Nambiar and Rajeev B. R., 'Nested Marginalities: Women in Healing in South India', draws on data collected over a period of two years (2014–16) in the three southern states of Tamil Nadu, Karnataka and Kerala. It discusses how the process of identification of 'women healers' is gendered, thus limiting women either to the role of dais and occasionally, as exceptions, to a few others who have stood apart due to their age, family tradition and other related support. Thus, while women's knowledge on food, nutrition and childbirth practices are valued (as grandma's knowledge), it is not enough to take on the role of healer even if such knowledge is practised outside the immediate family context. Yet, the healers in the authors' study have spoken in much more ambivalent ways than subscribing to the stereotypical notions of gender. The much-discussed gender binaries (nature/culture, public/domestic) may help, but do not adequately capture the nuances of everyday realities of the women's experiences in healing. The chapter shows that while in some cases gender norms seemed reinforced through their supporting role in healing (women supporting their husbands in medicine preparations while the men take the front-stage of patients consultations), subscribing to rules of biology (younger women are barred from entering sacred spaces, including the forest or healing shrine, during menstruation), in other instances these norms are redrawn to reverse gender roles or allow fluidity in performing such roles within the family sphere. The chapter explains why a gender lens is necessary to decode the nuances of diverse trajectories and life experiences of women in healing.

Janet Chawla in Chapter 10, 'Ritual Pollution and Women's Blood: Listening to Dais', draws on her 25 years of work with dais in different parts of India. Revisiting the evident association of pollution as necessarily a marker of oppression and hierarchy (of caste and gender), she discusses how the knowledge and skills on childbirth held by lower-caste women (dais) offer a renewed understanding of the maternal bodily events and processes. As the chapter demonstrates, an approach of 'active listening' to dais (and community knowledge) enables the understanding of the underlying philosophical, ontological, symbolic and social bases of knowledge and practice related to childbirthing. The knowledge and practices related to postpartum care, for example, not only corroborate how birthing is as much a physical as a social process, but also point towards an epistemology of body that needs to be in harmony with the five elements of earth and social relations. For the author, relooking at ritual pollution through the dai's worldviews is an entry point to convey that we need a critical and reflexive gaze to make sense of community health knowledge. Liberating ourselves from the rudimentary science/ritual, traditional/modern dichotomies would help us uncover the values of knowledge systems, both in terms of its scope and limitations. Thus, understanding how dais and community birthing traditions are learned, retained and adapted may make it possible for the State to make use of dais effectively.

Reinforcing such a feminist lens, Renu Khanna in Chapter 11, 'Dais: Transforming the Traditions', seeks to make a convincing case for a community model of childbirth with an important role played by dais. Based on her organisation's work with dais for three decades, she argues for explicit policy support for the recognition of dais' knowledge. The chapter narrates two sets of stories of dais set in Gujarat in the late 1980s (when the health system was weak with limited resources, poor roads and communications in the rural parts of Gujarat) and present times (when the state is active in intervening in maternal health through a spate of measures). The narratives from the 1980s point to a comprehensive role played by the dai and an elaborate birthing system with components like spacing, nutritional advice, practices including massages and manipulation, birthing positions, dealing with the placenta and postpartum rituals, helping the vulnerable body regain its strength. This body of knowledge has systematically been derecognised by the State in the name of safe delivery associated with institutional delivery. In the current context, with interventions from grassroots NGOs like SAHAJ (Society for Health Alternatives) and ANANDI (Area Networking and Development Initiatives), dais in this part of Gujarat have emerged as community leaders. Thus, the emerging narratives of dais are seeking to straddle the traditional and modern worlds (reflected in the state's maternal health practices) and expanding their remit to negotiate for women's health, both in community and State spaces. Khanna explains at length how the dais' role could be utilised by the health system not in opposition, but complementary to the existing maternal health regime. A more sustainable community model of maternal health needs to foreground the role of the community women—beginning with dais—in making childbirth a more humane, empowering process. The dismissive role of dais has always resulted from an inadequate understanding of their knowledge and skills (thus, their training focuses on the five cleans alone), and Khanna shows how reorienting our own lens to adopt a reflexive cooperative enquiry would help us identify the strengths—'good practices' of the dais, which can complement and strengthen maternal health through 'safe' delivery.

Cecilia Coale Van Hollen's contribution to the narrative account of a lady homeopathic practitioner in Tamil Nadu is an interesting addition to this volume. Though homeopathy is an officially recognised system of medicine, it does not share the connotation of 'indigeneity' as the other systems of medicine within the AYUSH umbrella. Focusing on homeopathy in everyday practice, Chapter 12, 'May the Vital Force Be With You: An Indian Homeopathic Doctor's Approach to the Gendered Ills of Our Time', discusses the narrative of a woman homeopathic practitioner who orients homeopathy to address issues of gender inequality and its impact on health. Drawing on her training in homeopathy (Bachelor of Homeopathic Medicine and Surgery or BHMS) and psychology, Dr Radha[6] positions homeopathy as a form of social service for the poor, and a remedy for the physically and mentally 'deranged' modern era. She is based in an NGO clinic providing health care and health service education to lower-caste women in Tamil Nadu. As the chapter illustrates, the narrative draws sharp distinctions between homeopathy and both allopathy and siddha (thus trying to position homeopathy as a unique body of knowledge illustrated through her own variant of practice). Dr Radha insists that understanding the relationships among the mind, the inner 'vital force' and the body is key to health, pharmacology and cure for any ailment, including depression, cancer, tuberculosis and rheumatism. She locates the cause of diseases in larger social and economic factors (unequal gender relations, increased competition and environmental degradation), which can, however, be treated through individual bodily interventions by controlling minds and homeopathic medicines. Locating homeopathy as a remedy for the deranged 'vital force' in the body caused due to the increasing stress disproportionately impacting women (changing lifestyles, increasing competition, double burden of managing work and home), she orients homeopathy to suit such gendered needs. She considers the core concepts in homeopathy to be particularly beneficial to women in India. Dr Radha's narrative on the unique position of homeopathy as a form of service catering to the specific needs of women is an expression of her desire to gain better recognition and elevate the status of homeopathy in a highly competitive plural medical therapy arena.

Together, the 12 contributions in this volume have sought to offer a layered understanding of a body of knowledge, practices and practitioners that are at the margins of the State. Anthropologists have argued how rich ethnographies are needed to understand such margins. A focus on marginality brings in new perspectives on understanding marginality and centrality (Das and Poole 2004; Ecks and Sax 2005). The chapters in the volume enrich our understanding of such margins, local health traditions, in two important ways. First, they unravel the amorphous category of 'local health traditions' as these unfold in different empirical settings. The chapters show how local health traditions exist as plural categories with varying internal logics and relationships based on local frames of reference as well as symbolic, political and pragmatic connotations. Thus, the references of local health tradition as siddha tradition in Tamil Nadu, paramparikavaidyas (traditional healing emphasising the familial/lineage links) in Karnataka, *nattuvaidaym* (local/indigenous medicine) in Kerala or folk ayurveda in Uttarakhand have their own significance. In other places, the specific traditions and their practitioners remain important on their own (dais in Gujarat, Himachal Pradesh and Jharkhand; homeopathic practitioners in an NGO clinic in Tamil Nadu), without any reference to a unified category. It is important to capture the plural forms of traditions, practices and experiences within the local health traditions, as State logic has been to categorise bodies of knowledge and practice by system, thus grouping the diverse local health traditions into the single category of non-system. This has resulted in the single category of local health traditions being homogenised although, as the contributions to the volume show, local health traditions are diverse.

Second, as is already argued, marginality is about a perceived 'relation' and not a given fact (Ecks and Sax 2005). This volume explicates the layered and shifting relations of local health traditions with individual institutionalised systems of medicine (while siddha medicine is the reference point in one state, it is ayurveda in another; epistemology of ayurveda in one context while individual AYUSH practitioners in other), the State, NGOs and different communities where these are practised. These are relations of power whose directions, nature and extent are neither uniform nor constant. The contributions together highlight the 'dialectics' (power at stake in different bodies of medical knowledge and practices) and the 'dynamics' of local health traditions in the debates on medical pluralism.[7]

Notes

1. Thanks to persistent civil society advocacy, specifically that steered by the network of LSPSS in the early 1990s and subsequent work by the FRLHT. For details of such advocacy, see Karnataka Knowledge Commission (2009) and Mishra, et al. (2018).

2. 'Litotes' comes from a Greek word meaning 'plain or simple', and is used to refer to something by stating what it is not.

3. See Bhasin (2007), Joshi (2016) and Hussain (2008) for references to studies in ethno-medicine/tribal health. In the Indian context, also see Basu (1994), Hussain (2008) and Nair (1994).

4. See Unnikrishnan and Suneetha (2012) for a summary of these related international conventions on traditional knowledge.

5. Physicians with expertise in eight branches of ayurveda as mentioned in classical texts; this is practised by select groups of families in Kerala.

6. Pseudonym.

7. Fassin and Fassin (1988) highlight these terms in their discussion on modes of legitimacy in traditional medicine in Senegal.

References

Ahlin, T., M. Nichter and P. Gopukrishnan. 2016. 'Health Insurance in India: What Do We Know and Why is Ethnographic Research Needed?' *Anthropology and Medicine* 23(1): 102–24.

Attewell, G., D. Hardiman, H. Lambert and P. Mukahrji. 2012. 'Agendas'. In *Medical Marginality in South Asia: Situating Subaltern Therapeutics*, eds D. Hardiman and P. Mukharji, 1–5. London: Routledge.

Balasubramanian, A. V. and M. Radhika. 1989. *Local Health Traditions: An Introduction*. Madras: Lok Swasthya Parampara Samvardhan Samithi.

Banerjee, M. 2002. 'Public Policy and Ayurveda: Modernising a Great Tradition'. *Economic and Political Weekly* 37(12): 1136–46.

______. 2009. *Power, Knowledge, Medicine: Ayurvedic Pharmaceuticals at Home and in the World* (New Perspectives in South Asian History). Hyderabad: Orient BlackSwan.

Basu, S. (ed.). 1994. *Tribal Health in India*. Delhi: Manak Publications.

Basu, H. 2014. 'Davaa and Duaa: Negotiating Psychiatry and Ritual Healing of Madness'. In *Asymmetrical Conversations: Contestations, Circumventions, and the Blurring of Therapeutic Boundaries*, eds H. Naraindas, J. Quack and W. Sax (Series: Epistemologies of Healing), 162–99. New York: Berghahn Books.

Bhasin, V. 2007. 'Medical Anthropology: A Review'. *Studies on Ethno-medicine* 1(1): 1–20.

Bode, M., and P. Unnikrishnan. 2013. 'Evidence Based Traditional Medicine: For Whom and To What End?' *eJournal of Indian Medicine* 6: 1–20.

Bodekar, G. 2001. 'Lessons on Integration from the Developing World's Experience'. *British Medical Journal* 322: 164–67.

Bodeker, G., and F. Kronenberg. 2002. 'A Public Health Agenda for Traditional, Complementary and Alternative Medicine'. *American Journal of Public Health* 92(10): 1582–91.

Bodeker, G., F. Kronenberg and G. Burford. 2007. 'Policy and Public Health Perspectives on Complementary and Alternative Medicine: An Overview'. In *Traditional, Complementary and Alternative Medicine Policy and Public Health Perspectives*, eds G. Bodeker and G. Burford, 9–38. London: Imperial College Press.

Cant, S., and U. Sharma. 1999. *A New Medical Pluralism?: Alternative Medicine, Doctors, Patients and the State*. London: UCL Press.

Chan, Margaret. 2008. 'Address at the WHO Congress on Traditional Medicine'. World Health Organisation. Available at https://www.who.int/dg/speeches/2008/20081107/en/ (accessed 18 March 2015).

Chandra, S. 2011. 'Status of Indian Medicine and Folk Healing'. Commissioned Report, Department of AYUSH, Ministry of Health and Family Welfare, Government of India.

Chauchan, Anjali. 2014. 'Ethno-medicine of Bhotia Tribe in Mana Village of Uttarakhand'. *International Journal of Sociology and Anthropology* 6(10): 296–304.

Convention on Biological Diversity. 1992. United Nations. Available at https://www.cbd.int/doc/legal/cbd-en.pdf (accessed 30 March 2016).

______. 2010. 'COP 10 Decision X/20: Cooperation with Other Conventions and International Organizations and Initiatives'. Available at http://www.cbd.int/decision/cop/?id=12286 (accessed 16 April 2016).

Convention on Biological Diversity. 2012. 'Workshop on the Interlinkages between Human Health and Biodiversity, Workshop Summary'. Secretariat of the Convention on Biological Diversity, Montreal, Canada, 2 April.

Das, V., and D. Poole. 2004. 'State and its Margins: Comparative Ethnographies'. In *Anthropology in the Margins of the State*, eds V. Das and D. Poole, 3–34. New Delhi: Oxford University Press.

Ecks, S., and W. S. Sax. 2005. 'The Ills of Marginality: New Perspectives on Health in South Asia'. *Anthropology and Medicine* 12(3): 3, 199–210.

Fassin, D., and E. Fassin. 1988. 'Traditional Medicine and Stakes of Legitimation in Senegal'. *Social Science and Medicine* 27(4): 353–57.

Flueckiger, J. B. 1997. 'There Are Only Two Castes: Men and Women: Negotiating Gender as a Female Healer in South Asian Islam'. *Oral Tradition* 12(1): 76–102.

Girija, K. P. 2017. 'Interface with Media and Institutions: The Reordering of Indigenous Medical Practitioners in Twentieth-century Kerala'. *History and Sociology of South Asia* 11(1): 1–8.

Government of India. 1975. 'Srivastava Committee Report—Health Services and Medical Education: A Programme for Immediate Action'. Ministry of Health and Family Planning, New Delhi. Available at https://www.nhp.gov.in/sites/default/files/pdf/Srivastava_Committee_Report.pdf (accessed 17 April 2016).

———. 2002. 'National Policy on Indian Systems of Medicine and Homoeopathy'. Ministry of Health and Family Welfare, New Delhi.

———. 2005. 'The National Rural Health Mission: Mission Document'. Ministry of Health and Family Welfare, New Delhi. Available at http://www.nird.org.in/brgf/doc/Rural%20HealthMission_Document.pdf (accessed 2 May 2015).

———. 2007. 'Eleventh Plan Document'. Planning Commission, New Delhi. Available at http://planningcommission.nic.in/plans/planrel/fiveyr/11th/11_v1/11th_vol1.pdf (accessed 2 May 2015).

———. 2009. 'Report of Steering Committee on AYUSH'. Planning Commission, New Delhi. Available at http://planningcommission.gov.in/aboutus/committee/strgrp12/st_ayush0903.pdf (accessed 2 May 2015).

———. 2012a. 'Report of the Working Group Steering Committee on AYUSH for 12th plan'. Planning Commission, New Delhi. Available at http://planningcommission.nic.in/aboutus/committee/wrkgrp12/health/WG_7_ayush.pdf (accessed 2 May 2015).

———. 2012b. 'Twelfth Plan Document'. Planning Commission, New Delhi. Available at http://planningcommission.gov.in/plans/planrel/12thplan/welcome.html (accessed 2 May 2015).

———. 2015. 'Draft National Health Policy'. Ministry of Health and Family Welfare, New Delhi. Available at http://www.mohfw.nic.in/showfile.php?lid=3014 (accessed 2 May 2015).

Government of India. 2017. 'National Health Policy'. Ministry of Health and Family Welfare, New Delhi. Available at http://cdsco.nic.in/writereaddata/National-Health-Policy.pdf (accessed 30 April 2017).

Halliburton, Murphy. 2009. *Mudpacks and Prozac: Experiencing Ayurvedic, Biomedical, and Religious Healing*. Walnut Creek, CA: Left Coast Press.

Hardiman, D., and P. Mukharji. 2012. *Medical Marginality in South Asia: Situating Subaltern Therapeutics*. London: Routledge.

Hughes, Charles C. 1968. 'Ethno-medicine'. In *International Encyclopedia of Social Sciences*, eds David L. Shills and Robert K. Merton, 87–93. New York: Macmillan.

Hussain, Azmal. 2008. *Ethno-medicine: Indian Perspectives and Practices*. Hyderabad: ICFAI University Press.

Jagadisha, T., L. Zhou, K. Kumar, J. Gao, H. Vaid, H. Liu, A. Hankey, G. Wang, N. Gangadhar, J-B. Nie and M. Nichter. 2016. 'Traditional, Complementary, and Alternative Medicine: Approaches to Mental Health Care and Psychological Wellbeing in India and China'. *Lancet Psychiatry* 3(7): 660–72.

Joshi, P. 2016. 'Emergence of Medical Anthropology in India'. *Eastern Anthropologist* 69(1): 1–11.

Karnataka Knowledge Commission. 2009. 'January 1–March 31, Sixth Quarterly Report'. Available at http://www.jnanaayoga.in/document/quartely_reports/QR_6.pdf (accessed 2 May 2015).

Kruske, S., and L. Barclay. 2004. 'Effect of Shifting Policies on Traditional Birth Attendant Training'. *Journal of Midwifery* 49(4): 306–11.

Lambert, H. 2012a. 'Medical Pluralism and Medical Marginality: Bone Doctors and the Selective Legitimation of Therapeutic Expertise in India'. *Social Science and Medicine* 74(7): 1029–36.

———. 2012b. 'Wrestling with Tradition: Towards a Subaltern Therapeutics of Bone Setting and Vessel Treatment in North India'. In *Medical Marginality in South Asia: Situating Subaltern Therapeutics*, eds D. Hardiman and P. Mukharji, 109–25. New York: Routledge.

Latour, Bruno. 1987. *Science in Action: How to Follow Scientists and Engineers through Society*. New York: Harvard University Press.

Leslie, Charles. 1976. *Asian Medical Systems: A Comparative Study*. London: University of California Press.

Lohokare, M., and B. V. Davar. 2010. 'The Community Role of Indigenous Healers'. In *Health Providers in India: On the Frontlines of Change*, eds K. Sheikh and A. George, 161–81. New Delhi: Routledge.

McClain, C. S. (ed.). 1995. 'Introduction'. In *Women as Healers: Cross-cultural Perspectives*, 1–20. New Jersey: Rutgers Press.

Mishra, A., and D. Nambiar. 2017. 'Revitalization of Local Health Traditions'. *Deccan Herald*, 27 February.

Mishra, A., D. Nambiar and H. Madhavan. 2018. 'The Making of Local Health Traditions: Revitalization or Marginalization'. *Economic and Political Weekly* 53(30): 41–49.

Mukhopadhyay, A. 1992. *State of India's Health*. Delhi: Voluntary Health Association of India.

Nair, Vishwanath N. 1994. 'Anthropology of Tribal Health and Medicine in Forest Environment'. Calicut: KIRTADS.

Nambiar, D., and A. Mishra. 2017. 'In Defense of Traditional Healers: Not What They Are Quacked Up To Be'. *eSSay* (esocialscience.com), 30 January: 1–5.

Naraindas, H., J. Quack and W. S. Sax. 2014. *Asymmetrical Conversations: Contestations, Circumventions, and the Blurring of Therapeutic Boundaries* (Series: Epistemologies of Healing). New York: Berghahn Books.

Nichter, M. (ed.). 1992. *Anthropological Approaches to the Study of Ethnomedicine*. Switzerland: Gordon and Breach Science Publishers.

Nichter, M., and Margaret Lock (eds). 2002. 'Introduction'. In *New Horizons in Medical Anthropology*, 1–34. London: Routledge.

Patel, Vikram. 2011. 'Traditional Healers for Mental Health Care in Africa'. *Global Health Action* 4: 7956.

Pfeiffer, J., and N. Nichter. 2008. 'What Can Critical Medical Anthropology Contribute to Global Health? A Health Systems Perspective'. *Medical Anthropology Quarterly* 22(4): 410–15.

Pigg, S. L. 1995. 'Acronyms of Effacement: Traditional Medical Practitioners in International Health Development'. *Social Science and Medicine* 41(1): 47–68.

Pordie, Laurent. 2007. 'Presentation: Ethnographies of Folk Healing'. *Indian Anthropologist* 37(1), special issue: 1–12.

Priya, R. 2012. 'AYUSH and Public Health: Democratic Pluralism and the Quality of Health Services'. In *Medical Pluralism in Contemporary India*, eds V. Sujatha and Leena Abraham, 103–29. New Delhi: Orient BlackSwan.

Quack, J. 2012. 'Ignorance and Utilization: Mental Health Care Outside the Purview of the Indian State'. *Anthropology and Medicine* 19(3): 277–90.

———. 2014. 'Porous Dividuals?: Complying to a Healing Temple (Balaji) and a Psychiatric Out-patient Department (OPD)'. In *Asymmetrical Conversations: Contestations, Circumventions, and the Blurring of Therapeutic Boundaries* (Series: Epistemologies of Healing), eds H. Naraindas, J. Quack and W. S. Sax, 56–84. Oxford: Berghahn Books.

Raguram, R., A. Venkateswaran, J. Ramakrishna and M. G. Weiss. 2002. 'Traditional Community Resources for Mental Health: A Report of Temple Healing from India'. *British Medical Journal* 325: 38–40.

Raje, Gauri. 2012. 'The Modernizing Bhagat'. In *Medical Marginality in South Asia: Situating Subaltern Therapeutics*, eds D. Hardiman and P. Mukharji, 152–70. London: Routledge.

Ranganathan, Shubha. 2014. 'Healing Temples, the Anti-superstition Discourse and Global Mental Health: Some Questions from Mahanubhav Temples in India'. *South Asia* 37(4): 625–39.

Richter, M. 2003. 'Traditional Medicines and Traditional Healers in South Africa: Discussion Paper Prepared for the Treatment Action Campaign and Aids Law Project'. Available at www.tac.org.za/documents/researchpapers/traditional_medicine_briefing.pdf (accessed 20 April 2005).

Sadgopal, Mira. 2009. 'Can Maternity Services Open Up to the Indigenous Traditions of Midwifery?'. *Economic and Political Weekly* 44(16): 52–59.

Sax, W. H., and Bhaskar Nair. 2014. 'A Healing Practice in Kerala'. In *Asymmetrical Conversations: Contestations, Circumventions, and the Blurring of Therapeutic Boundaries* (Series: Epistemologies of Healing), eds H. Naraindas, J. Quack and W. S. Sax, 200–36. Oxford and New York: Berghahn Books.

Sébastia, Brigitte (ed.). 2009. *Restoring Mental Health in India: Pluralistic Therapies and Concepts*. New Delhi: Oxford University Press.

Shankar, D., and P. Unnikrishnan (eds). 2004. *Challenging the Indian Medical Heritage*. Ahmedabad: Centre for Environment and Education.

Shodhini Collective. 1997. *Touch Me, Touch Me Not: Women, Plants and Healing*. New Delhi: Kali for Women.

Society for Medical Anthropology. 2017. 'Complementary and Alternative Medicine (CAM) and Integrative Medicine (IM) Group'. Available at http://www.medanthro.net/interest-groups/camim/ (accessed 13 June 2014).

Storeng, K., and A. Mishra. 2014. 'Politics and Practices of Global Health: Critical Ethnographies of Health Systems'. *Global Public Health* 9(8): 858–64.

Sujatha, V. 2007. 'Pluralism in Indian Medicine: Medical Lore is a Genre of Medical Knowledge'. *Contributions to Indian Sociology* 41(2): 169–202.

Sujatha, V., and L. Abraham. 2009. 'Medicine, State and Society'. *Economic and Political Weekly* 44(12) (special issue on Indian systems of medicine): 35–43.

——— (eds). 2012. *Medical Pluralism in Contemporary India*. New Delhi: Orient BlackSwan.

United Nations. 2002. 'Report of the World Summit on Sustainable Development'. Available at http://www.unmillenniumproject.org/documents/131302_wssd_report_reissued.pdf (accessed 21 March 2015).

Unnikrishnan, E. 2004. 'Materia Medica of the Local Health Traditions of Payyannur'. Discussion paper, KRPLLD, Centre for Development Studies, Thiruvananthapuram.

Unnikrishnan, P. 2011. 'Traditional Medicine in Health System Development: A Case Study of Kerala State, India'. *Yokohama Journal of Social Sciences* 15(3): 77–101.

Unnikrishnan, P. M., H. P. Lokesh Kumar and D. Shankar. 2010. 'Traditional Orthopedic Practitioners' Place in Contemporary Health'. In *Health Providers in India: On the Frontlines of Change*, eds Kabir Sheikh and Asha George, 182–200. London: Routledge.

Unnikrishnan, P., and M. A. Suneetha. 2012. 'Biodiversity, Traditional Knowledge and Community Health: Strengthening Linkages'. UNU-IAS policy report, Yokohama, Japan.

Wilder, Richard. 2000. 'Protection of Traditional Medicine'. Working paper no. 66, ICRIER, Delhi. Available at http://icrier.org/pdf/wilder66.PDF (accessed 18 June 2015).

World Health Organization. 1978. 'Alma Ata Declaration'. Presented at the International Conference on Primary Health Care, 6–12 September, Alma Ata, USSR. Available at https://www.who.int/publications/almaata_declaration_en.pdf (accessed 1 April 2016).

———. 2002a. 'Traditional medicine: Growing needs and potential'. WHO Policy Perspective on Medicines. World Health Organization, Geneva, May. Available at http://apps.who.int/medicinedocs/en/d/Js2293e/ (accessed 2 May 2015).

———. 2002b. 'Traditional Medicine Strategy (2002–2005)'. World Health Organization, Geneva. Available at http://www.wpro.who.int/health_technology/book_who_traditional_medicine_strategy_2002_2005.pdf (accessed 2 May 2015).

———. 2003. 'Traditional Medicine Report by the Secretariat'. Fifty Sixth World Health Assembly, Geneva. Available at http://apps.who.int/gb/archive/pdf_files/WHA56/ea5618.pdf (accessed 4 June 2015).

———. 2008. 'Beijing Declaration, Adopted by the WHO Congress on Traditional Medicine'. World Health Organisation, Beijing. Available at http://www.who.int/medicines/areas/traditional/TRM_BeijingDeclarationEN.pdf (accessed 4 June 2015).

World Intellectual Property Organisation. 2007. 'Intergovernmental Committee on Intellectual Property and Genetic Resources, Traditional Knowledge and Folklore', eleventh session. Available at http://www.wipo.int/edocs/mdocs/tk/en/wipo_grtkf_ic_11/wipo_grtkf_ic_11_12.pdf (accessed 1 March 2016).

Wreford, J. 2005. 'Missing Each Other: Problems and Potential for Collaborative Efforts between Biomedicine and Traditional Healers in South Africa in the Time of AIDS'. *Social Dynamics* 31(2): 55–89. University of Cape Town: Centre for African Studies.

Legitimacy and Recognition

one

Authenticity, Alliances and Results

Notions of Legitimacy Held by Traditional Healers in South India

Devaki Nambiar, Arima Mishra,
Harilal Madhavan, Sarika Kadam, Shrish N. R.,
Steffy Dhayalan and Pooja Venkatesh

The Dialogue

In January 2016, we had organised a dialogue on the 'revitalisation of local health traditions' in Azim Premji University (APU), Bengaluru, India, that saw the participation of representatives from governmental and non-governmental organisations (NGOs), academic and research institutions and public-health practitioners, including traditional healers.[1] A panel discussion with the traditional healers was held as part of the dialogue. It was an unusual sight (see Image 1.1). Facing the crowd, occupying a single file of chairs were eight traditional healers from the three southern Indian states of Karnataka, Kerala and Tamil Nadu. They ranged in age from 28 to over 80 years, representing myriad areas of specialisation, experiences and perspective. Facing them, seated in semi-circles, sequestered by linguistic preference, were representatives of NGOs, academic institutions and government agencies. At the opposite end of the room, like a bold underline highlighting the proceedings, was a file of young students of the APU Masters in Development programme, listening ardently to the polyglot discussion. This was not quite the assemblage any one group was familiar with—it was not class, a meeting of an organisation or association, or conference, or an official delegation in petition.

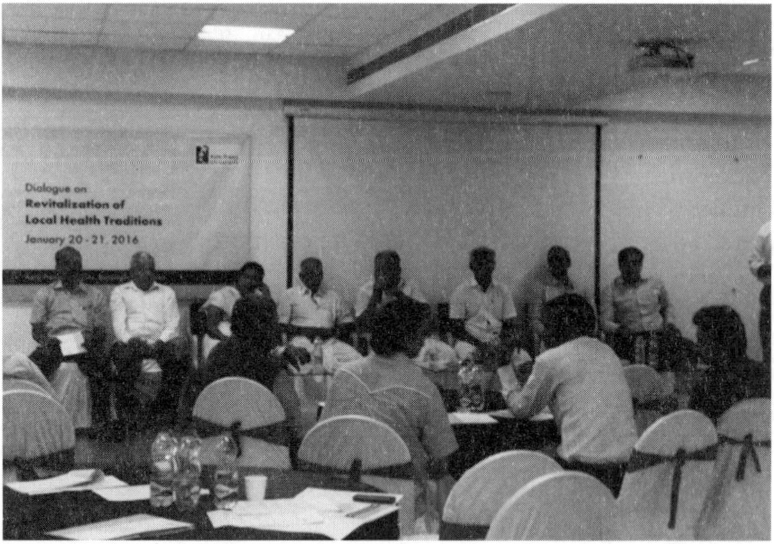

Image 1.1: Traditional Healers in the 'Dialogue on the Revitalisation of Local Health Traditions', 20–21 January 2016, Bengaluru.

Photo Credit: Azim Premji University.

A question was asked in English, and then translated into three regional languages (Kannada, Tamil and Malayalam): 'How can local health traditions be revitalised?'. Each of the healers spoke in turn, pausing for volunteer translators to render their thoughts in the various other languages spoken in the room. A healer from Karnataka underscored that the very survival of the officially recognised systems of ayurveda was contingent on the knowledge and practices of *paramparikavaidyas* like him. Traditional healers or paramparikavaidyas were far more authentic than those being awarded Bachelor in Ayurvedic Medicine and Surgery (BAMS) degrees, who very often took to practising allopathic quackery after getting their degrees. The contributions of such healers, he felt, should be encouraged rather than suppressed. Another healer, from the Western Ghats bioreserve region of Tamil Nadu, talked about monthly meetings of their association (*sangams*). He encouraged the government to acknowledge and support such efforts. This had unique salience in his home state, where traditional practitioners and those accredited with Bachelor in Siddha Medicine and Surgery (BSMS) degrees have substantial interaction, in most cases mutual respect, and are, in fact, widely seen to be in a continuum, where codified siddha knowledge has organic links with the heritage of traditional practice.[2] Another healer called upon the stakeholders sitting in front of him to create pressure on behalf of healers and advocate for them with government and other authorities (this includes the AYUSH community) to understand and acknowledge the richness of traditional medical knowledge. The next healer, seated by her father and *guru* (teacher), was the only woman healer present. She described a case of blood cancer that came to their multi-generational practice after being diagnosed by allopathic doctors. The patient came to her, too poor to afford care in the allopathic hospital. He was healed and yet the healer responsible received no 'official' recognition, though this certainly resulted in patients' reaffirmation of their practice, as many patients were inspired by such successful healing experience and came to seek care. As the remaining five healers took their turns, we, the organisers of the dialogue, sat up in our seats and nodded. We were not in each others' line of sight, but jointly sensed a culmination.

We had sought to understand the 'revitalisation of local health traditions' in Karnataka, Kerala and Tamil Nadu. The dialogue underway in front of us, with its mix of languages, narratives, stakeholders and perspectives, was synecdochic to our study—chaotic and yet there were moments of poignant clarity. Implicit in the statements being made by the healers were their understandings of the strengths of their practice. For one, the authenticity of practice was emphasised by healers either through affiliation with or distinction from codified systems of non-allopathic medicine (ayurveda in particular). Second, peer affiliation was a mechanism by which healers built their reputations and advanced their practice. Finally, the capability of healers, in dealing with complex cases with success, was deemed worthy of acknowledgement.

These statements represented to us the centrality of the issue of legitimacy in answering the question posed, even as the word 'legitimacy' was of our own construction, and there wasn't much of an idea of what colloquial terms could be used to describe this notion and its manifestations.[3] Notwithstanding the different languages and registers, there was a kind of echoing of this central idea. They were akin to 'resonances', redefined by Sleeboom-Faulkner (2015: 579) as 'the shared experiences and understandings of a practice among different parties, interest groups, and cultures forming a driving force in the continuation of that practice'. She goes on to say that,

> Resonances are communications that make sense in a certain context, so that their translation into an international language, in this case English, is difficult to achieve ... [and yet] collectively created resonances are crucial to our understanding of what the researcher presents as 'how medical systems work out there' and their implied moral economies. (ibid.: 580)

This chapter seeks to describe the collective resonances related to the notion of legitimacy echoing not just in this dialogue, but in our repeated interactions with 51 healers from across the three Indian states over the course of a two year-long ethnographic study on the 'revitalisation of local health traditions' in India (2014–16).

As already discussed in the Introduction, local health traditions have been seen largely as functioning far beyond the remit and purview of the State (Hardiman and Mukharji 2012; Lambert 2012; Quack 2012). This situation, as is well documented, arose through the mechanism of registration of practitioners via the Medical Practitioners Acts (1938–62), which in effect created the very category of non-codified, illegitimate practitioners, cast into permanence by the Indian Medicine Central Council Act of 1970 (Unnikrishnan and Harirammurthi 2012: 283–84). A tautology of professionalisation has since endured, described by Lambert (2012) as the only path towards legitimation, which places healers into a 'terminology distinct speciality'. Healers are then subject to the disciplinary power exercised by the State onto its people, and react by engaging in subaltern practice on the fringes of the law. However, as others have observed (Banerjee 2000; Hardiman and Mukharji 2012; Lambert 2012; Sax and Nair 2014; Weiss 2009), there are frames larger than the State for battles over legitimacy, not least among which is the epistemological tussle between biomedicine and alternative sciences, various categories of market-linked, pharmaceuticalised medicine, as well as a legion of practices and beliefs where divine providence as well as professional skill and expertise intercalate not only among providers, but also seekers of healing. From the perspective of the healers present at our meeting, there were multiple sources of and pretexts for legitimacy.

Our methodology of identifying the healers itself drew us to sources of legitimacy. We sought to understand these features in the experiences and understandings of healers, where possible linking to directions for action, including that of the State, on local health traditions. We followed events, people and places—including observations of the Siddha Marma conference in Kanyakumari with 300 healers, as well as government and non-governmental organisations working on local health traditions—that led us to many traditional healers. We reached out to members of the healers' associations. In other cases, the healers themselves directed us to their own peers, informed us about their meetings and other events, where we were able to locate more participants. In other cases, our hosts, contacts and participants in field sites—including a cab driver—led us to 'popular healers'. Thus, our understanding of sources of legitimacy drew not only from the in-depth interviews we had with healers, but was also informed by interactions with members of healers' collectives, and patients visiting the healers at their places of practice or attending health camps organised by them. The narratives that we present here are, thus, co-created by the healers, their peers, patients and us, the researchers, who made sense of these narratives to understand legitimacy that is beyond State acceptance/non-acceptance.

Our ethnographic project, thus, took us from Thiruvananthapuram to Wayanad to Palakkad in Kerala, Kanyakumari to Coimbatore to Gudalur in Tamil Nadu, and Chamrajnagar to Kanakpura to Belgaum, Ankola and Shimoga in Karnataka. Of the 51 healers, 12 were women and the rest were men; their ages ranged from 28 to 80 years. A majority (33) were paramparikavaidyas whose learning and practice was linked to a specific family lineage. The healers had diverse expertise of treating ailments ranging from snake bites, bone-setting, maternal and child health, jaundice and many others. The diversity was not only in the nature of expertise and practice, but also in the participants' understanding and expectations in terms of a revitalisation of their traditions (implicit or explicit). For instance, for tribal healers in Gund in Karnataka and Gudalur in Tamil Nadu, the revitalisation agenda sounded alien, while healers in Belgaum were indifferent and those in Thiruvananthapuram (Kani tribal healers), Kanyakumari and Shimoga explicitly spoke of what the government should do or not do in connection with keeping such traditions alive. It is important to be mindful of this diversity among the healers themselves to situate their perspectives and experiences.

Healers' Voices

Echoed in the January meeting were themes from interviews conducted beforehand, that spanned various explications and interpretations of the legitimacy of the knowledge and practice of local health traditions. These included, but were not limited to: the *authenticity* and longevity of the local health traditions practice, *affiliation* with peers through associations and *reputation* of healers and their patients, manifest through proud narratives of healing diseases like cancer and diabetes, exampling the limitations of biomedicine.

Authenticity and Longevity

The precedence and primordial nature of healing practice was a major frame for healers; a kind of traditional legitimacy as seen among African traditional healers as well (Fassin and Fassin 1988). This was manifest through a series of distinctions made by comparing their practice to others, whether in terms of its sacred character relative to biomedicine, the distinction between *parampara* (tradition) and *nati* (native/indigenous) healers, or the articulations or disarticulations of traditional healing in relation to codified systems like ayurveda.

For healers in Tamil Nadu (who are called siddha *vaidyars* or *paramapari vaittiyar*), 'perfect knowledge [wa]s to be found in the teachings of the past, not in the discoveries of the future' (Weiss 2009: 35). A traditional healer from Thiruvallur explained: 'Herbs were found by the Siddhars long back and still they are there. They were not destroyed by Siddhars, or anyone else. It is the allopathy (biomedicine) people who destroyed them thinking that they are very learned.' Thus, the legitimacy of practice is already established in nature and is to be sustained and preserved, in effect threatened by the approach of biomedicine, which is not just prospective, but also (bio-) prospects destructively.

For tribal healers in Tamil Nadu, the act of passing on the knowledge had to have divine endorsement:

> **Interviewer:** What are the criteria for choosing a *shishya* (student)?
>
> **Male tribal healer from Coimbatore, Tamil Nadu:** I should get permission from the Goddess Amman Arul, then only I will teach the person.
>
> **Female tribal healer from the Nilgiris, Tamil Nadu:** It is very difficult to learn the tradition from anyone. You have to go and ask the healers in far tribal settlements. They will teach only when they get permission from God.

For the siddha vaidyars, the timeless and divine nature of siddha therapeutic knowledge was essential to the tradition. A 57-year-old healer explained thus:

> There is no threat to siddha *vaidyam* (traditional medicine). It cannot go away and it is something that cannot be wiped off. We are alive because Shiva is in each one of us. Even the reason you [referring to the researcher] have come to me is because of him. You are doing without this awareness. He is in every one of us. Can god destroy a god? Only our bodies are different.

The divine reference to Shiva is widely reflected in the writings and verses of Agastya, a well-known siddhar, and most of the contemporary vaidyas practise his knowledge, which has been widely documented in texts and verses (Weiss 2009). Efforts underway in Tamil Nadu to validate and document such knowledge under the auspices of AYUSH Traditional Knowledge documentation projects were challenged on these grounds. It is, in fact, felt that, 'There is no need to protect this medicine. It will not become extinct as it was not created by humans. It was told by God. It may become useless to us but it will never become extinct' (male healer, Vadalur, Tamil Nadu). Whether in relation to documentation or the diffusion of therapeutic knowledge, the immortality of siddha—given its divine origins—was underscored. This, admittedly, did not concord with the epistemologies of modern medicine or even statehood, for that matter.

While the divine nature of tradition was more explicitly expressed by the healers in Tamil Nadu, for those in Karnataka and Kerala, it was *parampara* (lineage or tradition) and the intergenerational, extensive and embedded knowledge, training and practice that parampara inheres that was underscored. The evoking of parampara functioned, at times, as a qualification in introductions, serving as a professional legimitiser. Most healers, in their introductions, would indicate how many generations of their family had passed on their therapeutic knowledge: 'I am a fourth-generation healer', 'My family has been practising for 25 years', 'We are paramparikavaidyas', 'We belong to Sri Putrumaharshi's *paramaparai* (lineage)'. This was an important identifier and marker of the precedent set by their practice.[4]

Following from this, in Karnataka, one healer made a distinction between *nati vaidya* (native/indigenous healers)[5] and paramparikavaidya (traditional healers):

> **Male healer from Gavnal, Karnataka:** People are considering themselves nati vaidya but they are giving anything. Nati vaidyas are banned from practice by government.

> **Interviewer**: How do you differentiate from nati vaidya?
>
> **Healer**: We are paramparikavaidyas (proudly). I am the fifth-generation healer. These nati vaidyas know only superficial things and give medicine. They do not possess systematic knowledge on plants and herbs, how to identify, collect and prepare medicines. We have a parampara (tradition).

Thus, the generational/hereditary (and traditional) nature of local health traditions was seen as being more authentic than the superficial knowledge and practice (read quackery) espoused by healers who were local, but not traditional. The gaze was in this way trained onto the local health traditions community itself by these healers and such distinctions made on the very grounds of legitimacy. Parampara was evoked to draw attention to the rigorous nature of transmission of knowledge from one generation to another and the apprentice mode of learning during this process of transmission (essentially, learning by observing and doing). In this regard, traditional healers underscored the divine qualities of a learner—sincerity, devotion, piety, commitment, perseverance and honesty (this was contrasted with the profit motive of others who claim themselves as traditional healers). The requirements and demands of paramparik training included careful and systematic observation and understanding of the local ecology—water, air, soil, temperature, specific techniques of identification, collection and replenishment of herbs and plants (including the use of senses like smell, touch and taste), prescriptions of bodily interventions in harmony with nature, relationships between food and medicine, and so on (Nambiar and Mishra 2017).

Elaborating on the expansive nature of local health traditions, a 70-year-old healer explained:

> It is not just about medicine. It is *sanskriti*, the kind of culture that we are part of. Just the fact that we are finding it difficult to find words in another language to describe traditional medicine shows the depth and breadth of these words. Traditional knowledge is holistic and is integrated with *jalshastra* (the science of water), metallurgy, astronomy, geography, astrology.

When thanked for sharing his experiences, he quickly remarked, 'Nothing is mine. It is the *prakriti* (nature) that has offered this to us and we must remember prakriti for what we learn. Nothing is ours and I have only shown what prakriti has given us.'

Healing necessarily mandated sensitivity to ecological sustainability, as one traditional healer from Karnataka laid out for us: 'We are trained not to cut from all sides of the bark of the same tree. The tree will die. We cut a little and then move on to the next tree .... We are the ones who collect and use, so we should take care that the trees do not die. You cannot simply cut anywhere.' There were elaborate processes that younger healers would have to go through before they became eligible to practice on their own. Decades-long and apprentice-based models of selection, training and practice were described, which were in many ways more stringent and expansive than what a typical biomedical imagery would allow. But for the healers, these models demarcated authentic practice from quackery, which they saw as a menace to their professions. It is important to note here that some paramparikavaidyas have some sort of 'official' legitimacy as well. For example, in response to a complaint by the Indian Ayurvedic Association about quackery, the Kerala High Court passed an order allowing only paramparikavaidyas with 20 years of family practice to continue the tradition. Similarly, the grants-in-aid scheme of KIRTADS (Kerala Institute of Research, Training and Development Studies of Scheduled Castes and Scheduled Tribes) is extended to paramparikavaidyas alone.[6]

In some of the family traditions, authenticity was represented in the multiplicity of knowledge and reinterpretation of texts through experiential knowledge. Kerala astavaidyas (traditional physicians belong to a Brahmin community in Kerala), despite being forbidden to conduct Brahmin rituals because they regularly attended to surgical treatments, received social esteem because of their command over traditional logic (*tarka*), Sanskrit poetry (*kavya*), traditional Sanskrit grammar (*vyakaraṇa*) and astrology (*jyotsyam*), in addition to vaidyam. Expertise in special treatments (for example, in *hastayurveda* or medicine for elephants) and reinterpretation of many texts like Ashtangahridaya or the older books with great details (like Prayogasamuccaya) have clearly established legitimacy for healers in these traditions (Yamashita and Ram Manohar 2013).

Distinctions were also made, by many healers, between local health traditions and codified AYUSH systems, stating that the former are more authentic, a finding that resonated in other studies too (Sébastia 2012; Sieler 2013). A male healer from Gund, Karnataka, explained it thus: 'Ayurveda is *shashtriya vidhuna* (textual learning). The doctors do not have the *vanshik* (generational) and practical knowledge. Thirty per cent of people get the official degrees only to display their certificate. Their knowledge is limited.' Another healer in family practice in Karnataka, whose brother had completed BAMS, explained the limited significance of this degree. The degree certificate was posted in their place of practice, ostensibly a marker of legitimacy, and yet neither healer drew on ayurveda for his practice: 'People are coming from distant places to avail of our family treatment. So, how could I give them the smaller ('*chota*') treatment of ayurveda?' (male healer, Belambar, Karnataka). So traditional healing, passed down generations, was seen as the big (and authentic) treatment specifically sought by the patients. Any certification, they clarified, was for 'official/legal protection'. A reputed octogenarian traditional healer from south Kerala noted that he supported his son in pursuing a Bachelors in Ayurveda degree. He deemed this 'necessary for the time' and yet noted that even with this training, he did not find his son capable enough to be taught some of his unique experiential knowledge. Thus, codified systems did not necessarily serve to expand, enhance or support the local health traditions knowledge, apart from conferring some legal protection from harassment.

The authenticity of local health traditions as distinct from codified ayurveda was also said to be reflected in the preparation of medicines. A 70-year-old healer said:

> Your [referring to the researcher who had training in ayurveda] way of approaching medicine is *shastriya* (textual) while ours is *deshi* (local). We ourselves collect the herbs, crush it and prepare the medicines. That is why it is effective. While in ayurveda they procure medicines from pharmacies, which are not that effective.
>
> Ayurveda is rooted in *parampara nattuvaidyam* (traditional local medicine). If the branches (referring to Ayurveda) are considered legitimate and these are allowed to flourish, how can the roots be (referring to local health traditions) considered redundant? (A 58-year-old male healer serving as the secretary of a State Healers' Association)

This tension between local health traditions and codified ayurveda was manifest particularly in Kerala, where efforts had been underway to create a role for traditional healers in pedagogy. From the perspective of one healer, in this effort, ayurveda was seen to draw its legitimacy, somewhat exploitatively, from local health traditions:

> When they started Ayurveda College in Thiruvananthapuram, the *marmavaidya* (massage healer) expert teachers were not there. So they appointed paramparikavaidyas for teaching. It was a temporary

> appointment. They learned marmavaidya from the vaidyas within six months. After few months, the Ayurveda Medical College students conducted a strike against the appointment of traditional vaidyas. It was with the support of senior doctors. They demanded the appointment of 'qualified doctors' as teachers. As a result, paramparikavaidyas were out. They are trying to demolish our traditions. (Male healer from Poovar, Kerala)

In this case, we see lamentation over the exploitative nature of ayurveda *vis-à-vis* local health traditions, which derives from the motivations of 'qualified' practitioners. These tensions continue in Kerala even while the community-academia-industry linkages thrive to document tribal community knowledge to innovate pharmaceutical products.[7]

For healers, there appears to be a clear—in fact, sacred and divine—basis for the authenticity and value of traditional knowledge and practice of healing, one that is distinct from *ad hoc*, native practice, involves the rigorous and systematic transfer of knowledge through the apprentice mode of learning and has a vexed relationship with codified systems of non-allopathic medicine, specifically ayurveda. This served to distinguish traditional healing in important ways for healers, and accordingly its legitimacy, by specifying both what it is and what it is not.

Affiliations and Alliances

In multiple states, especially for those linked to siddha practice, peer membership in associations represented an opportunity to build solidarity and refine practice, enabling its sustenance. Starting in the 1970s and especially in the early or mid-2000s, many sangams/*sangh*s (associations/consortia), *sanghatana*s (unions) and *parishad*s (boards) were created across all three states. A lot of them have since run into financial difficulties and are inactive, but many remain active. In almost all cases, sangams offered certification to healers (for which they typically have to pay a fee), which legitimated their practice to a certain extent. Certificates indicated that the holder was a 'siddha medical practitioner'. Most such sangam member-groups would meet once a month and for special seminars a few times a year. Techniques of practice would be shared and debated, herbs and herbal preparations brought and exhibited. These collective forums served as platforms for recognition and affirmation of the practice.

The 2014 National Siddha Varma Conference, for example, was organised by the Siddha Vaidyargal Mahasangam, a network of siddha sangams, with the support of a private religious charitable organisation. Close to 300 traditional healers were in attendance at the three-day event, hailing from Tamil Nadu, Puducherry, Kerala and Andhra Pradesh. The chief guest of this congregation was a senior functionary in the defence ministry who spoke about his traditional-healer father, and many celebrities who had gained from local health traditions. Another sangam leader and traditional healer noted that the WHO was soon going to recognise *varma/marma* therapy[8] and that this branch of local health tradition ought to receive greater government recognition as well. In a recent meeting of the Healers' Association in Palakkad, Kerala, more than 200 traditional healers gathered to felicitate 10 senior healers/vaidyas including a woman bone-setter, and deliberate on the future of their knowledge and practice. A retired high court judge was the guest of honour who handed over the awards and endorsed local health traditions by speaking about his own positive experiences of being healed.

The discussions in this meeting centred around the modalities of sharing knowledge among the healers' community in more systematic and robust ways. A member of a large collective of healers clarified, 'Mere registration of healers, as happens for many individual associations, should not be the goal of this collective.' Reinforcing this line of thinking, members of the Karnataka Healers' Association said that the ultimate goal of the association is to revive the *gurukula*[9] systems of learning that can do justice to the rich and composite nature of local health traditions and not any *ad hoc* documentation of knowledge without ensuring sustenance of its practice.

Apart from associations, allying with academic organisations, civil-society institutions, government research institutes and other powerful votaries of local health traditions has been useful for healers. Botanic and entomological institutes across the south have long worked closely with tribal healers to understand ethno-medical practices and products, which continues to this day. For these collaborations, gatekeeper healers worked closely with universities (in one case in Tamil Nadu, a healer's brother was a botanist), while those providing the knowledge were paid honoraria. These partnerships also involved the forestry department, which acted as the main gatekeeper for sharing information on 'legitimate', 'popular' healers for the purpose of documentation by government research institutions. Alliances also involved participation in workshops/seminars/conferences organised by academic institutions.

From the 1990s onwards, civil-society organisations too entered the fray. At this time, the Foundation for the Revitalisation of Local Health Traditions was among the most active allies of healer associations, helping to form them (sometimes as founder members) and advocate for their causes at the national and sub-national levels.[10] Two central mechanisms identified for this were (a) documentation and validation of traditional health practices, and (b) certification of healers as *gramvaidyas* (village doctors) through an elaborate participatory methodology.[11] Apart from this, other organisations like the Jawaharlal Nehru Tropical Botanic Garden and Research Institute (Kerala), Centre for Traditional Medicine Research (Tamil Nadu) and Indian Council of Medical Research (ICMR), Regional Centre (Belgaum, Karnataka) have been actively involved in documenting traditional health knowledge in close and continued collaboration with various healers. The Karnataka Biodiversity Board has organised public meetings with traditional healers as part of the documentation of traditional knowledge. Invitation to such meetings is widely advertised in newspapers, including the vernacular ones. As an official of the board explained, 'Since the information about the meeting is advertised by a Government agency, healers see this as an opportunity to get 'official' recognition and hence many of them have come to attend and share their knowledge voluntarily.' Healers have turned to several such events hoping to gain official recognition and affirmation, a process similar to that observed in African contexts (Amoah, et al. 2014).

The involvement of State agencies like ICMR, TBGRI and National Ayurveda Dietics Research Institute (NADRI), and the endorsement of elected representatives as well as individual State actors, through felicitation or reaching out to them to document their knowledge suggest not a very strict separation of boundaries between the State and players in the field of local health traditions. Rather, the healers' testimonies have drawn attention to the intercalated, enmeshed nature of the State—former senior functionaries would endorse them in public fora, government institutes would invite them to dialogues and platforms and electoral parties would negotiate with them to grant certain conditional privileges, like certification for those in paramparik practice.

While at one level the healers wanted such alliances and affiliations, given their inherently *ad hoc* and sometimes hierarchical nature, there was, for some, a disenchantment with such alliances and what healers got back from them: 'Even founders are interested in growing their own NGOs. What is the meaning of an association if it does not provide facilities to the vaidya?' (male healer from Karnataka). 'People from cities come to document our knowledge, but we have no idea what they do with it as they don't come back and share with us. Documentation is of no use if this does not lead to recognition of healers themselves' (a healer from Kanakpura, Karnataka). These resentments have led many associations/ sangams to think of other sustainable models of self-organisation.

The performative aspects of alliances—in sangam meetings/healers' exchange, in exercises of documentation, participation in seminar/ conference organised by academic institutions—were seen by multiple stakeholders as critical to legitimacy.[12] In many cases, the methodologies of documentation used in these alliances have been replicated and extended, wherever finances allow, and disseminated through association periodicals, flyers and even in media appearances, extending the performative dimensions of legitimacy. In Kerala, for instance, a traditional healer rose to fame due to his public appearances in the media on his fight against adulteration in food products. He continues to serve as a consultant on issues related to adulteration in the state, claims to offer herbal alternatives for adulterated medicines and is a spokesperson in the movement against the irrational use of antibiotics.

Results and Reputation

Legitimacy was asserted through the therapeutic prowess of healers. Put simply, 'the Government can't take any action against paramparikavaidyas because we are successful vaidyas. We successfully treat, so people are with us' (male traditional healer from Kattakkada, Kerala).

One healer spoke about his father's proficiency and how the reputation of their practice grew, translating eventually into legitimacy:

> We treat all patients who come to our doorstep. But my father's specialty was AIDS. He cured a patient of AIDS by 90 per cent. A book has been published on this. A researcher like you from another medical college came to document my father's practice.
>
> Actually, what happened in the past is that we treated cancer of an advocate. After that we got publicity about being able to treat cancer. This was word-of-mouth publicity: if we cure one patient, then he will come back with 10 more patients. But the advocate mentioned this to Dr A...,

> the dean of [a famous hospital in another state]. She called my father asking him to give her medicine for cancer and HIV. You know, na, that hospital? It is famous! They studied how our medicine helped the patient. He was all over the newspapers and the radio....
>
> My patients are ministers, Central Intelligence Department officials. When I ask them about the legal status [of our practice], they say, 'We are not giving legal status as you don't have degree, but we are not banning you either.' We are in between these two. (Male traditional healer from Gavnal, Karnataka)

In Karnataka and Kerala in particular, there were many narratives detailing the care given to celebrity patients—film actors, politicians, civil servants, senior police functionaries and members of the judiciary—and accolades being received thereafter. One healer talked about how some of his patients could not afford 'English medicine' and came to him instead: 'Initially ... most of the patients were local but after we treated a famous personality, we became very famous and patients started to come from other parts of Karnataka, Maharashtra and Goa' (male traditional healer from Santibastiwad, Karnataka). Such proud narratives were reinforced by local organisations and associations felicitating healers for their contribution to the health and healing of marginalised communities, the documents of which were prominently displayed in consultation spaces.

The healer from Gavnal, Karnataka, practised out of a luxury hotel on a monthly basis; his travel expenses were compensated for by his hosts and patrons. One of the owners of this group of hotels had personally benefitted and had since extended this opportunity and various other forms of support to this healer and his family practice. This healer treated patients in his own village and those coming from other places in Karnataka and the region, but also conducted regular, free health camps in the villages 'adopted' by the aforementioned group of hotels. Coverage in the media was a manifestation of legitimacy, to which the healers proudly drew our attention during the course of our conversations (see Images 1.2 and 1.3).

In these narratives of reputation and results, we see implicitly the limitations of biomedicine, observed in other works in India (Bhardwaj 2013; Lambert 2012), on the one hand, and the faith that many patients have in relation to the practice of local health traditions on the other. This faith was itself a source of legitimacy that healers were well seized of—something that allowed their practice to flourish, even as it may have been unrecognised by formal state institutions and agencies.

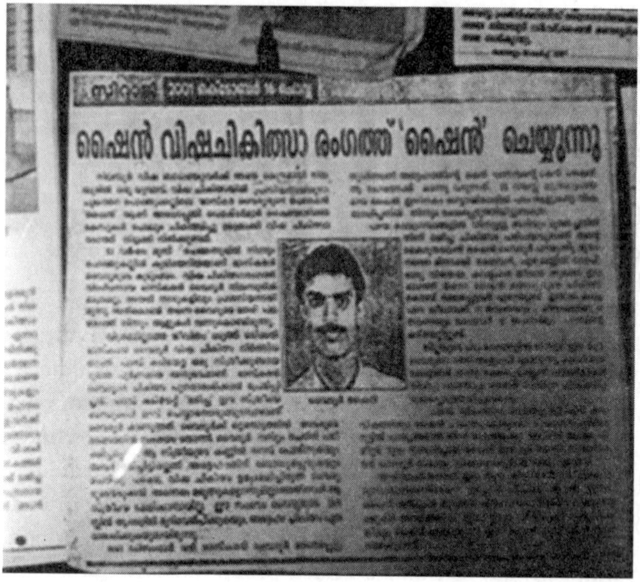
ഷൈൻ വിഷചികിത്സാ രംഗത്ത് 'ഷൈൻ' ചെയ്യുന്നു

Image 1.2: Media coverage of practice of Shine Vaidyar

Source: *Siraj Daily*, 16 October 2001.

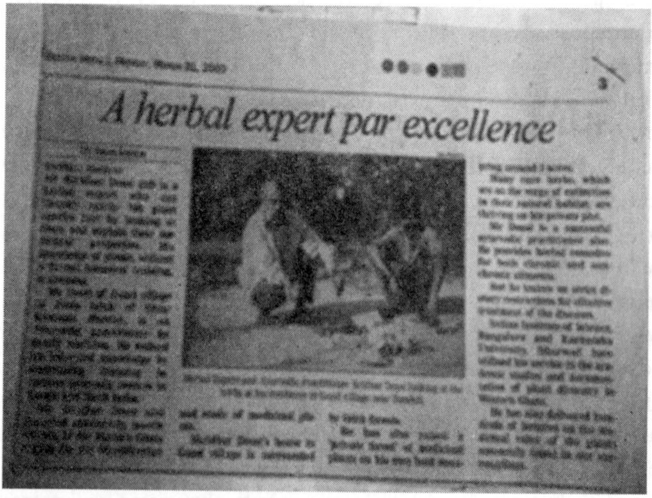
A herbal expert par excellence

Image 1.3: A herbal expert par excellence

Source: *Deccan Herald*, 31 March 2003.

While prowess and ability were a shared source of legitimacy, the healers with whom we spoke accorded varying emphasis and priority to authenticity and the alliances among healers' associations, collectives and sangams. For example, those in a generational family practice emphasised authenticity and generational transfer more than affiliations and alliances. In fact, many such healers whom we spoke to in north Karnataka were not members of any association. Their huge patient base was more indicative of their social legitimacy than peer affirmation through a sanghathana. On the other hand, healers who had learnt from a guru or master (thus acquired knowledge) or were first-generation healers drew more on the legitimacy of collective strength through association, a feature also seen in studies of Senegalese healers (Fassin and Fassin 1988). It followed that the lack of legal or State recognition/certification for legitimacy was also given varying priority across healers. For many popular, in many cases tribal, healers in the Nilgiris, Wayanad, Kerala or north Karnataka, this barely received mention.

Healers' Narratives: Lessons for the Study of Pluralism

This chapter, in line with the thrust of the volume, has sought to explore medical pluralism by consciously privileging the perspectives and experiences of the traditional healers themselves as well as the various arguments put forward by them when reflecting upon their practice and its vitality. While for the State, institutionalised training, registration, codification and other modes of standardisation have been the only means to define a legitimate body of medical knowledge and practice, healers' experiences decouple the notion of legitimacy from automatically referring to the gaze and rituals of statehood and of biomedicine. Healers spoke of longevity and precedence, the ethos and rigour of the apprentice mode of learning and experientially acquired skills, modes of collective sharing and social legitimacy through patients' experiences. In doing so, they drew our attention to the many notions of legitimacy that contribute as much to understanding the vitality of the traditions as to potential threats by the State and codified systems of medicine. In the same vein, these pretexts of legitimacy have also drawn our attention to the enmeshed nature of the State where, despite not according legal recognition, State actors (formally and informally) have endorsed and recognised traditional healers and their practices (Nambiar and Mishra 2019).

The claims to legitimacy emerging from our dialogue and fieldwork demonstrate the construction of therapeutic identities—as healers, involving a web of comparisons and associations drawn by healers. Elsewhere, describing antiretroviral therapy (ART) patients in the Ivory Coast and Burkina Faso, Nguyen (2010) describes 'informal and formal procedures, protocols, and policies' governing the treatment and lives of people living with HIV that operate at multiple scales (individual and transnational) and parallel the (therapeutic) state, or government-sanctioned apparatus of care. He calls this the 'Republic of Therapy'. The creation of these rituals and claims to legitimacy are isomorphic to, and enmeshed in, the State, looping through and beyond it—but chiefly, these claims are made by those who are outside of the State's purview.

We see something not identical, of course, but perhaps similar in the case of healers in the Indian context who represent a republic of healing. Healers' claims to legitimacy draw from a series of rituals, processes and, critically, from relationships with famous others, peers and therapeutic selves. These notions of legitimacy—indeed, a republic of this sort—do not necessarily suggest that State recognition (a more explicit legal/official recognition) does not matter to the healers; it certainly does. These narratives, however, contest the typical parameter of legitimacy that the Sate recognises. Through drawing attention to the rigorous nature of acquiring knowledge, healers' narratives offer us an alternative construction of quackery, a concern that is collectively shared by the healers. The healers' narratives and the discussions in our dialogue further question legitimacy itself—legitimacy for whom and why? One of the participants in our dialogue in January 2016, who is a researcher studying his own community's traditional knowledge, thought aloud:

> If we are talking about legitimisation, who will/should legitimise local health traditions and its practitioners? Is it the healers themselves, the local association, or the peer group? Or is it the State? Or the AYUSH department? Local health tradition is not just a list of herbs and plants, it is a culture. We have to understand this composite body of knowledge, its sources, practices and what hold these traditions before speaking about legitimacy or documentation.

Another senior public health activist participating in the same dialogue added:

> Should we be talking about legitimacy at all? Why should an indigenous local health tradition now establish itself to be legitimate? Local health

> traditions have always existed, which people have used in different forms. How does it continue to survive otherwise in the absence of any legitimacy? Instead of legitimacy, we should be talking about de-legitimating strategies of the State, professional associations of codified systems of medicine and biomedicine.

These discussions point towards a reorientation of the lens of medical pluralism itself. India is characterised by what Priya (2013) calls 'undemocratic pluralism', where through policy (in)attention or budgets, the State tends to nest systems of medicine and knowledge in a hierarchy. This hierarchisation assumes a logic of legitimacy that, in turn, obfuscates the strengths and limitations emanating from any one body of knowledge or domain of practice (Mishra and Nambiar 2017). The agenda of the revitalisation of local health traditions needs to have a lens of plurality, whereby, rather than being construed in terms of what and how local health traditions are not (not biomedicine, not AYUSH), they may be understood for what they mean to people—what kinds of cultural expressions they engender and therapeutic identities they reflect. 'Revitalisation' would benefit significantly from such reframing, leading us to several possibilities and critical conversations across different medical systems and traditions, plural modes of defining and achieving legitimacy and vitality of medical traditions, and different ways of understanding the processes of learning and practice of medicine. Listening to the healers and their experiences, for us as researchers, has been the first step in this direction.

Notes

1. The two-day dialogue was organised as part of the research study on policy lessons *of* and *for* the revitalisation of local health traditions from 2014 to 2016. The project was funded by the Azim Premji University (Grant #RC 00016). Four chapters (Chapters 1, 6, 8 and 10) in this volume are based on this research study. The dialogue aimed to create a space for practitioners of different systems of medicine including traditional healers, NGOs and government representatives to collectively deliberate on the issues and concerns around local health traditions. Such a spirit of dialogue was important to the ethos of pluralism as local health traditions are always spoken of either through the AYUSH lens or through representatives of the various NGOs claiming to be the allies of local health traditions knowledge and its practitioners; however, rarely have healers themselves shared the stage with others to voice their concerns.

2. It is a common practice among siddha graduates (BSMS) in Tamil Nadu to intern with traditional *siddha vaidyas* (traditional healers) as part of their learning.

3. Colloquial terms refer more to the sources of legitimacy implying *gyana/ parampara shakti* (power of hereditary knowledge), *siddhi shakti* (reputation) or *lok/sambandh shakti* (power of people/affiliations/associations).

4. And yet almost all healers, when asked about the future, lamented the lack of interest and rigour among younger generations to pursue practice. They were mindful of the fact that this was vitiating the premise of intergenerational transfer of knowledge, and some healers were ensuring its preservation through partnerships with academic and civil-society organisations, while others took to documenting the knowledge themselves.

5. The term *nattu vaidyas* originally referred to all traditional medical practitioners, including registered as well as folk healers. The government department was called *nattur chikitsa vakupu* (indigenous medicine department) until the early 1990s in Kerala. The government renamed the department Indian Systems of Medicine, drawing a distinction between those systems of medicine which are codified, practitioners who are registered and those who are not. This distinction became politically significant as this was seen as a conscious process of distanciation by practitioners of AYUSH from the nattu vaidyas (Unnikrishnan and Harirammurthi 2012). The latter have sought to reassert the authenticity of their knowledge and practice through highlighting the generational nature of knowledge through reconfiguring the terms of reference as *parampariya vaidyas* or *parampariya nattur vaidyas*. See Girija (2017) for details on politics of identification and how the media played an important role in the reconfiguration of nattuvaidyam.

6. For more details, see www.kirtdas.kerala.gov.in (accessed 10 March 2017).

7. Jeevani is one such product based on the systematic documentation of the knowledge of the Kani tribal community through the benefit-sharing model.

8. *Marma chikitsa* (therapy) refers to a system of therapy where the afflictions of the physical body are healed through the systematic stimulation of the vital points.

9. A *gurukula* is where trainees apprentice with more experienced practitioners for years in order to hone and acquire skills through oral transfer of knowledge, learning by doing and developing relationships with patients alongside their mentors.

10. It facilitated the National Healer's Conference in Karnataka in April 2017.

11. See Bode and Unnikrishnan (2013) for more details on the methodology of documentation.

12. The healers participating in the dialogue saw APU too as an ally. The invitation from the university establishes their legitimacy as 'healers'. In addition, they also expected this dialogue to be of a similar nature as the sangam meetings,

where healers are encouraged to share their knowledge, display herbs/plants or anything else they wish to showcase. In an explicit feedback session, one of the healers, who is also a secretary of a healers' association, said, 'You as a university can do a lot. Please organise a healers' exchange and call all traditional healers and also the officials of the Department of AYUSH/Health and Welfare. We are ready to offer free health camps and let the officials see what our practice entails.'

References

Amoah, S. K. S., L. P. Sandjo, S. N. Leite and M. W. Biavatti. 2014. 'Herbalists, Traditional Healers and Pharmacists: A View of the Tuberculosis in Ghana'. *Revista Brasileira de Farmacognosia* 24(1), January–February: 89–95.

AYUSH. 2002. 'National Policy on Indian Systems of Medicine and Homoeopathy'. Department of Ayurveda, Yoga and Naturopathy, Unani, Siddha and Homoeopathy, Ministry of Health and Family Welfare, Government of India, New Delhi.

Banerjee, M. 2000. 'Whither Indigenous Medicine'. *Seminar* 480, May: 44–48.

———. 2009. *Power, Knowledge, Medicine: Ayurvedic Pharmaceuticals at Home and in the World, New Perspectives in South Asian History*. Hyderabad: Orient BlackSwan.

Bhardwaj, R. 2013. '"No one medicine is enough": Accounts of Complementary Therapy Practitioners in Delhi'. In *Multiple Voices and Stories: Narratives of Health and Illness*, eds A. Mishra and S. Chopra Chatterjee, 46–74. New Delhi: Orient BlackSwan.

Bode, M. 2008. *Taking Traditional Knowledge to the Market: The Modern Image of the Ayurvedic and Unani Industry, 1980–2000*. Hyderabad: Orient Longman.

Bode, M., and P. Unnikrishnan. 2013. 'Evidence Based Traditional Medicine: For Whom and to What End?' *eJournal of Indian Medicine* 6: 1–20.

Cant, S., and U. Sharma. 1999. *A New Medical Pluralism?: Alternative Medicine, Doctors, Patients and the State*. London: UCL Press.

Charles, L. 1980. 'Medical Pluralism in World Perspective [1]'. *Social Science and Medicine* 14(4), November: 191–95.

Fassin, D. and E. Fassin. 1988. 'Traditional Medicine and Stakes of Legitimation in Senegal'. *Social Science and Medicine* 27(4): 353–57.

Girija, K. P. 2017. 'Interface with Media and Institutions: Reordering of Indigenous Medical Practitioners in Twentieth-century Kerala'. *History and Sociology of South Asia* 11(1): 1–18.

Hardiman, D., and P. B. Mukharji. 2012. *Medical Marginality in South Asia: Situating Subaltern Therapeutics* (Intersections: Colonial and Postcolonial Histories Series). Abington: Routledge.

Harrison, M. 2006. *Legitimacy, Meaning and Knowledge in the Making of Taiwanese Identity*. New York and Basingstoke: Palgrave Macmillan.

Lambert, H. 1992. 'The Cultural Logic of Indian Medicine: Prognosis and Etiology in Rajastani Popular Therapeutics'. *Social Science and Medicine* 34: 1069–76.

———. 2012. 'Medical Pluralism and Medical Marginality: Bone Doctors and the Selective Legitimation of Therapeutic Expertise in India'. *Social Science and Medicine* 74(7): 1029–36

———. 2013.'Introduction: Plural Forms of Evidence in Public Health: Tolerating Epistemological and Methodological Diversity'. *Evidence and Policy* 9: 43–48.

Lohokare, M., and B. V. Davar. 2011. 'The Community Role of Indigenous Healers'. In *Health Providers in India: On the Frontlines of Change*, eds K. Sheikh and A. George, 161–81. New Delhi: Routledge.

Mishra, A., and D. Nambiar. 2017. 'Revitalization of Local Health Traditions'. *Deccan Herald*, 27 February.

Mishra, A., and S. Chopra Chatterjee. 2013. *Multiple Voices and Stories: Narratives of Health and Illness*. New Delhi: Orient BlackSwan.

Mishra, A., D. Nambiar and M. Harilal. 2018. 'The Making of Local Health Traditions: Revitalization or Marginalization'. *Economic and Political Weekly* 53(30): 41–49.

Nambiar, D., and A. Mishra. 2017.'In Defense of Traditional Healers: Not What They Are Quacked Up To Be'. *eSSay* (esocialsciences.com), 30 January.

———. 2019.'A Light Inside a Pot: Sources and Sites of Power Emerging from an Ethnography of Traditional Healing in South India'. *Global Public Health* 14: 515–27.

Naraindas, H., J. Quack and W. S. Sax. 2014. *Asymmetrical Conversations: Contestations, Circumventions, and the Blurring of Therapeutic Boundaries* (Series: Epistemologies of Healing). Oxford and New York: Berghahn Books.

Nguyen, V. K. 2010. *The Republic of Therapy: Triage and Sovereignty in West Africa's Time of AIDS*. Durham: Duke University Press.

Nichter, Mark, and Margaret Lock (eds). 2002.'Introduction'. In *New Horizons in Medical Anthropology*, 1–34. London: Routledge.

Pati, B., and Harrison M. 2001. *Health, Medicine and Empire: Perspectives on Colonial India*. Hyderabad: Orient BlackSwan.

Priya, Ritu. 2013. 'The Status and Role of AYUSH and Local Health Traditions in Public Health: The Focus'. International Institute for Asian Studies, Leiden. Available at https://iias.asia/sites/default/files/IIAS_NL65_2425.pdf (accessed 18 March 2016).

Quack, J. 2012. 'Ignorance and Utilization: Mental Health Care Outside the Purview of the Indian State'. *Anthropology and Medicine* 19(3): 277–90.

Sax, W. and Hari Kumar Bhaskar Nair. 2014. 'A Healing Practice in Kerala'. In *The Asymmetrical Conversations: Contestations, Conventions, Circumventions and the Blurring of Therapeutic Boundaries*, eds Harish Naraindas, Johannes Quack and William Sax, 200–36. London: Berghahn Books.

Sébastia, B. 2012. 'Competing for Medical Space: Traditional Practitioners in the Transmission and Promotion of Siddha Medicine'. In *Medical Pluralism in Contemporary India*, eds V. Sujatha and Leena Abraham, 165–85. New Delhi: Orient BlackSwan.

Sieler, R. 2013. 'From Lineage Transmission to Transnational Distance Education: The Case of Siddha Varma Medicine'. *European Journal of Transnational Studies* 5(1): 112–43.

Sleeboom-Faulkner, M. 2015. 'Translating "Asian" Modes of Healing and Biomedicine'. *Medical Anthropology* 34(6): 572–85.

Sujatha, V. 2009. 'Patient as a Knower: Principle and Practice in Siddha Medicine'. *Economic and Political Weekly* 44(16), 18–24 April: 76–83.

Sujatha, V., and L. Abraham (eds). 2012. *Medical Pluralism in Contemporary India*. New Delhi: Orient BlackSwan.

Unnikrishnan, P., and G. Harirammurthi. 2012. 'Local Health Practitioners in India: Resilience, Revitalization and Reintegration'. In *Medical Pluralism in Contemporary India*, eds V. Sujatha and Leena Abraham, 280–303. New Delhi: Orient BlackSwan.

Weiss, R. S. 2009. *Recipes for Immortality: Medicine, Religion and Community in South India*. New York: Oxford University Press.

Yamashita, T., and P. Ram Manohar. 2013. 'Memoirs of Vaidyas: The Lives and Practices of Traditional Medical Doctors in Kerala, India'. *Indian Journal for History of Science*, Indian National Science Academy 6(2): 1–23.

two

Accreditation, Certification and Self-regulation

An Innovative Approach for Strengthening and Reintegrating Traditional Community Health Care Providers

Unnikrishnan Payyappallimana,
Hariramamurthi Govindaswamy,
Sarin Sasikumar and Debjani Roy

Focused efforts over the past three decades by civil-society organisations and healers' networks have brought considerable attention to local health traditions in the country, both in the policy space and in communities of practice. This has resulted in a series of developments including nation-wide networks of traditional community health care providers (TCHPs), promoted by NGOs and community-based organisations, initial policy guidance from the central government, increased resource allocation and even the setting up of a North Eastern Institute for Folk Medicine (NEIFM) based in Arunachal Pradesh. There have also been considerable advances with respect to strengthening specific aspects of local health traditions over the years through the network of TCHPs, self-regulatory mechanisms, regular state- and *taluka*-level[1] meetings, *nattuvaidyarathna* (local traditional community-based health care provider/folk healer of excellence) awards[2] at the state level, establishing documentation and training centres, capacity-building programmes, pilot models of integration in public health programmes, networking through community to community-level exchanges as well as participation in national, regional and international events (Payyappallimana, et al. 2010).

While there is increasing focus on documentation and promotion of local health traditions, carriers of such knowledge—the TCHPs—are at a crossroads due to certain persistent challenges such as formal recognition and lack of a legitimate space for continued practice. There is rapid erosion of knowledge and expertise as the community of expert TCHPs are ageing fast. Intergenerational learning interests are challenged by the livelihood options available for young entrants. Although the older generation of TCHPs provided free services as a non-livelihood function in a subsistence society, the prospects of practice for the younger generation do not meet the livelihood needs in increasingly market-driven rural societies. Social legitimacy is also at risk as more and more TCHPs are moving out of their mainstream profession, that is, local health traditions, resulting in an increased reliance of patients on institutionalised care. Migration of TCHPs away from their communities to semi-urban contexts for better financial prospects has been another trend. Growing unethical commercial interests within the tradition has become a self-defeating factor. Dominance of formalised AYUSH and modern biomedical systems, and the consequent conflicts, have further marginalised TCHPs. Formalised systems of medicine enjoy credibility and legitimacy in the health policy domain and the wider population, while TCHPs who provide informal services are often equated with quacks by the health system, and are often subjected to targeted harassment through the legal framework. While the internal challenges are multifaceted, regrettably, policymakers have also not fully realised the urgency, importance and relevance of recognising and strengthening TCHPs and, in turn, contributing to the formal health system. Overall, there seems to be a strong promotional bias in the way the traditional knowledge for the health sector is valued (in the new 'herbal' medicine age), as compared to how TCHPs are recognised (Payyappallimana 2010).

Health System Challenges

Though nationwide data on TCHPs is still unavailable, it is estimated that their numbers are nearly the same as those of AYUSH practitioners for ayurveda, unani, siddha and *sowa-rigpa*[3]—around 7.5 lakhs (AYUSH 2015)—or of biomedical physicians. The depth and spread of local health traditions is evident in the large number of medicinal species that have been recorded on a continued basis across the country. Studies on the so-called 'informal health service providers' in low- and middle-income countries have continually suggested that there is a widespread presence of informal health service providers in most countries, which is a considerable resource for primary health care and presents a good opportunity for the health sector to expand access to care (Shah, et al. 2011).

There is an increasing concern in India about the inadequacy of the health workforce, especially in rural and inaccessible areas. The discussion regarding strengthening of the trained paramedical workforce has been on the rise, partly because of the lack of expected impacts of the ambitious Accredited Social Health Activists (ASHA) strategy (Garg, et al. 2013; NHSRC 2011). The health care system in India currently has a three-tier strategy—primary, secondary and tertiary institutional machinery for the delivery of health care, the primary health centre being the first institutional contact point for a medical doctor or paramedic. TCHPs exist within communities as informal health care service providers in most rural communities. A recent idea proposed by health care activists is that by making appropriate use of TCHPs and home-level caregivers as the fourth tier of community-supported human health workforce available at no additional cost, we could in turn make access to universal health care possible to every village in the country.[4] The selective integration of TCHPs to increase the health care workforce has been an approach in many low and middle-income countries, especially in areas like mental health, reproductive health, HIV/AIDS and tuberculosis treatment (Payyappallimana 2010). Some researchers argue that there is a clear disparity in their health care integration across the population, based on socioeconomic development and in priority disease areas, that is, in inaccessible areas where mediocre services are provided by integrating 'non-qualified' health workforce (Sheehan 2009). 'Right-based advocates' of health have insisted that having the best health care across the population, irrespective of levels of socioeconomic development, has to be a human right. From an ethical angle, they also express concerns related to the setting of standards of the skills and health care management provided by TCHPs (Cash 2005). This raises a number of concerns in relation to regulation, capacity building, quality of health care, safety, pedagogical approaches and institutionalisation, among others, regarding TCHPs.

In this paradoxical context, an important point being discussed about and among TCHP networks and promoters is the future of these traditions and the specific priority needs and focus for their revitalisation agenda. Within TCHP communities, there are experts with very specialised unique knowledge and skills for specific disease/health areas. This is a relatively small segment, yet it can make a significant contribution to health care if appropriately integrated. A large section of the younger TCHPs are new entrants to the field with relatively less skill or expertise. A significant number of new entrants among TCHPs are from the *guru-shishya parampara*,[5] unlike in earlier times, when the traditions were carried forward within the family. When knowledge is transmitted within the family, the younger generation learns it from a very young age and with as many as 10–15 years of continuous perseverance and observation. This experiential mode of learning from a young age is progressive and practical hands-on learning. Unless the learner clears one level of learning, she or he is never introduced to the next, higher level. It requires the learner to demonstrate their skills and its improvement before being allowed to independently provide health care services. But in recent times, since the past two decades or more, new entrants into the field come from the guru-shishya parampara, having studied from local manuscripts and books than from family traditions. In some of the more financially stable TCHP families, the younger generation learns one of the AYUSH systems of medicine and becomes a qualified health care service provider.

However, a common trend is that younger generations within the TCHP family are increasingly less inclined to carry forward the tradition due to lack of State legal recognition and the increasing livelihood challenges of continuing with service-based health care. The period of learning too begins much later in life for learners for the guru-shishya tradition. Hence, the new entrants have relatively fewer skills and expertise in their respective streams when compared to the transmission of cumulative skills and expertise from within the family tradition. But there are exceptions, too. For example, with respect to streams such as jaundice or traditional bone-setting, the new entrants from within the family are still not uncommon since the practice is relatively more reassuring and rewarding in economic terms. Hence, the younger generations show interest in carrying forward the family traditions in such streams. The younger generation of TCHPs with less expertise would require focused training to advance their knowledge and skills. In terms of priorities, a key question has been whether the unique skills of traditions such as *marma chikitsa* (healing of the afflictions of the physical body through the systematic and therapeutical stimulation of the vital points), *nadi pariksha* (assessment and diagnosis of the clinical state of an individual by a trained and careful examination of his/her pulse), etc., should be the focus of the revitalisation agenda, or if the effort should be towards filling the vacuum of the health workforce by mass training of TCHPs and informal providers, irrespective of the levels of expertise. Development researchers also suggest applying market-based approaches in addition to skill training and capacity building (Ahamed, Boom and Sweeney 2011). Contextually, relevant strategies will have to be designed based on systematic research, given the resource constraints confronting the field.

Integration of TCHPs: A Policy Overview

From the early 1970s, the integration of TCHPs in primary health care has been discussed actively. Integration and utilisation of TCHPs, including birth attendants, in national health systems was a key topic in the 1977 World Health Assembly and the Alma Ata Conference of WHO on primary health care in 1978 (WHO 1978). These discussions continued actively for two to three successive decades and a lot has been written about the potential and challenges of the integration of TCHPs in health systems. There have also been several pilot models where attempts have been made to introduce TCHPs in specific areas of health system planning. This received a further impetus with the various WHO traditional medicine strategies, such as the 2003–05 strategy and the subsequent 2005–14 strategy (WHO 2002). The global traditional medicine strategy for traditional medicine (2014–23) continues to acknowledge the need for the appraisal of TCHPs based on contextual relevance and the creation of self-regulatory systems (WHO 2013). Certification of TCHPs has attracted new interest in many regions in the recent past, especially in countries with rich traditions, yet a relatively shorter history of regulating and formalising traditional medicine. Quality, safety, efficacy and rational practices continue to be in discussion with respect to the integration of traditional medicine in the science and policy domains. In countries like Thailand, Philippines, Nigeria, Ghana, Kenya, Burkina Faso, Burundi and South Africa, this is reflected in the national policies in synergy with WHO policies (ibid.).

As an example, Thailand, according to the 4th National Social and Economic Development Plan (1977–81), which received worldwide attention for its comprehensive and inclusive development approach, discusses three strategic areas. They are: (a) indigenous systems of health and wellness maintenance; (b) indigenous self-health care (self-care and household care, including aspects such as antenatal and postnatal care); and (c) indigenous medicine practised by TCHPs. In the third dimension, the identified policies serve as a crucial link between social, cultural, economic and ecological contexts as an important component in the community health culture. The Thailand National Health Act of 2007 stipulated the development of legal and other standards for certification of the status of TCHPs. A national regulation for issuance of certificate was passed in 2010 which allows screening and certification to integrate TCHPs in community health as part of reforming and decentralising the health sector. A local health fund was established under the National Health Security System in 2006 to promote self-reliance in health for the public and to integrate local health traditions in community health. Indigenous medicine learning centres have been established in several provinces. In 2015, a total of 55,475 TCHPs were identified and registered under six categories such as medicine, pharmacy, massage, birth attendants, bone healers and ritual performers. A national database has been created. Of these, nearly one-third have more than 20 years of experience. Based on a systematic method, 165 have been certified as per the Thai Traditional Medicine Protection Act 1999 and 2,075 are being assessed under the scheme. A knowledge-management project linked with the colleges that offer Thai traditional medicine degree courses has been started to document and impart the knowledge to the young traditional medicine graduates (Ministry of Public Health, n.d.). Evidently unique features of the strategy are the bottom-up process of integration of healers in community health; linkages with formal academic institutions and students for intergenerational and value-based traditional medicine learning; comprehensive scheme for certification; creation of the local health fund and centres of learning at the provincial level; and, above all, even integration of non-material aspects such as spiritual healing and rituals.

More recently at a broader level, policy perspectives on health are slowly moving away from the curative, vertical, institutionally centred health services to wider perspectives including social and environmental drivers and determinants, preparedness, preventive care and community wellbeing. With the introduction of new perspectives such as Eco-social Health, One Health, Planetary Health and so on, it has further widened in scope (CDC 2017; WHO 2017). Though these perspectives have been currently focused more on academic and theoretical work rather than on actual community-level engagement, these present a new opportunity in the future to integrate TCHPs and other indigenous and local knowledge-holders in building holistic development in communities. It is noteworthy that, unlike private practitioners, a large part of TCHPs still maintain a prominent, yet unrecognised, holistic health appeal due to their selfless community service as well as focus on preventive and promotive health care.

On the multilateral environmental policy side, a strong link with biodiversity, ecosystem services and associated cultural diversity also offers significant opportunity for the integration of traditional, indigenous and local knowledge-holders and practitioners in the development policy context. From a non-health sector perspective, policies such as the CBD reflect the importance of the integration of traditional knowledge holders in conserving and sustainably utilising biodiversity and ecosystem resources. It states that traditional knowledge should be valued and considered like other forms of knowledge relevant for development. Article 8(j) of the CBD (1992) states:

> Each contracting Party shall, as far as possible and as appropriate: Subject to national legislation, respect, preserve and maintain knowledge, innovations and practices of indigenous and local communities embodying traditional lifestyles relevant for the conservation and sustainable use of biological diversity and promote their wider application with the approval and involvement of the holders of such knowledge, innovations and practices and encourage the equitable sharing of the benefits arising from the utilization of such knowledge innovations and practices. (ibid.)

Additionally, the policy emphasises, 'Full and effective participation of indigenous and local communities in all stages of the identification and implementation of the elements of the programme of work.' It also asserts the rights of traditional knowledge holders on their knowledge, innovations and practices and highlights the need for a holistic approach and equity in development consistent with the spiritual and cultural values and customary practices of indigenous and local communities. Relevant activities under the work programme of CBD include capacity building of indigenous and local communities (ILCs); development of appropriate guidelines and mechanisms to foster effective participation; mechanisms to involve women specifically with respect to accessing, documenting and conserving resources, and learning exchanges; assessment of status and trends of knowledge, innovations and practices of indigenous and local communities; equitable sharing of benefits-guidelines; appropriate legislation for the protection of intellectual property rights; and so on (CBD 1992).[6]

There are several other sustainability areas where traditional knowledge has been considered important. Though currently there is no health focus, in the Intergovernmental Platform on Biodiversity and Ecosystem Services work programmes on indigenous and local knowledge have assumed high significance. These also form new opportunities for integrating TCHPs in development discussions. On the flip side, the bias reflected in the way traditional knowledge is handled as compared to the support and recognition received by the TCHPs is evident in the policies. With the formulation of national biodiversity regulations, knowledge associated with biological resources is the sovereign right of the State. There is increasing recognition of biocultural knowledge, which is being safeguarded through various processes of *sui generis* documentation systems, yet the holders of knowledge get less prominence or protection on their individual rights (Payyappallimana 2010).

TCHP Integration Efforts in India

Studies have highlighted the hierarchy that exists in medical pluralism in India not only between biomedicine and AYUSH practices, but also between AYUSH and local health traditions. This is amply evident in the way resources are allocated (AYUSH 2017). Following the Indian Medicine Central Council Act of 1970, TCHPs who did not have prior registration with any state medical council and were not formally educated are not allowed to practise as medical practitioners (Government of India 1977). Though different states followed diverse approaches, the national regulation impacted the practice in due course.

Following the strong revitalisation movement from the 1980s, there have been efforts to integrate TCHPs through different pilot models in health systems. Several NGOs across the country have done considerable work to strengthen community-level practices. Since the past two decades, as a leading organisation in the sector, the FRLHT has been involved in the documentation and rapid assessment of local health traditions (DRALHT) in association with TCHPs across the country, to bring about the revitalisation and mainstreaming of TCHPs to serve the primary health needs of the community outside the home and institution-based care as a first response. This procedure employed a systematic, participatory research methodology for the documentation of knowledge and skills, along with a social learning-based approach towards the assessment of practices at the community level. The strategy has made significant impacts in identifying key community priority health needs and appropriate traditional community health care practices that are effective and relevant for fulfilling the local community health needs. The first author of this chapter has been involved in the creation of tools for DRALHT and application of the same in community settings, and has worked with TCHP associations for over 20 years.[6] Other diverse approaches such as home and community herbal gardens, community health interventions in areas such as malaria, anemia, etc., as well as linking with the value chain for developing local community-owned enterprises and livelihoods through quality certified products and services have also been important elements of the revitalisation agenda (Shankar and Unnikrishnan 2004; Harirammurthi et al. 2007).

As discussed in the Introduction to the volume, in the 2002 national AYUSH policy the term 'local health traditions' was used for the first time, which triggered increased attention towards the whole sector within the AYUSH department. As a central government policy directive, a report of the Task Force on Health and Family Welfare by the Government of India in 2002 acknowledged that folk health culture had been generated over centuries and had select elements drawn from the classical codified stream. The National AYUSH Policy of 2002 also acknowledged, again for the first time, the need for revitalising local health traditions for improving primary health care. It was observed that TCHPs enjoyed a definite social legitimacy in their own localities. It also recognised the fact that local health traditions, overall, were being eroded, resulting in a loss of community-supported human resources that are very important to the realisation of a long pending goal of health for all. Against this backdrop, a task force that was formed recommended that household health traditions and folk medicine be revitalised, folk practitioners be recognised and utilised as part of the primary health care system, and research into these traditions and cultures be supported. In different states, the support received for the strengthening of TCHPs has been different. Some states like Karnataka have been very proactive, where the department of health has created a task force to address the issue of regulation, training and integration of local health practitioners in the state health system. A Task Force on Traditional Health Practices and Practitioners, Department of AYUSH, Ministry of Health and Family Welfare, Government of India, was constituted in November 2009 with two agendas. It had the mandate to consider and suggest ways and means of officially and legally recognising and developing traditional health practices and practitioners within the framework of the AYUSH Policy Statement of 2002, the NRHM statement of 2005, the Eleventh Five-Year Plan document of 2007 and the National Health Bill that was under discussion at that time. The task force was also asked to propose a suitable scheme to integrate traditional health practices and practitioners into official national health care policy and programmes such as the National Health Mission, within the framework of the approach paper of the Planning Commission.[4]

The Task Force recommended a number of measures to enable and facilitate the functioning of traditional practitioners and practices, and stated that none of these was intended to control or regulate them. These included:

1. Documentation of traditional health practices and providers in all the districts.
2. Enlisting of the traditional health providers by the local elected bodies (panchayats), supported by the traditional health providers' associations, NGOs, voluntary health service centres and any other community-based organisation.
3. Development of a procedure for the accreditation and certification of the prior knowledge and skills of providers and practices (as suggested by UNESCO's initiative on traditional knowledge). The certification procedure must consider the experience of the users of the traditional health providers' services as well as be verified by (a) the local peer organisation of traditional health providers, (b) principles of the locally practised codified AYUSH systems, and (c) the modern public health perspectives. It should not be a mandatory requirement for a traditional health provider to obtain the certification, this remaining a voluntary process.

4. Constituting state (that is, the province in the Indian context) and district resource centres for local health traditions, which may be anchored in existing reputed AYUSH colleges or NGOs. The tasks of these Resource Centres would be to:
   (a) document local health practices for primary health care,
   (b) collate the list of providers and practices enlisted with the panchayats,
   (c) locate an accreditation body of traditional local health practitioners who have been certified by the approved procedure,
   (d) promote interaction among the traditional providers for sharing of skills and practices,
   (e) promote the knowledge and use of local health traditions among the population, and
   (f) ensure the availability of natural resources required by the local health traditions, restore local medicinal plants and herbs and undertake any other activity that will strengthen local health traditions.

The Centre for Traditional Knowledge Systems (CTKS) of IGNOU,[5] New Delhi, taking inspiration from the United Nations Educational, Scientific and Cultural Organization's (UNESCO) conceptualisation of 'prior learning', worked on covering the rich traditional and non-codified forms of traditional knowledge in various disciplines such as the performing arts, fine arts and craft, textiles, museology, metallurgy, agriculture, horticulture, forestry and veterinary practices, natural resource management, environmental protection, architecture and housing, customary law and health science and practices. Besides other initiatives, a major one was the conception and designing of the system for the Accreditation and Certification of Prior Learning (learned knowledge or prior knowledge) (ACPL), based on an innovative adaptation of modern principles of personnel certification guidelines as per ISO 17024 in order to give the local health tradition knowledge pool and the bearers of the knowledge wider recognition.[7*]

CTKS was sanctioned a grant for the implementation of a pilot project proposal to the Department of AYUSH, Ministry of Family Welfare and Health, Government of India, to certify traditional health practitioners in one district in each of the six states of Chhattisgarh, Odisha, Rajasthan, Gujarat, Tamil Nadu and Karnataka. The pilot project was implemented in collaboration with FRLHT, Bengaluru, and the Quality Council of India (QCI), New Delhi. The pilot was conducted in 2010–12, and 517 TCHPs were certified following the norms of the International Best Practices for the Personnel Certification under ISO 17024. The detailed report was submitted to the mentoring and funding agency that funded the pilot project under their local health traditions scheme.

The National Health Policy of 2017 articulates the need for developing mechanisms for the certification of 'prior knowledge' of traditional community health care providers and creating opportunities for enhancing their skills as well as engaging them in the conservation and generation of natural health care resources.

Accreditation, Certification and Training of TCHPs: An Innovative Approach

In line with the developments mentioned earlier, the ACPL of TCHPs has been considered an important strategy to appraise the knowledge and skills of TCHPs as well as to develop minimum standards of competence (MSC) for the practice. It is envisaged that this could, in turn, facilitate integration of their services in local health care in a more formal manner in the future. As mentioned earlier, in the pilot project for the ACPL of TCHP as per the requirement of ISO 17024, the minimum standards of competence in selected streams of traditional health practice were developed. In each state, a nodal NGO was entrusted with the responsibility of carrying out the assessment and certification process as per the protocols devised for the same. In Karnataka, FRLHT carried out this certification programme. The second author has been interfacing with various TCHP associations across the nation for over 20 years. All the three organisations, including CTKS, FRLHT and QCI, were responsible for the implementation of the pilot phase of the certification of prior learning, while the third author undertook a process evaluation of the said programme in Karnataka.[8] The fourth author has played a central role in the operationalisation of the ACPL methodology along with the QCI. Other states like Chhattisgarh, Gujarat, Odisha, Rajasthan and Tamil Nadu also piloted the programme.

Although the pilot was implemented in six states across the country and uniform procedures were followed, for the sake of understanding, this chapter highlights the experiences of Karnataka as a case study. As a prelude to the initiation of the ACPL programme in Karnataka, a stakeholder's consultation meeting was initially convened and attended by representatives of NGOs working in the field of community health and representatives of the state TCPHs' association of Karnataka, Paramparika Vaidya Parishat. Based on the inputs provided by the TCHP association on the density of the presence of TCHPs, the Shimoga district was selected to pilot the scheme in Karnataka. The ACPL programme that was implemented in Karnataka involved the following steps:

Step 1: As a first step, a rapid village survey was carried out in 10 randomly selected villages each of Shimoga and Soraba Taluks of the Shimoga district to identify the most common streams of traditional community health care practices prevalent in the district. Based on the findings of the survey and in consultation with the TCHPs of the Shimoga district, three streams, namely jaundice, common ailments and traditional bone-setting, were chosen as streams for certification.

Step 2: A Subject Expert Committee comprising expert TCHPs and ayurveda physicians was constituted to develop a minimum standards of competence (MSC) document in the selected streams, which was essentially to be used as an interview schedule or tool for evaluation of the TCHPs during the process of an oral assessment.

Step 3: The MSC document developed by the Subject Expert Committee was put forward to a specially constituted collegium comprising expert and senior TCHPs, ayurveda physicians and project-implementation partners for the ratification of the same.

Step 4: Advertisements in the vernacular newspapers of the Shimoga district calling for applications from TCHPs in the notified streams of practice for the ACPL programme were put up by FRLHT on behalf of CTKS, IGNOU.

Step 5: The endorsement of their application and the facts therein by the president or secretary of the village panchayat was mandated to establish authenticity of the applicant. On receipt of the same, to shortlist them for the evaluation, applications were then scrutinised as per the formulated eligibility criteria.

Step 6: An evaluation committee was constituted for evaluating competence in terms of awareness, knowledge and skills of the applicants. The committee consisted of at least three senior TCHPs from the respective stream, with at least one amongst them from a different pilot district (other than where the assessment is conducted) as well as having at least one AYUSH practitioner.

Step 7: The evaluation committee assessed the competence of the TCHPs by an oral interview with the help of the MSC document that was developed for the stream concerned. After satisfactorily assessing the competency of the candidate, a practical demonstration of skills and a field visit were carried out at the place of work of the candidate to evaluate their technical skills and expertise.

Step 8: Once the candidate was found to be satisfying the MSCs in the given stream based on detailed evaluation, the evaluation committee would recommend for certification under the ACPL programme for that stream concerned.

Step 9: Candidates who were not found to satisfy the requisite MSCs were recommended for training by the evaluation committee to provide them a chance to improve their skills and re-apply for certification at a later stage.

Table 2.1: Details of Applicants of the ACPL Programme in Karnataka

Header	*Total number*
Total applicants	507
Applicants recommended for field visit	151
Applicants not available during field visit	20
Applicants recommended for certification:	
Common ailments	36
Jaundice	61
Traditional bone-setting	14
Candidates recommended for training	20

Reflections

Over the past two decades, various methodologies have been developed and implemented for strengthening TCHPs and the rich community knowledge traditions of health and wellbeing. The ACPL process had demonstrated that processes with sufficient rigour can be adopted to establish the MSCs amongst TCHPs. This has potential, in the long term, to motivate the TCHPs to improve their theoretical and practical knowledge-base and generate confidence in the community with respect to specific streams of knowledge and skills. A vital learning from the process is that only a section of expert TCHPs would complete the certification process without any form of training. In a way, this provided a legitimate opportunity for the TCHPs to address the issues of lack of official recognition and policy legitimacy and enhance the shrinking social legitimacy. For example, the fact TCHP applicants were endorsed for certification by their Gram Sabha or Gram Panchayat is in itself a bottom-up approach confirming the immediate social recognition and legitimacy. The assessment of competency of the healers was done bearing their standing as community-supported TCHPs as the primary health care providers, and as such the ability to deliver safe and efficacious services based on knowledge, skills and experience, in light of their envisioned role, was defined to be most critical. It was understood that there would be a need towards systematic gradation of knowledge, competency and skills of the practitioners based on their expertise in order to prepare them for the process. This also highlighted the critical need for systematic documentation and regular, focused training programmes for further implementation of the scheme. Rigorous research is required to identify levels of key skills and expertise of local health traditions and their gradation.

Yet another important learning was that to create a collegium of experts, it was important to identify local expert TCHPs and familiarise them with the entire process. Care was taken to assure that there is no absolute domination of AYUSH experts qualified through formal learning. Since the methodology involved all key stakeholders such as the community, TCHPs, AYUSH practitioners, QCI, university and NGOs, it provided an opportunity for collective learning for all stakeholders. The codified system of ayurveda as existing today has, to a large extent, evolved from indigenous community-based health practices. This makes them amenable to an understanding of each other, though this attempt is not necessarily and wilfully exercised from either side. Hence, a very conscious attempt was made to include members who were sensitive to views dissimilar to their tenets of practice in the collegium. This exercise aided in creating sensitisation and awareness of expectations from different stakeholders and the need to accommodate varied perspectives towards building a consensual framework for assessment. Though the forum was present for the previous ACPL programme, the degree of actual interaction between the stakeholders is a question that is sensitive and merits further consideration. In order to assess impact, there is also a need for systematic evaluation to capture the experiences of TCHPs who have already been certified. A situational analysis of those who were certified is yet to be carried out. What has been done so far is only a process evaluation of the erstwhile ACPL programme which was conducted almost a year after the completion of the same. The overall reaction to the process was positive, based on the TCHP perception that the assessment methodology was fair and had the depth to gauge their competencies.[9]

The TCHPs do not have a government-run system to regulate their practice. In fact, the collective arrangements of the TCHP association provided the first opportunity for self-regulation. For example, the TCHPs who are desirous of becoming members are required to be endorsed as TCHP with certain minimum years of experience by their village panchayats, in order to be conferred with the association membership. Every state-level association has a memorandum of association and clear guidelines on the membership and a broad code of conduct. Though the self-regulatory frameworks have not been well-defined by the respective associations, there is a laudable attempt towards the same. These are works in progress, yet clearly in the right direction. Not every genuine expert in the TCHP community is willing to assume the role of a guru. It is important to also consider (though this is yet to be substantiated) the commercial interests at play in taking up such roles.

A few pertinent questions are: What should the specific content for training of TCHPs for optimal services in health care delivery be? Does it need to be based partly on the theory of the AYUSH codified systems as well as the basics of traditional community health care, including ethics of health care? Does the provision of such training affect, alter or contaminate their pristine and traditionally rooted concepts of health services? How can the patients be assured that the TCHPs have recognition and legitimacy to continue their service? Can the health system integrate or recognise these health care providers within the current institutional mandates? Does such integration or recognition ensure that the identity of these health care providers will remain protected, or would they be subsumed within a larger codified system of medical discipline? Could there be a possibility for a national institute for folk medicine?

An important reflection of the process is regarding the creation of a new and distinct field of traditions like the recent introduction of sowa-rigpa. This will require critical thinking in terms of organising the knowledge in a systematic manner and creation of a pedagogy that would be suitable for various knowledge practices like herbal medicine, physical therapies and spiritual aspects of healing, including specialised knowledge of tribal healing, and so on. It is needless to say that there is insufficient theorising in the field of local health traditions so as to prepare it as an independent field/discipline. There are experiences, like in the case of *nuad thai*[10] in Thailand (Ministry of Public Health, Undated) or *judo seifuku*[11] in Japan, that could provide some guidance for the process (Payyappallimana and Serbulea 2013). Similarly, unique knowledge and skills such as in marma should be strengthened and integrated. Otherwise, these region-specific practices would get subsumed under the pan-Indian codified traditions in the future or be perpetually considered a subset of AYUSH practices. Creation of an independent department for folk medicine would be a prerequisite for the creation and strengthening of such an innovative knowledge stream. One of the major challenges here is to club the wide array of knowledge practices under one category. Based on the experience of the pilot and the positive response received from the various stakeholders, a national scheme was launched in March 2017—Voluntary Certification Scheme for the Traditional Community Healthcare Providers, which has been implemented across the country. The certification of TCHPs has been done in the states of Tripura and Chhattisgarh by the QCI-approved Third Party Personnel Certification Bodies—EticaClinpharm Private Limited, Raipur, Chhattisgarh and North East Christian University, Dimapur, Nagaland under the Scheme following the principles of ISO 17024 for Personnel Certification.

Conclusion

The critical challenge of access to basic health care remains an unresolved glaring promise in many regions of the country. At the same time, TCHPs continue to be a central part of the primary health care system in the country. The role of TCHPs has been well-acknowledged in the global strategy on traditional medicine as well as various national policy documents in the country. Sadly, the current three-tier system of health delivery as well as the biomedical-centred health system has not been able to fructify this into a reality. An innovative approach developed for accreditation and certification of prior learning has had the positive impact of improving the confidence of the TCHPs and has the potential for creating State and strengthened social legitimacy for local health traditions in the future.[12] Such a pool of primary health care providers offers a great resource for sustainable health outcomes in the population, derived from resources which represent the cultural ethos of said communities. If acknowledged justly, they constitute a potential fourth-tier to the current organised delivery of health services that is in vogue in the nation today.[13]

In March 2017, the QCI, an autonomous body under the Ministry of Commerce, in collaboration with FRLHT launched the Voluntary Certification Scheme for Traditional Community Healthcare Providers (VCSTCHP), a name given after much deliberation, taking a cue from the National Health Policy 2017. It is a National Scheme, the first worldwide, that provides competence standards presently for six streams, namely jaundice, management of common ailments, traditional bone-setting, traditional birth practices, management and treatment of poisonous bites and arthritis, and sets out the evaluation and certification process following the worldwide concept of competence, which involves defining knowledge and skills for a particular job and evaluating them through appropriate means like oral interview, demonstration and onsite observations.

The genuine concept of universal health coverage (UHC) in a multicultural nation like ours rests only with a bottom-up approach of empowering the community and revitalising household- and village-level health traditions. Recent efforts towards innovative means of formal recognition to the community health providers could go a long way in strengthening community-based knowledge.

Notes

1. A *taluka* is an administrative division in India which denotes a sub-district.
2. FRLHT (now Trans-disciplinary University) gives nattuvaidyarathna awards to one male and/or one female folk healer selected by a committee. Healers and the wider public have been invited to put forward nominations at the state level in Karnataka, Tamil Nadu and Kerala since 1995. The selection committee screens the nominations and shortlists the five best healers. Then,

a subcommittee visits the shortlisted candidates and selects one female and/or male healer to be awarded. So far, 27 folk healers have been awarded with the nattuvaidyarathna award, which consists of a *panchaloha* (alloy of five metals, namely gold, silver, copper, zinc and iron) statue of Dhanwanthari accompanied by a cash award of Rs 10,000.

3. *Sowa-rigpa*, the Tibetan system of medicine, believed to have originated in Tibet, is widely observed in the northeastern states of India, Nepal, Bhutan and Mongolia.

4. Personal communication with Darshan Shankar (2015).

5. The fourth author was entrusted with the setting up of the Centre, formulating and implementing all the projects for the promotion, preservation and protection of the various traditional knowledge systems of the country.

6. *Guru-shishya parampara* denotes a tradition where there is a transmission of knowledge from an expert teacher (*guru*) to a disciple (*shishya*), through an oral and practical mode. The shishya lives with the family of the guru for the purpose of learning. The relationship between the two is marked by trust, devotion and respect, and is such that the guru not only performs the role of a knowledge provider, but also one of a mentor.

7. The first two authors contributed to the recommendations of the aforesaid task force.

8. The fourth author was Director of CTKS, IGNOU, and is currently Advisor (TCHP), QCI, New Delhi.

9. The third author is a graduate in the ayurveda system of medicine with close to 15 years of professional experience.

10. FRLHT, along with QCI, has currently launched a voluntary national scheme for the certification of TCHPs that would strictly adhere to the ISO 17024 specifications. This scheme will assist TCHPs living in rural communities, including the far-flung and difficult terrains, to get themselves assessed against a MCS framework, which has the flexibility to accommodate a diversity of knowledge and skills of the TCHPs across the country in various streams of traditional health care practices.

11. A traditional Thai massage which integrates pressure points, stimulation, energy manipulation and postures, widely used for therapeutic purposes.

12. A therapeutic procedure developed from Japanese martial arts for treating injuries resulting in bone fractures or dislocations, contusions or sprains. This is a legally recognised form of traditional practice in Japan.

13. The National Biodiversity Authority (NBA), Government of India, also has in its Acts the provision of recognising the services of the 'local vaidyas and hakims.' The scheme owners of the VCSTCHP have approached the NBA to (a) adopt and promote VCSTCHP as the Scheme that fits in with the NBA agenda for Access and Benefit Sharing (ABS); (b) issue an advisory to the state biodiversity boards to register certified TCHPs under the Biodiversity

Management Committee (BMC) and maintain the data of certified and non-certified local vaids and practitioners; (c) to train and facilitate the use of traditional knowledge to enhance the livelihood and health security of village-based community traditional knowledge holders under the ABS of NBA.

14. The Government of India, for the first time in recognition of the services being provided by the TCHPs, on Republic Day, 26 January 2018, conferred the prestigious Padma Awards to three TCHPs from Kerala, Karnataka and Tibet. It was a well-deserved recognition for the TCHPs who are the first points of contact for the rural and tribal areas for any sort of primary health care issues.

References

Ahamed, S., A. Boom and R. Sweeney. 2011. 'Analysing Relationship between the State and Non-State Health Care Providers, with Special Reference to Asia and the Pacific'. Health Policy and Health Finance Knowledge Hub, working paper series no. 10, March. Nossal Institute for Global Health, University of Melbourne.

AYUSH. 2015. 'Medical Manpower AYUSH 2015'. Available at http://ayush.gov.in/sites/default/files/Medical Manpower Table 2015.pdf (accessed 5 June 2017).

———. 2017. 'Notes on Demands for Grants Expenditure of the Centre Central Sector Schemes/Projects Strengthening of AYUSH Delivery Systems 2017–18'. Ministry of Finance, Government of India. Available at http://indiabudget.nic.in/ub2017-18/eb/sbe5.pdf (accessed 5 June 2017).

Cash, R. 2005. 'Ethical Issues in Health Workforce Development'. *Bull World Health Organ*. 83(4): 280-84. Available at http://www.scielosp.org/pdf/bwho/v83n4/v83n4a11.pdf (accessed 5 June 2017).

CBD. 1992. 'Article 8(j)'. United Nations. Available at https://www.cbd.int/doc/legal/cbd-en.pdf (accessed 5 June 2017).

CDC. 2017. 'One Health'. Centre for Disease Control. Available at https://www.cdc.gov/onehealth/index.html (accessed 5 June 2017).

Garg, P. K., A. Bhardwaj, A. Singh and S. K. Ahluwalia. 2013. 'An Evalutation of ASHA Workers' Awareness and Practice of their Responsibilities in Rural Haryana'. *National Journal of Community Medicine* 4(1): 76–80. Available at http://njcmindia.org/uploads/4-1_76-80.pdf (accessed 5 June 2017).

Government of India. 1977. Indian Medicine Central Council Act 1970. Available at http://ayush.gov.in/sites/default/files/The%20Indian%20Medicine%20Central%20Council%20Act%2C%201970.pdf (accessed 5 June 2017).

Harırammurthi, G., P. Venkatasubramanian, P. M. Unnikrishnan and D. Shankar. 2007. 'Home Herbal Gardens: A Novel Health Security Strategy Based on Local Health Knowledge and Resources'. In *Traditional, Complementary and Alternative Medicine: Policy and Public Health Perspectives*, eds G. Bodeker and G. Burford, 167–84. London: Imperial College Press.

Ministry of Public Health. n.d. 'Knowledge Management of Thai Indigenous Medicine: A Decade of Experience to Revive the Folk Wisdom'. Department of Thai Traditional and Complementary Medicine, Ministry of Public Health, Thailand.

NHSRC. 2011. 'ASHA: Which Way Forward ...?' Available at http://poshan.nic.in/sites/default/files/e-library-docs/Evaluation_of_ASHA_Program_2010-11_Report.pdf (accessed 5 June 2017).

Payyappallimana, U. 2010. 'Knowledge and Practitioners: Is There a Promotional Bias in Traditional Knowledge in Policy and Practice?' In *Approaches to Development and Well-being*, eds Suneetha Subramanian and Pisupati B., 194–208. Tokyo: UNU Press.

Payyappallimana, U., and M. Serbulea. 2013. 'Integration of Traditional Medicine in the Health System of Japan: Policy Lessons and Challenges'. *European Journal of Integrative Medicine* 5(5): 399–409.

Payyappallimana, U., G. Hariramamurthi and Wim Hiemstra. 2010. 'Celebrating Healing Heritage'. Summary of the Proceedings of International Healers Exchange and Conference on Traditional Medicine for Sustainable Healthcare, Bangalore, India, 8–22 November. Jointly organised by Department of AYUSH, Government of India, FRLHT, Compas, UNDP Equator Initiative and UNU-IAS.

Shah, N. M., W. R. Brieger and D. H. Peters. 2011. 'Can Interventions Improve Health Services from Informal Private Providers in Low and Middle-income Countries? A Comprehensive Review of the Literature (Key Messages)'. *Health Policy Plan* 26(4): 275–87. Available at https://oup.silverchair-cdn.com/oup/backfile/Content_public/Journal/heapol/26/4/10.1093/heapol/czq074/2/czq074.pdf?Expires=1496731048&Signature=finIQbjye7z6~sAPRBQBPtXShsA0Qybo43-HGTwzzQ0Gd0OwqdV3uqVyjzWkp8jqerTY9DGf-a9a1y2jkQe0aav0oA9JQi6v3EolTHlcb5g4FBG (accessed 5 June 2017).

Shankar, Darshan, and P. M. Unnikrishnan (eds). 2004. *Challenging the Indian Medical Heritage*. New Delhi: Foundation Books.

Sheehan, Helen. 2009. 'Medical Pluralism in India: Patient Choice or No Other Options?' *Indian Journal of Medical Ethics* 6(3), July–September: 138–41.

WHO. 1978. 'Primary Health Care'. Report of the International Conference on Primary Health Care, Alma-Ata. Available at https://www.unicef.org/about/history/files/Alma_Ata_conference_1978_report.pdf (accessed 5 June 2017).

WHO. 2002. 'Traditional Medicine Strategy 2002–2005'. Available at http://www.wpro.who.int/health_technology/book_who_traditional_medicine_strategy_2002_2005.pdf (accessed 5 June 2017).

______. 2013. 'WHO Traditional Medicine Strategy 2014–2023'. Available at http://apps.who.int/iris/bitstream/10665/92455/1/9789241506090_eng.pdf (accessed 5 June 2017).

______. 2017. 'One Health' Available at http://www.who.int/features/qa/one-health/en/ (accessed 5 June 2017).

three

Whom Do the Rural Poor Consult for Health Care and How Much Do They Spend in India's Pluralistic Health Care Arenas?

Mark Nichter*

In much of the world, people have access to multiple therapy systems, types of practitioners and distribution points for pharmaceuticals in what medical anthropologists have termed pluralistic health care arenas (Nichter and Quintero 1996). When, how and why populations utilise health care resources as they do is a core concern for medical anthropologists as well as health planners. In this chapter, we summarise findings from a study conducted in 1979–80 that looked closely at patterns of practitioner consultation among the poor in the pluralistic health care arenas of two districts of Karnataka in south India. The study focused on rural households as a means to better understand who they consulted about non-catastrophic health problems and how much they spent on various types of diagnosis/divination and treatment.[1] The study was designed to consider differences in health care seeking patterns by caste (a marker of cultural variance as well as structural vulnerability) in one district, and proximity and access to towns as health care hubs in the other district. Health care needs were defined as encompassing the

* Project Community Diagnosis was funded by an Indo-US Sub-commission on Education and Culture grant to the author. I would like to acknowledge the vital role played by H. K. Bhat, Srinivas Devadigas and Mimi Nichter in training and supervising local teams of researchers in North Kanara and South Kanara. Lauren Pring assisted in quantitative data analysis and Charla Dain in the editing of the final manuscript. Finally, my thanks goes to Arima Mishra for encouraging me to revisit this study and reflect on lessons learned.

curative, palliative, protective and promotive needs of individual members of households as well as households as a unit of analysis when the illness of one member was interpreted as a sign that the entire household was vulnerable. The health care needs of afflicted household members and the way illness affects the household production of health (Berman, et al. 1994) are core concerns of medical anthropologists engaging the field of health policy and system research (Gilson, et al. 2011). A core concern of medical anthropologists investigating ethno-medicine is household response to illness as a sign of misfortune beyond the individual, and the politics of responsibility associated with reinstating wellbeing within households, kin networks and communities (Nichter 1992).

Two things are distinctive about this study. First, it was attentive to the full range of practitioners actually consulted by households over a typical year. Most studies conducted in India (prior to the study and even today) focus on health care consultations for particular types of health conditions (for example, diarrhoea, pneumonia, tuberculosis, childbirth), specific segments of the population (for example, women of reproductive age, children, those with chronic illness) or consultations with broad categories of practitioners (modern *versus* traditional, biomedical/ allopathic *versus* indigenous). Many of these studies are projective and seek to identify patterns of resort by asking informants who they would consult if they had a particular problem or what system of medicine they would prefer.[2] This study looked at actual behaviour. Second, the study examined intracultural variation in practitioner consultations and health care expenditure among the poor as well as intercultural (regional) differences in populations with access to a similar range of practitioners.

The data from this study are somewhat dated. We would argue, however, that they offer valuable lessons, provide a baseline against which we can measure changes in health care seeking over time, help us identify key research questions and generate hypotheses worthy of testing. Relevant to this volume, the study leads us to consider how widely different types of traditional practitioners are consulted by the poor in India's complex and evolving health care arenas. We first present quantitative survey data (in the results section) and then turn to ethnographic observations that address what is not revealed by the statistics in the chapter's discussion section.

Methods

The research upon which this chapter is based was collected during Project Community Diagnosis (Nichter 1997). Household-level data were compiled on health-related consultations with the full range of health care providers available in local health care arenas. This included ritual specialists when specifically consulted for health-related concerns and offerings to deities if directly related to an illness event. Data were also collected on self-care, but this lies beyond the scope of the current chapter and is only mentioned in passing.

Site Selection

Field sites in two adjoining districts in the state of Karnataka, India—north and south Kanara districts—were selected as a means to explore two working hypotheses: (a) Caste differences in practitioner consultation exist in locations where nucleated caste settlements exist,[3] and (b) distance from towns as centres of medical treatment influences patterns of health care seeking. Site selection was based on differences in residence patterns in the two districts as well as differences in the general health status of these districts as determined by the Karnataka State Population Centre (Population Centre 1978). The field site selected in north Kanara was located 300 km from the site selected in south Kanara. In 1971, the population density of north Kanara was estimated to be 83 persons per square kilometre, and settlements were predominantly nucleated caste hamlets with each village typically consisting of one to two patrilineal caste groups. North Kanara ranked 11th out of 19 districts in Karnataka with respect to overall health status. The north Kanara district health officer identified the cluster of villages selected for study as lying in one of the least developed areas of the district. Most of the population was agriculturalists and fishermen. The literacy rate in the district was 56 per cent for males and 26 per cent for females.

South Kanara district, by comparison, ranked first out of 19 districts in the state of Karnataka based on an aggregate of basic health indicators. Population density in the district was 230 persons per square kilometre (nearly three times the density of north Kanara). The region historically comprised small feudal kingdoms ruled by a dominant caste having agricultural fields and gardens tended by the tenant castes. These castes pledged loyalty to the landowner (*dani*—literally, lord of the land) and deities protecting the kingdom. Following land reform (which came late to the region—just 10 years before the study), former tenants received small landholdings. Many former tenant households were still compelled to work as day agricultural laborers or *beedie* (local cigarette) rollers for survival. The literacy rate in south Kanara (52 per cent males and 35 per cent females) mirrored that of north Kanara.

Presence of cosmopolitan and traditional practitioners in the two field sites

Prior to the study, the distribution of cosmopolitan practitioners in the taluks selected for study were mapped.[4] The category 'cosmopolitan practitioners' includes both institutionally trained Bachelor of Medicine, Bachelor of Surgery (MBBS) allopathic doctors and non-institutionally trained registered medical practitioners (RMP) dispensing allopathic medications.[5] The two were both called doctor and not distinguished by poor households. The following practitioner to population ratios were calculated (Table 3.1).

Table 3.1: Cosmopolitan Practitioner Distribution in the North and South Kanara Study Sites

	Ankola Taluk, North Kanara			*Puttur Taluk, South Kanara*		
	Town	*Rural*	*Total*	*Town(s)**	*Rural*	*Total*
MBBS	9	6	15	11	11	22
MBBS: Population Ratio*	1:1333	1:4667	1:2667	1:1590	1:7096	1:4344
RMP	2	6	8	11	8	19
RMP: Population Ratio*	1:6000	1:4667	1:5000	1:1590	1:9757	1:5029
MBBS & RMP Ratio*	1:1091	1:2333	1:1739	1:800	1:3579	1:2300

Note: *In south Kanara, the study area encompassed one large crossroads town and two smaller towns.

In both field sites, there was roughly one practitioner recognised by the local population as a 'doctor' (be they institutionally trained or RMP) per 2,300 population.

Mapping traditional practitioners proved challenging, given that some practitioners only received a few clients a month and others several a day. Many practitioners also had hybrid practices. Divided into two broad categories and only counting practitioners that served at least three clients a week, we estimated that in north Kanara, 44 diviners/exorcists and 22 herbalists served the population under study. In south Kanara, 70 diviners/exorcists and 57 herbalists served the population under study. The larger number of practitioners in south Kanara reflects a much higher population density, and the presence of several practitioners who migrated to south Kanara from Kerala, which was only 20 km from the field area. We would estimate that in both north and south Kanara there was roughly one herbalist for every 1,700–1,800 people. In north Kanara, there was roughly one diviner/exorcist (broadly defined) for every 900 people and in south Kanara one diviner/exorcist per every 1,300 people.

Household Sample

All households included in the study were poor with a per capita income below $100; many had an income below $50. Inclusion criteria required that all participating households have (a) six to eight inhabitants (the mode in both districts), (b) one or more children under the age of six (the majority of households), and (c) fall within three sub-categories of relative poverty on an economic class continuum. Panels of local advisors were tasked with differentiating levels of poverty based on estimated yearly household income, landholding and house construction. Households from the following three categories were included in the study: the very poor (under $300 annual income per year), poor ($300–$400 annual income) and low middle class ($401–$600 annual income).

Sample selection was purposive. In north Kanara, samples of households were selected from nucleated caste hamlets following a directional protocol where households meeting the study criteria were selected from each side of chosen hamlets. Household heads of 225 agricultural, fishing (sea and river) and service (carpenters, smiths, potters, scavenger) castes agreed to participate in the study. One hundred and eighty-eight households (84 per cent retention) completed all six rounds of survey interviews (Appendix 1). All hamlets selected for study were situated within 10 km from a small crossroads town with a taluk-level government hospital, a church-run missionary hospital, nine qualified allopathic doctors (five of whom had private practices), two RMPs prescribing allopathic medication without formal institutional training, and two chemist shops. All households were also within 5 km of either the government hospital or a primary health centre, at least one RMP and a wide range of indigenous practitioners.

In south Kanara, 90 households hailing from multi-caste settlements agreed to participate in the study and 82 households (91 per cent retention) completed all six rounds of interviews. All households were located within 10 km of one bustling crossroads town (population of 18,000) and/or two smaller towns (population less than 5,000) with a total of six pharmacies, a taluk-level government hospital, two private hospitals (termed nursing homes), 11 qualified doctors (all of whom had a private practice even if employed by the government) and 11 RMPs (including three institutionally trained ayurvedic practitioners dispensing allopathic medicine).[6] As in north Kanara, all households were also situated within 5 km of a government hospital or primary health care centre, 3 km from at least one popular RMP and a wide range of traditional practitioners. Sub-samples of 30 households were originally drawn from communities located at different distances from a town. The 82 households that remained in the study (Appendix 2) hailed from interior villages not accessible by paved road (N = 25), villages connected to the town by a paved road and bus service (N = 30) and neighbourhoods located within 1 km of the town (N = 27).

Survey Implementation

A team of trained local investigators interviewed household members over a six-month period. Interviewers visited each participating household once per month for an in-depth interview focusing on health care seeking and expenditure.[7] During the first interview, the interviewers collected retrospective data on all practitioner consultations and expenditure over the previous six months. To enhance recall, we employed a local calendar constructed around meaningful events such as rituals and agricultural operations. Six-month recall data was independently cross-checked with two adult household members. We found a high degree of recall concordance (over 80 per cent) between household members for consultations involving expenditures greater than Rs 10 (1979: $1.25). Given reasonable concordance about consultations involving expenditure, we pooled retrospective and prospective data to generate a year-long treatment consultation profile for each household to account for seasonal variance.[8] Recall for small amounts of money used to purchase herbal medicines at a provision shop or a few pills at a chemist shop was poor and this data are not presented in the survey data that follow.

Results

Descriptive statistics are presented on a variety of health care utilisation and expenditure variables. We begin with aggregate data from the two districts and broad categories of practitioners and then turn to more fine-grained data. Tests of statistical significance were run on some variables, using Fisher's Exact Tests (FET) to determine statistical significance for small sample sizes.

Total Health Care Consultations and Expenditures in North Kanara and South Kanara

Over the course of a year, 8,695 health care consultations were reported by the 270 households sampled in north and south Kanara to the following types of practitioners: cosmopolitan practitioners (MBBS, RMPs and pharmacy staff when directly consulted as dispensing practitioners)[9] and traditional practitioners (herbalists, priests, exorcists, diviners, astrologers and oracles when consulted for health problems). In Tables 3.2 and 3.3, we call attention to the percentage of total consultations and expenditure to two broad categories of practitioners: cosmopolitan and traditional practitioners.

Four patterns stand out. First, the pooled data for total health care consultations and expenditures reveal that while north Kanara households had twice the number of practitioner consultations as households in south Kanara (38:19), households in south Kanara spent 64 per cent more on practitioner consultations ($21.50:$33.60). Second, consultations with cosmopolitan practitioners in north and south Kanara were roughly the same, but mean expenditure to cosmopolitan practitioners was 61 per cent higher in south Kanara (Rs 178: or $22.25) than in north Kanara (Rs 109 or $13.6). Third, north Kanara households consulted traditional practitioners almost five times more often than south Kanara

Table 3.2: Total Annual Health Care Consultations and Expenditures in North and South Kanara

	Consultations				*Expenditures*			
	North Kanara (n=188)		*South Kanara (n=82)*		*North Kanara (n=188)*		*South Kanara (n=82)*	
	n	*Mean*	*N*	*Mean*	*Rs*[a]	*Mean (Rs)*	*Rs*	*Mean (Rs)*
Total	7,145	38	1,550	19	32,852	175 ($21.6)	22,300	272 ($33.6)

Notes: [a] The exchange rate in 1979 was Rs 8.1 per $1.

Mean consultations and expenditures per household.

Table 3.3: Total Annual Health Care Consultations and Expenditures per Broad Category of Health Care Provider in North and South Kanara

	Consultations						*Expenditures*					
	North Kanara (n=188)			*South Kanara (n=82)*			*North Kanara (n=188)*			*South Kanara (n=82)*		
	n	*%*	*Mean*	*n*	*%*	*Household mean*	*Rs*	*%*	*Household mean (Rs)*	*Rs*	*%*	*Mean (Rs)*
Cosmopolitan	2,818	40	15	1,170	75	14	20,561 $2538	63	109 $13.5	14,600 $1803	65	178 $22
Traditional	4,327	60	23	380	25	5	12,291 $1517	37	65 $8	7,700 $9506	35	94 $11.6

Note: Mean consultations and expenditures per household.

households (23:5). Despite this huge difference in mean consultations, households in south Kanara spent 55 per cent more on traditional practitioners and offerings to illness-related deities. Fourth, inter-district differences between mean number of consultations and mean expenditure suggests significant differences in cost per consultation in north and south Kanara; the cost per contact in south Kanara is much higher than that in north Kanara. Table 3.4 presents more fine-grained data on percentages of total consultations to particular types of cosmopolitan and traditional practitioners in the two districts.

TABLE 3.4: Percentages of Total Consultations to Specific Types of Practitioners in North and South Kanara

Total Consultations by Practitioner Type	*Government Doctor*	*Private Allopath and RMP*	*Dispensing Pharmacy Staff*	*Herbalist*	*Exorcist and Temple Priest*	*Astrologer and Oracle*	*Total*
North Kanara (N=188)	662 (9%)	2,156 (30%)	—	410 (6%)	2,422 (34%)	1,495 (21%)	7,145 (100%)
South Kanara (N=82)	275 (18%)	610 (39%)	275 (18%)	200 (13%)	85 (5%)	105 (7%)	1,550 (100%)

Four patterns are once again noteworthy. Private allopathic doctors were consulted far more than government doctors in both north and south Kanara—three times more often in north Kanara and twice as often in south Kanara. The mean household expenditure for private consultations was $10 in north Kanara and $13 in south Kanara. The mean cost per private practitioner visit in north Kanara was $1.03 while in south Kanara it was $1.8 (80 per cent more). Second, in south Kanara, 18 per cent of all cosmopolitan practitioner consultations were to dispensing pharmacy staff, many with no formal training. This was not the case in north Kanara at the time of the survey.[10] Third, in both districts only a small percentage of total practitioner consultations (north Kanara: 6 per cent; south Kanara: 13 per cent) were with herbal practitioners (trained ayurvedic practitioner or hereditary/folk practitioner, both termed a 'vaidya'). Fourth, the percentage of total consultations to exorcists and diviners was five times greater in north Kanara than in south Kanara (55 per cent:12 per cent).[11]

Two other inter-district points of comparison are briefly worth highlighting before presenting intra-district data: mean health expenditure as a percentage of household income and household debt related to health care expenditure. We assessed mean household expenditures as a percentage of mean household income levels in the three sub-categories of very poor, poor and low middle class. We estimate that households spent 4–7 per cent of total household income on direct health care related expenses in north Kanara and 7–11 per cent of household income in south Kanara (more precise economic class data from south Kanara is offered later).

We also collected data on debt related to HC expense (Image 3.1). Sixty-seven per cent of north Kanara households reported debt due to health care expenses while in south Kanara, only 36 per cent of households reported such debt. The median amount of debt in both districts for non-catastrophic illness was Rs 51–100 ($6.30–$18.5).[12] Eighty-seven per cent of debt was related to out-of-pocket expenses on cosmopolitan practitioners and allopathic medicines. The source of loan reported in the two districts varied considerably. In north Kanara, it was commonplace to receive treatment on credit from private practitioners. Here, 40 per cent of households had outstanding debt to private cosmopolitan practitioners, 18 per cent to moneylenders and the rest to friends or relatives. In south Kanara, only 10 per cent of households had health care debts to private practitioners. Ten per cent had taken health care related loans from former landlords, 20 per cent from moneylenders, 10 per cent from banks, 10 per cent from rotating credit groups, 10 per cent from the beedie cottage industry branch managers (their employers) and 40 per cent from friends and relatives.[13]

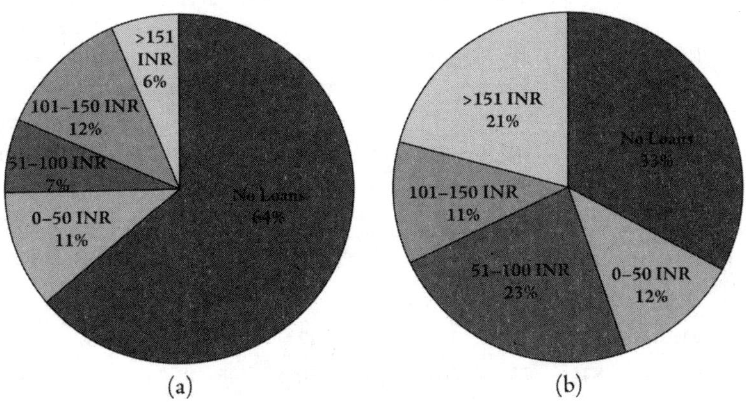

Image 3.1: Loans Related to Health Care in (a) North Kanara and (b) South Kanara

Intra-district Differences: Caste, Class and Distance from a Town

Caste differences: North Kanara

Data from North Kanara illustrates the importance of studying caste differences in practitioner seeking in the regional pluralistic health care arena. Table 3.5 highlights broad variation in the percentage of households consulting broad categories of practitioners. Differences across caste clusters is significant for agricultural castes ($p = 0.000$, FET), but not for service or fisherman castes. It is insufficient, however, to merely examine health care seeking by broad category of practitioner as this obscures important inter-caste differences. Table 3.6 provides a disaggregated look at practitioner consultation among the agriculturalist and fishermen castes. Presented is the percentage of households consulting each type of practitioner over the course of a year.

Table 3.5: Mean Annual Practitioner Consultation Rate by Caste: North Kanara

		Agricultural Castes				*Service Castes*			*Fisherman Castes*	
		AGR	*HLK*	*NMR*	*NDV*	*SON/ VSH*	*MDL/ KLS/ ACH*	*CHM/ HOL*	*AMB/ KRV*	*HRI*
		(*n*=25)	(*n*=40)	(*n*=30)	(*n*=21)	(*n*=14)	(*n*=13)	(*n*=7)	(*n*=18)	(*n*=20)
Cosmopolitan	Mean	10	15	16	6	14	20	20	16	15
	%*	56	73	90	100	85	100	100	22	30
Traditional	Mean	19	21	18	5	17	12	32	57	48
	%	84	73	60	19	50	46	71	83	95

Note: *Percentage of households consulting over the course of a year (for example, 56 per cent of Agers consulted modern practitioners).

Table 3.6: Annual Household Consultations by Selected Castes: North Kanara

			Private	*Government*	*Herbalist*	*Exorcist*	*Priest/ Diviner*	*Astrologer*	*Oracle*
Agricultural Castes	AGR (n=25)	n	14	13	16	18	21	10	14
		%	56	52	64	72	84	40	56
	HLK (n=40)	n	29	27	14	29	29	18	22
		%	73	68	35	73	73	45	55
	NMR (n=30)	n	27	7	3	14	18	12	6
		%	90	23	10	47	60	40	20
	NDV[a] (n=21)	n	21	4	5	1	3	3	4
		%	100	19	24	5	14	14	19
	Total (116)	n	91	51	38	62	71	43	46
		%	78	44	33	53	61	37	40
p-value (FET)			0.000	0.000	0.000	0.000	0.000	0.100	0.001
Fisherman Castes	AMB/ KRV (n=18)	n	15	4	8	11	15	10	12
		%	83	22	44	61	83	56	67
	HRI (n=20)	n	17	3	17	14	19	13	14
		%	85	15	85	70	95	65	70
	Total (38)	n	32	7	25	25	34	23	26
		%	84	18	66	66	89	61	68
p-value (FET)			0.016	0.687	0.016	0.734	0.328	0.741	1.00

Clear caste differences in practitioner consultation emerge. For example, 100 per cent of Nadava agriculturalist households consulted private practitioners, while only 19 per cent consulted government doctors. By comparison, many households from other large agriculturalist castes—52 per cent of Ager (a Scheduled Caste) and 68 per cent of Halakki Gowda (a tribal group)—consulted government practitioners. However, low percentages of Namdahri agriculturalists and fishermen households consulted government health facilities, although 80–90 per cent consulted private practitioners. A larger percentage of Agers and Harikant fishermen households also consulted herbalists than other castes.

FETs were run to compare castes in the same socioeconomic cluster. Differences emerged. For example, among samples of Halakkis, Namdharis and Harikants (all with a 50 per cent:50 per cent very poor:poor ratio), significant differences were found for consultation with government practitioners (p = 0.000), herbalists (p = 0.000), priests/diviners (p = 0.021) and oracles (p = 0.001). Among very poor households (80 per cent of Agers, and 100 per cent of washermen, smiths and scavengers), significant caste differences in practitioner consultations were documented for exorcists and diviners (p = 0.007).

Disaggregated data for health care expenditures is also revealing (Table 3.7). Across all castes, the lion's share of household health practitioner expenditure was for consultations with private cosmopolitan practitioners. This general finding is hardly surprising and is well-documented by scores of studies conducted all over India. It is worth highlighting, however, that caste-specific mean expenditure on private practitioners varied considerably, from Rs 80 to 180. Notably, the very poorest caste samples in the survey (AGR, MDL/KLS/ACH) reported the highest mean spending on private practitioners. This observation was more closely examined in south Kanara.

Table 3.7: Mean Annual Health Care Expenditures by Selected Castes: North Kanara

		Private	*Government*	*Herbalist*	*Exorcist*	*Priest/ Diviner*	*Astrologer*	*Oracle*	*Offerings*
AGR (n=25)	Rs*	102	54	11	15	27	10	8	23
HLK (n=40)	Rs	80	49	24	26	10	17	7	33
MDL/ KLS/ ACH (n=13)	Rs	180	27	17	7	38	11	4	7
AMB/ KRV (n=18)	Rs	84	28	18	76	32	24	14	56

Notes: *Annual household mean expenditure in rupees ($1 = Rs 8).

Percentages are across rows and represent the percentage share of mean expenditures by type of practitioner.

Also notable is the substantial amounts of money spent on types of practitioners that are not typically captured in health expenditure surveys. For example, among AMB/KRV fishermen households, mean expenditures on exorcists approached that on private doctors. There was a greater tendency among these castes to view individual episodes of illness as possible signs of witchcraft that might affect the entire household as well as make fishing more precarious. This resulted in the high aggregate expenditures on various forms of divination (diviners/astrologers/oracles) and offerings to deities.

Practitioner consultation and median health care expenditure by class and proximity to a town: South Kanara

In Table 3.8, we present data on the percentages of households in south Kanara consulting different types of practitioners disaggregated by economic status and residence and group mean practitioner expenditures.

Seven consultation patterns may be highlighted. First, in south Kanara a statistically significant inverse relationship exists between level of income and the percentage of households consulting private practitioners. A lower percentage of low-middle class households (67 per cent) consulted private practitioners than poor (80 per cent) and very poor (94 per cent) households. Second, low-middle households also consulted fewer government practitioners, suggesting that their overall health status may be better than that of the other two groups. Third, a higher (but not statistically significant) percentage of village (80 per cent) and satellite village (93 per cent) households consulted private practitioners than town-based households (74 per cent). Fourth, a higher percentage of town-based households visited government health facilities than village households, in part because it is more convenient to do so. Fifth, 49 per cent of all households consulted pharmacy staff as dispensing practitioners. Sixth, few town-based households consulted exorcists, although about a quarter consulted astrologers. On the other hand, nearly half of all village-based households consulted exorcists and/or astrologers. Seventh, the mean number of consultations with any practitioner was fairly similar (interior village: 15; satellite village: 17; town: 17).

An examination of health expenditure found that expenditures to cosmopolitan practitioners varied only slightly across economic groups, with the very poor spending 65 per cent of their total health care budget

Table 3.8: Percentage of Households Consulting Different Types of Practitioners and Median Expenditure: South Kanara

				Private Doctor	*Government Doctor*	*Chemist*	*Herbalist*	*Exorcist*	*Astrologer*	*Offerings to Deity*	*Total*
Class	Utilisation	Very poor (n=32)	n	30	17	15	6	12	11		
			%	94	53	47	19	38	34		
		Poor (n=38)	n	30	23	19	13	15	8		
			%	80	60	50	34	40	21		
		Low-mid (n=12)	n	8	5	6	4	4	4		
			%	67	42	50	33	33	33		
		p-value (FET)		0.050	0.518	0.955	0.315	0.999	0.394		
	Expenditure	Very poor (n=32)	Rs	60	5	82	29	20	20	10	226
		Poor (n=38)	Rs	63	14	32	37	15	15	29	205
		Low-mid (n=12)	Rs	130	37	69	31	13	15	32	327
Locale	Utilisation	Town (n=27)	n	20	18	14	8	3	7		
			%	74	67	52	30	11	26		
		Satellite village (n=30)	n	28	12	13	6	14	13		
			%	93	40	43	20	47	43		
		Interior village (n=25)	n	20	11	13	8	13	5		
			%	80	44	52	32	52	20		
		p-value (FET)		0.126	0.115	0.757	0.577	0.002	0.159		
	Expenditure	Town (n=27)	Rs	40	4	32	30	10	10	17	143
		Satellite village (n=30)	Rs	100	20	47	27	20	19	20	253
		Interior village (n=25)	Rs	50	17	76	52	9	19	65	288

on doctors and dispensing pharmacy staff, the poor 53 per cent and the low-middle class 72 per cent. Interior village households spent twice as much on practitioners and rituals to deities as households located near the town. Interior village and town households spent 50–53 per cent of their total practitioner budget on cosmopolitan practitioners and satellite villages 66 per cent. The sub-samples spending the most on consultations with private and government doctors were low-middle class households and satellite village households, and the sub-samples spending the most on dispensing chemists were the very poor and interior village households.

Turning to traditional practitioners, interior village households spent the most on herbalists and offerings to deities. Interior village households spent more than thrice as much on offerings to deities as households in satellite villages and towns, and almost as much on offerings to deities (Rs 65) as their combined expenditure on private and government doctors (Rs 67). Table 3.9 presents data on health as a percentage of annual income. Notably, the very poor and poor households spent a greater proportion of their yearly income on consultations with practitioners than the lower-middle class. Curiously, the estimates generated by this study were close to those offered by three pharmaceutical representatives (working for top-tier companies) serving the district for more than five years. When interviewed, they estimated that 6–8 per cent of the household income of the poor was spent on health care. Officials at the district health office offered the opinion that 3–4 per cent of the poor's household income was health related.

Table 3.9: Out-of-pocket Practitioner Expenditures as a Percentage of Household Income: South Kanara

Class	*n*	*Yearly Income*	*Median Expenditure*	*Percentage of Income*
Very poor	32	< 2,500	226	9
Poor	38	2,500–4,000	205	5–8
Low middle	12	4,100–6,000	327	5–6

Discussion

In this chapter, we demonstrated the importance of considering interregional as well as intraregional differences when assessing patterns of practitioner consultation and expenditure among the poor in India. In this section, we highlight some of the main findings of the survey and present ethnographic observations that provide additional insights into health care seeking patterns, and raise issues for future research. In keeping with the focus of this volume, we pay particular attention to consultations with traditional practitioners. As a heuristic process, we present data as a response to nine core research questions that both inspired the study and emerged while it was being conducted.

1. *How much regional variation exists in practitioner consultation among the 'rural poor'*: There have been several general descriptions of health care seeking among the 'rural poor' in India based on national surveys that typically ask respondents about consultations in the public and private health sector as well as with practitioners of ayurveda, unani and homeopathy during the past few weeks or months.[14] State-wide aggregate data are then compared. While they are a useful exercise to get at general trends, these descriptions gloss over intraregional differences at both the state and district levels, miss differences in consultation patterns among different reference groups and are based on consultation data from a limited range of traditional practitioners providing care within India's pluralistic health care arenas. Moreover, it is important to consider the percentages of households consulting different types of practitioners over the course of a year in addition to percentages of total consultations with cosmopolitan *versus* traditional practitioners. Each indicates something quite different with respect to how the needs of the poor are being met. For this reason, it is important to complement large national surveys with small surveys, like the one presented here, in addition to qualitative research that provides a contextual analysis of patterns that emerge (Hentschel 1999).

Consider, for example, the case of north Kanara, where 62 per cent of all practitioner consultations were with traditional practitioners compared to 28 per cent of consultations in south Kanara. Does this mean that traditional practitioners are less important health care resources for the poor in south Kanara? A closer look at consultation rates provides a more nuanced picture. A significant percentage of households in south Kanara do in fact consult a range of traditional practitioners, albeit not as often as households in north Kanara. While it is true that only 5–7 per cent of all consultations are for some form of exorcism or divination (compared to 21–34 per cent in north Kanara), one-third of households from all three economic subgroups in south Kanara and almost half of all households located in interior or satellite villages consulted one or both types of these practitioners.

Consultations with herbalists offer another case in point. In south Kanara, consultations with herbalists as a percentage of consultations with any practitioner was double that of north Kanara (13 per cent: 6 per cent). Looking more closely, however, one finds that herbalists are consulted by 33 per cent of all households in south Kanara (with some notable economic group and residence differences). A third of all agricultural castes in north Kanara also consult herbalists, and among fishermen castes, two-thirds reported consulting herbalists.

Ethnographic data suggest reasons for these differences. The two regions have quite different cosmologies and types of caste and village rituals. In south Kanara, if an illness is seen as a possible sign of witchcraft or supernatural intervention, the rural population often makes offerings to a household or village *buta* (diety) during a possession ritual. These rituals provide an opportunity for divination and secure protection by patron deities in exchange for offerings (*hareke*). Such rituals do not exist in north Kanara. And one reason why fishermen consult herbalists more than other castes in north Kanara is because their local fund of knowledge of herbal medicines is less elaborate than most agricultural castes, the Agers being a notable exception. Our response to the question posed is that considerable interregional and intraregional variation exists in the consultation of different types of practitioners as well as in practitioner expenditure. A more in-depth picture of what is going on within local health care arenas demands more fine-tuned research attentive to historical and changing contexts.

2. Do impoverished households with access to both traditional and cosmopolitan practitioners have general preferences for medical systems, or do they consult a mix of practitioners? In both north and south Kanara, the poor consulted a variety of traditional and cosmopolitan health practitioners. In many cases, herbal home care was tried first and then allopathic medicine. In other cases, allopathic medicine was used for fast symptomatic relief, enabling one to return to work and then herbal medications were consumed to reestablish bodily rhythms (such as digestion or defecation) associated with health. In still other cases, cosmopolitan and traditional medicine was used (and prescribed by

RMPs) concurrently. We identified few illnesses with specific preferences for one system of medicine over another. Notable exceptions included a preference for herbal medicine for rheumatoid arthritis, digestive problems, 'woman's complaints' and sexual disorders among men.

We found that most poor households adopted a pragmatic approach to dealing with health problems. When asked about general preferences, some informants stated that while they might prefer herbal treatment to cosmopolitan medication for a particular ailment, herbal medication took a long time to be effective, leading them to take cosmopolitan medication for fast relief. Among this group, several study participants (especially in south Kanara) noted that once their body became habituated to allopathic medicines, it no longer responded to herbal medicine as well as it had in the past. This idea was supported by herbalists who told patients that it was necessary for them to take purification medicines to purge their body of the residue of allopathic medicine and to increase their body's receptiveness to herbal medications before their treatment would be effective.

Based on the findings of this study, we question the utility of general practitioner preference studies. Such studies give the impression that health care decision-making is driven by static preferences instead of real-world contingencies. Preference data does not predict actual behaviour. Take, for example, a large 35-district (33,666 households; 45,000 sickness episodes) study conducted by the ICMR. The survey recorded treatment preferences for 45,000 minor and serious illness episodes (Singh, et al. 2005) and paid special attention to preferences for indigenous systems of medicine. The study found a 33 per cent preference rate for indigenous medicine for 'normal' health problems. However, only 14 per cent of respondents reported actually using indigenous medicine to treat their ailments.[15]

3. Do caste, class, and proximity to town influence who the poor choose to consult for routine health care needs? We identified distinct patterns of practitioner consultation correlated with caste, class and proximity to town. Ethnographic inquiry was required to understand how each variable influenced health care seeking. For example, in north Kanara, caste differences in consultation patterns were associated with several different factors. These ranged from a predisposition of particular castes to suspect that illness was a sign of malevolence to caste identity associated with tradition or modernity, and from practitioner demeanour towards patients based on their position in the local caste hierarchy to the mistrust of clinics based on past experience or circulating rumours.

For example, when we investigated why 100 per cent of the Nadava agriculturalist households consulted private practitioners when only 19 per cent consulted accessible government doctors, we found this caste to be highly invested in presenting itself as 'forward' (progressive) and better educated.[16] It viewed the use of government clinics as a sign of poverty. In this case, social distinction (Bourdieu 1984; Williams 1995) appeared to influence health seeking behaviour. High percentages of the Namdhari agriculturalists and fishermen households exhibited similar health seeking behaviour, but for different reasons. When queried why they did not visit government clinics, several reported that members of their caste were not treated well at these facilities. In short, they felt disrespected. The Halakki Gowdas, on the other hand, did not report this level of disrespect despite being a tribal group. The Namdhari and fishermen case draws attention to the importance of clinic staff-patient relations and acts as a factor influencing the use of government health services (see also Ergler, et al. 2011). In short, social relations matter.

Ethnographic data also help explain why, in south Kanara, distance from a town influenced which practitioners were consulted as well as patterns of practitioner expenditure. For example, the survey found that controlling for economic subgroup, interior households spent more at pharmacies than members of the same subgroup residing in satellite villages and towns. Distance and access to a town influenced medicine purchasing behaviour at pharmacies, both when medications were prescribed by practitioners and dispensed by pharmacy staff. Households with easier access to towns were more likely to try and see if a medication worked before purchasing a full prescription. If the medicine appeared to work, they purchased more of it. If there was no demonstration effect, they visited a different practitioner to try a different medication. Households from interior villages were more likely to purchase a larger (but not necessarily a full) portion of a prescribed or recommended medication unless it was very costly. They did so to save on the indirect and opportunity costs of travel. Two additional observations were made. Members of interior households often delayed visits to town-based practitioners or a pharmacy to piggyback a trip to a practitioner with some other work. They also delayed travelling to town until they felt they had enough money to pay for the kind of treatment they imagined they might need in keeping with lay-cost reckoning.[17]

4. Does access to cosmopolitan and institutionally trained ayurvedic practitioners replace the perceived need for traditional practitioners? An Indian health planner interviewed at the beginning of this study voiced the opinion that with greater access to qualified medical practitioners, local populations would stop seeking the services of traditional practitioners and RMPs, who dispensed both allopathic and ayurvedic medications. This assumption was not borne out by this study. Greater access to MBBS doctors did not appear to have diminished the popularity of either RMPs or herbalists in either district.[18] Access to an increasing number of institutionally trained ayurvedic doctors also did not reduce the popularity of ayurvedic practitioners who obtained their skills through apprenticeships with established healers (often family members).

In the case of psychosocial and mental health problems commonly expressed through a somatic idiom of distress (Nichter 1981), traditional practitioners and RMPs were consulted more often than MBBS practitioners.[19] And in cases where symptoms were interpreted as signs of spirit-based afflictions, exorcists and healing temples continued to be popular sources of treatment. A recognition of this health care seeking pattern has led some mental health researchers in India to seek collaborative working relationships with healers (see Thirthalli, et al. 2016 for an overview). Notably, we found that referrals of patients with psychological problems were already taking place in south Kanara. We documented astrologers, exorcists and Ayurvedic practitioners who referred these patients to each other. We also documented three MBBS doctors who referred patients with somatic complaints they could not effectively manage to ayurvedic practitioners renowned for treating such cases.

5. Do low numbers of consultations with herbalists indicate low use of herbal medications in general? We did not find this to be the case. Over 80 per cent of households in both districts commonly used five or more herbal medicines (beyond common spices) as home remedies for common complaints. Most herbs were harvested locally or purchased for small amounts of money from small provision shops. We found that knowledge and use of herbal medication varied by caste (for example, the Agers in north Kanara had poor knowledge of herbs while the Halakki Gowdas and Nadavas had far better knowledge) and whether a person over the age of 50 was present in the household. We further observed that knowledge of herbal medications often did not translate into home treatment practice. Many study participants could name herbs for a far broader range of ailments than those they felt comfortable treating. While they might be able to name and identify herbs, they did not know how to prepare them, how much to administer and what dietary restrictions specific herbal treatments required. Knowledge of herbal medicines, in general, was far greater in south Kanara than in north Kanara, as was access to herbal medications in local shops.

6. Does consultation of traditional practitioners decrease with a rise in the level of income or closer proximity to town? We found that in north Kanara, consultations with diviners and exorcists were fairly constant across economic subgroups except among the Nadava caste. In south Kanara, there was no statistically significant difference in the consultation of these practitioners between subgroups based on income or residence, with one exception. Far fewer households residing in towns consulted exorcists. Interior villagers also consulted herbalists more often than households in satellite villages and towns. Contrary to our expectations, we found that the poorest of the poor in south Kanara consulted herbalists less often than those with slightly more resources, although the difference was not statistically significant.

7. How important is 'treating the household' when an illness is suspected to be a sign of malevolence or unpaid debt to an ancestor or patron deity? We found that significant resources were expended in both districts to divine the cause of illness when it was deemed unusual, recurrent, or concurrent with other mishaps (*dosha*). The spiritual protection of households is a serious health care concern among the poor, especially in times of heightened social tension. For example, considerable social friction was experienced in south Kanara during our survey related to land disputes between neighbours and within families following land reform legislation. As a result of such disputes, there were lapses in household and village-level buta rituals. Prolonged or recurrent illness during this time of transition often led to the 'what if' subjunctive reasoning that indexed concern about malevolent forces and unfulfilled ritual obligations. Notably, the median yearly expenditure on healing rituals and offerings to buta spirits in interior village households approximated their median expenditure on private practitioners. We would argue that these protective activities at a time of perceived vulnerability need to be seen as forms of preventive and promotive health engagement.

8. How does access to government health facilities affect the use of private practitioners for routine health problems? The popularity of private practitioners among the rural poor in India has been well-documented for four decades, from 1980 to 2020.[20] We found that in both north and south Kanara, nearly all households that consulted government clinics also consulted private cosmopolitan practitioners. Five reasons the poor visited private practitioners, reported by study participants, were: (a) Government clinics have long waiting times and at rural clinics, one never knows if the doctor will report for duty; (b) little time (often 2–3 minutes) is spent with patients; (c) government clinics have low stocks of the required medicines, making it necessary for patients to purchase medicines from outside, while private practitioners offer one-stop care; (d) when medicine is available at government clinics, only one-to-two-day allotments of medications are doled out, requiring patients to revisit the clinic again and again; and (e) government doctors offer poor treatment during duty hours, but better treatment in their private practices.

We observed that two types of patients visited rural government outpatient clinics: those in dire straits using these clinics as a last resort safety net and those consulting a government doctor to find out if their illness was serious enough to warrant visiting a private doctor (or government doctor after duty hours in their private practice).[21] Notably, in the latter case, it was the quality of medication at government clinics, more than the competence of the doctor, that led patients to seek private treatment.

At the time the survey was being conducted, structural adjustment policies favouring fee for services at government outpatient clinics were being debated in India. Our interviews with patients suggested that it was very likely that the 'safety net group' of patients would consult inexpensive RMPs if requested to pay fees. We would hypothesise that the 'check and see if serious' group would be more likely to consult private MBBS doctors.[22]

9. *How much do the poor spend on non-catastrophic health care?* National Consumer Expenditure Surveys are periodically conducted in India to estimate the percentage of total household income spent on health care. In 1999–2000, the estimate for rural India was 4.8 per cent and in 2004–05 it was 6.1 per cent, with the state of Kerala being an outlier at 9.5 per cent (Joe and Mishra 2009).[23] These surveys cover a wide range of residential settings and economic groups, and focus primarily on out-of-pocket expenditures on allopathic doctors. One of these surveys' chief findings has been that over three-quarters of the out-of-pocket expenses are for medications, something difficult to disaggregate from consultation fees by dispensing doctors in rural India (see also Garg and Karan 2008).

Our survey only focused on non-catastrophic health problems among the poor and low middle class, and covered a much wider range of traditional practitioner consultations. We found that that the poor spent 4–11 per cent of their total household income on consultations with practitioners and health-related offerings to deities. We also documented significant inter- and intra-district variance in the amount spent on particular types of practitioners by class, caste and residence subgroups. Two findings stand out. First, in both districts, the poorest of the poor spend the highest percentage of their total household income on practitioner visits despite having access to 'free' government health facilities. Second, and of particular importance to this edited volume, in both districts roughly one-third of total practitioner expenditure was on traditional practitioners and health-related offerings to deities. The rural poor's expenditure in this broad health sector is hardly peripheral and should not be underestimated.

Limitations

Several limitations of the survey described in this chapter need to be noted, aside from its relatively small sample size, which renders its findings suggestive and not generalisable. First, it needs to be acknowledged that a practitioner's reputation influences consultation choice as much as and sometimes more than the therapeutic system. The importance of reputation and perceived 'power of the hand' (*kai guna*) for particular patients as well as for the treatment of particular types of ailments has been noted by past medical anthropological research (Ager and Pepper 2005; Kumar 1994;

Nichter 1978; Nichter and Nordstrom 1989). Another limitation is that several other variables are important to consider when assessing patterns of practitioner utilisation and expenditure. Consultation rates by age and gender, and whether an aliment is longstanding, recurrent or new, are also important to take into account. A third limitation is that the health care expenditure estimated in this study is conservative. We did not include catastrophic health expenditures, nor did we include small amounts of money spent for medications used in self-care. We also did not sample for nor did we compare households with elderly members. We did ask about recurring expenses for medications for chronic complaints, but none were reported outside of consultations with practitioners. Also not accounted for in the study were indirect costs incurred from transportation to practitioners and opportunity costs related to lost wages.

Conclusion

It is our hope that this study will inspire future research that takes into consideration shifting trends in health care seeking and expenditure among reference populations, changes in the composition of pluralistic health care arenas, and emerging government policies and programmes and their implications for pluralistic therapeutic practices. Pluralistic health care arenas are dynamic and subject to market factors influencing the supply of practitioners and the demand for particular types of goods and services, commodity chains and distribution networks, public health interventions (such as health insurance) and demographic and health transitions. Medical anthropologists engaged in health service and system research (Gilson, et al. 2011) will have their work cut out for them, studying how the poor respond to changes in India's health and health care environment. Trends in health care seeking among vulnerable populations also reflect psychosocial needs, perceived risks and social as well as structural insecurities, ways in which distress and concern are expressed and experienced culturally at the site of the body, and actions taken to both reduce harm and secure protection. These are issues that a broadly defined and critical ethno-medical lens brings into focus (Nichter 1992).

APPENDIX 3.1: Caste Demographics: North Kanara

Caste Type	*Caste*	*Caste Code*	*Sample (households)*	*Mean Family Size*	*Class*
Agriculturalists	Ager	AGR	25	6.2	80% very poor; 20% poor
	Halakki Gowda	HLK	40	6.9	50% very poor; 50% poor
	Namdhari	NMR	30	6.5	50% very poor; 50% poor
	Nadava	NDV	21	6.8	50% poor; 50% middle class
Fishermen	Harikant	HRI	20	7	50% very poor; 50% poor
	Ambiga and Karvi	AMB/ KRV	18	8.1	Poor
Scavengers and Tanners	Chamagar and Holeya	CHM/ HOL	7	7	Very Poor
Carpenters, potters, and washermen	Achari, Kelasi and Madivalla	ACH/ KLS/MDL	13	7.1	Very poor
Goldsmith merchants	Sonagar	SON	9	6.5	33% very poor; 67% poor
Small shopkeepers	Vaisha	VSH	5	6.4	40% low middle class; 60% poor
Total			188		

APPENDIX 3.2: Sample Characteristics: South Kanara

Locale	*Size*	*Mean Income*	*Very Poor*	*Poor*	*Low Middle*
Interior village	25	4,000	9	13	3
Satellite	30	4,000	12	13	5
Town	27	3,800	11	12	4
Total	82	–	32	38	12
Percentage of Total			39	46	15

Notes

1. Catastrophic health problems were defined in this study as those resulting in medical expenses constituting more than 25 per cent of the household yearly income. The definition is normed to household income and is not based on a set amount spent in rupees. Approximately 10 per cent of households originally sampled experienced catastrophic illness and were not included in this analysis.

2. Many studies have described general 'patterns of treatment resort', leaving one with the impression that durable preferences for particular types of health care sources exist and that general preferences are primary drivers of treatment seeking behaviour. The author's past research (Nichter 1978, 1980) and observations made during this study suggest that actual health care decisions among the poor are pragmatic as well as culturally informed. They involve far more than preferences. Decisions are subject to predisposing, enabling and service-quality related factors as well as the presence or absence of decision-makers in the household and the social status of the afflicted. Relevant factors include perceptions of illness causality and responsibility, duration and perceived severity, household economics and the cost of treatment, the seasonal availability of resources and lines of credit, and clinic and practitioner reputation, along with perceptions of quality of care. Decisions are also based on patients' short- and long-term agenda when seeking health care, given the resources at hand and real world contingencies, the social relations of illness labelling, and the extent to which an illness constitutes an idiom of distress and its treatment an idiom of concern. In sum, health care decisions are complex. It is beyond the scope of this chapter to present case studies illustrating how decisions are made, negotiated, rationalised and reassessed over time.

3. Other studies in India have considered caste when examining patterns of health care utilisation, but observations have often been limited to particular health issues or general comparisons of high:low caste or caste consultation of government *versus* private practitioners (Bhatia and Cleland 2001; Matthews et al. 2001; Mukherjee, et al. 2011; Navaneetham and Dharmalingam 2002; Rani and Bonu 2003). For example, a study in Uttar Pradesh found that women from lower castes were nearly three times less likely to use antenatal care and tetanus toxoid, and almost five times less likely to use a trained birth attendant after adjusting for socioeconomic status (Saroha, et al. 2008). In Orissa, Ager and Pepper (2005) found that almost 30 per cent more members of the Scheduled Castes used government hospitals than other castes, and nearly 20 per cent more general caste members used private practitioners than those in the Scheduled Castes.

4. For a more detailed mapping of the distribution of cosmopolitan and traditional practitioners in south Kanara, see Nichter (1978). This article provides information on a village-by-village basis of a larger study area that

overlaps with the area in which the survey was conducted. It also addresses the age profile of practitioners.

5. The term 'registered medical practitioners' (RMPs) is used to denote non-formally trained health care providers who provide a mix of treatments from Indian Systems of Medicine and Homeopathy (ISM&H, now referred to as AYUSH) and allopathic treatments. The origin of the term RMP dates back to 1933, when the colonial government introduced a state registration system for non-qualified medical practitioners having an established medical practice for 10 years or more, or evidence of apprenticeship with an experienced practitioner (George and Iyer 2013). Today, although only institutionally trained, qualified doctors are legally permitted to register and practise medicine, the term RMP has persisted. Some RMPs have acquired degrees and diplomas from non-authentic sources (Ashtekar and Mankad 2001; Kumar, et al. 2007). Others practise medicine after having acquired experience as compounders, traditional birth attendants or assistants to qualified physicians. It is estimated that RMPs account for about half of all health care providers in India (Sudhinaraset, et al. 2013). As they provide accessible, affordable and culturally sensitive care, they have a fair degree of acceptance by the community. RMPs are often more willing to defer payment or in some cases accept payment in kind (May, et al. 2014), which contributes to their popularity among the poor. Case studies suggest that patients visit RMPs with the same types of symptoms they present to formally trained practitioners, and in many cases believe them to be just as competent for common illnesses. See also Das and Mohpal (2016); Gautham et al. (2014); May, et al. (2014); Pinto (2004); and Ranga and Panda (2015).

6. The population density in south Kanara was far higher than in north Kanara. Some south Kanara study households were within 10 km of more than one town with doctors in residence and chemist shops.

7. A survey instrument was constructed, pretested and subsequently modified. Informed consent was obtained from heads of households orally. Initial interviews on health care seeking took 30–45 minutes and subsequent interviews 15–30 minutes.

8. We deemed the importance of accounting for seasonal variation in health care utilisation to outweigh the limitations of six-month recall in our efforts to capture a full year of health care seeking behaviour.

9. We follow Dunn (1976: 135) and Leslie (1976: 6) in our use of the term 'cosmopolitan' medicine. Cosmopolitan medicine characterises the global penetration of allopathic medicine into local health care arenas, such that it is a g/local phenomenon influenced by myriad factors. We choose to use this term instead of 'modern', 'scientific' and 'Western' medicine, all of which are based on assumptions that we find problematic.

10. In north Kanara, consulting of pharmacists was rarely reported in 1979. This changed by the late 1980s.

11. It was challenging to decipher when offerings to deities were specific for illness because offerings were often prompted by series of misfortunes (*dosha*) including, but not confined to, illness.

12. Annual debt due to health care is difficult to assess. We present debt incurred during the study year, and not debt carried over from previous years and compounding interest from past loans taken from moneylenders. None of the debt reported here is from catastrophic illness requiring a long hospital stay or major operation. Debt due to health care expenditures and practitioner willingness to extend credit are complex and important topics for future research.

13. Five MBBS practitioners serving the local population for more than eight years stated that they had been far more willing to extend credit in the past, but that debt recovery had become more difficult 'in these changing times'. Another shift we observed was a move away from taking loans from landlords. This was a common practice prior to land reform in the 1970s. Debts to landlords for health care were still found to be common among migrant labourers hired by small plantation owners who extended loans against wages, but migrant labourers were not included in this study.

14. For an overview of all India surveys conducted by the Institute for Research in Medical Statistics, National Sample Survey Organisation (NSSO), National Council of Applied Economic Research (NCAER) and National Family Health Survey (NFHS), and the differences in rural-urban sampling frames employed, see Singh, et al. (2005).

15. We also found that projective 'what would you do if' questions did not map well onto actual experience.

16. The research team did not get the sense that the Nadava caste was a trendsetter for other castes, and in fact a fair amount of friction existed between the Nadavas and several other castes in this study.

17. Lay-cost reckoning played a role in both health care decision-making and how much practitioners charged patients for their services, a fee that included the cost of medicines dispensed (Nichter 1983). When needed medications exceeded the amounts patients expected to pay, they were prescribed. This cost was figured into the private practitioner expenditure data as it was linked to a consultation.

18. This was particularly apparent in south Kanara where rising competition between doctors in the city of Mangalore and large towns led to a greater number of young MBBS doctors starting practices in smaller crossroads towns. This trend became more notable in the two decades post-1990, with large landowning households sending children for medical training at a time profitability from agriculture was falling. The demand for medical seats was in turn met by the opening of private allopathic and ayurvedic medical colleges. The age and experience of MBBS and institutionally trained ayurvedic doctors influenced their popularity. Some study participants stated that they preferred consulting an older RMP rather than a young MBBS or ayurvedic doctor, citing the Kannada

proverb, '*Hosa vaidya nigintha hale rogine melu*' (Better to consult an old patient than a young doctor).

19. Analysis of RMP prescription practices by Eks and Basu (2014) and symptom presentation to RMPs by Rao (2005) suggest that those afflicted with mental disorders often consult RMPs (Ranga and Panda 2016) as well as diviners, exorcists and temples renowned for healing.

20. See for example Ager and Pepper (2005), Basu (1990), Bhat (1993), Levesque, et al. (2006), Rani and Bonu (2003), and Rohde and Vishwanathan (1994).

21. We observed government doctors who had booming private practices after duty hours because patients perceived the medications they dispensed from their home clinics to be of superior quality. This impression was promoted by some doctors as a means to build their private practice.

22. When presenting survey data at United States Agency for International Development (USAID), New Delhi, and two health and development conferences in the United States, the author was asked by policymakers if, given the amount of money the poor currently spent on health care, they could afford to pay a fee for services at government clinics. In each instance, he responded that most of the poor consulting government clinics did so as a safety net and were in dire need. While it was true that the poor often consulted private practitioners, it was unlikely that they would pay for services at government clinics beyond what they already gave as small incentive payments to staff, unless the perceived quality of care (and medications) improved dramatically. Even a modest fee for services was likely to dissuade people from attending government clinics and lead to their seeking care from low-cost RMPs (whose fees were typically half those of MBBS doctors). Given the data presented on how much the poor spent on traditional practitioners and private cosmopolitan practitioners, they remained unconvinced. This raised an ethical dilemma for the author. Concern that the data might be used in a manner not intended, a decision was made not to disseminate the data, given the prevailing political climate.

23. For more recent data using the consumption expenditure data, National Sample Survey 2009–10, which is attentive to households with/without elders, see Mohanty, et al. (2014).

References

Ager, A., and K. Pepper. 2005. 'Patterns of Health Service Utilization and Perceptions of Needs and Services in Rural Orissa'. *Health Policy and Planning* 20(3): 176–84.

Ashtekar, S., and D. Mankad. 2001. 'Who Cares? Rural Health Practitioners in Maharashtra'. *Economic and Political Weekly* 36(5–6), 3 February: 448–53.

Basu, A. M. 1990. 'Cultural Influences on Health Care Use: Two Regional Groups in India'. *Studies in Family Planning* 21(5): 275–86.

Berman, P., C. Kendall and K. Bhattacharyya. 1994.'The Household Production of Health: Integrating Social Science Perspectives on Micro-level Health Determinants'. *Social Science and Medicine* 38(2): 205–15.

Bhat, R. 1993.'The Private/Public Mix in Health Care in India'. *Health Policy and Planning* 8(1): 43–56.

Bhatia, J. C., and J. Cleland. 2001. 'Health Care Seeking and Expenditures by Young Indian Mothers in the Public and Private Sectors'. *Health Policy and Planning* 16(1): 55–61.

Bourdieu, P. 1984. *Distinction: A Social Critique of the Judgement of Taste*. Cambridge: Harvard University Press.

Das, J., and A. Mohpal. 2016. 'Socioeconomic Status and Quality of Care in Rural India: New Evidence From Provider And Household Surveys'. *Health Affairs* 35(10): 1764–73.

Dunn, F. L. 1976. 'Traditional Asian Medicine and Cosmopolitan Medicine as Adaptive Systems'. *Asian Medical Systems: A Comparative Study*, ed. Charles Leslie, 133–58. Berkeley: University of California Press.

Ecks, S., and S. Basu. 2014.'We Always Live in Fear: Antidepressant Prescriptions by Unlicensed Doctors in India'. *Culture, Medicine, and Psychiatry* 38(2): 197–216.

Ergler, C. R., P. Sakdapolrak, H. G. Bohle and R. A. Kearns. 2011.'Entitlements to Health Care: Why is There a Preference for Private Facilities among Poorer Residents of Chennai, India?' *Social Science and Medicine* 72(3): 327–37.

Garg, C. C., and A. K. Karan. 2008.'Reducing Out-of-pocket Expenditures to Reduce Poverty: A Disaggregated Analysis at Rural-Urban and State Level in India'. *Health Policy and Planning* 24(2), 17 December: 116–28.

Gautham, M., K. M. Shyamprasad, R. Singh, A. Zachariah, R. Singh and G. Bloom. 2014. 'Informal Rural Healthcare Providers in North and South India'. *Health Policy and Planning* 29 (supplement 1): i20–i29.

George, A., and A. Iyer. 2013. 'Unfree Markets: Socially Embedded Informal Health Providers in Northern Karnataka, India'. *Social Science and Medicine* 96, 1 November: 297–304.

Gilson, L., K. Hanson, K. Sheikh, I. A. Agyepong, F. Ssengooba and S. Bennett. 2011.'Building the Field of Health Policy and Systems Research: Social Science Matters'. *PLoS Medicine* 8(8): e1001079.

Hentschel, J. 1999.'Contextuality and Data Collection Methods: A Framework and Application to Health Service Utilization'. *The Journal of Development Studies* 35(4): 64–94.

Joe, W., and U. S. Mishra. 2009. 'Household Out-of-pocket Healthcare Expenditure in India: Levels Patterns and Policy Concern'. Working paper no. 418, Centre for Development Studies, Thiruvananthapuram, Kerala, India. Available at http://opendocs.ids.ac.uk/opendocs/handle/123456789/3136 (accessed 27 May 2017).

Karan, A., S. Srivastava, A. Chakraborty and H. Matela. 2016. 'Key Indicators of Morbidity Utilization and Health Expenditure: Tamil Nadu'. Technical report, Public Health Foundation of India, New Delhi.

Kumar, R., V. Jaiswal, S. Tripathi, A. Kumar, and M. Idris. 2007. 'Inequity in Health Care Delivery in India: The Problem of Rural Medical Practitioners'. *Health Care Analysis* 15(3): 223–33.

Kumar, S. 1994. 'India's Health Care Utilization Survey'. *The Lancet* 344(8934): 1424–25.

Leslie, C. 1976. *Asian Medical Systems: A Comparative Study*. Berkeley: University of California Press.

Levesque, J. F., S. Haddad, D. Narayana and P. Fournier. 2006. 'Outpatient Care Utilization in Urban Kerala, India'. *Health Policy and Planning* 21(4): 289–301.

Matthews, Z., S. Mahendra, A. Kilaru and S. Ganapathy. 2001. 'Antenatal Care, Care-seeking and Morbidity in Rural Karnataka, India: Results of a Prospective Study'. *Asia-Pacific Population Journal* 16(2): 11–28.

May, C., K. Roth and P. Panda. 2014. 'Non-degree Allopathic Practitioners as First Contact Points for Acute Illness Episodes: Insights from a Qualitative Study in Rural Northern India'. *BMC Health Services Research* 14(1): 182.

Mohanty, S. K., R. K. Chauhan, S. Mazumdar and A. Srivastava. 2014. 'Out-of-pocket Expenditure on Health Care among Elderly and Non-elderly Households in India'. *Social Indicators Research* 115(3): 1137–57.

Mukherjee, S., S. Haddad and D. Naranyana. 2011. 'Social Class-related Inequalities in Household Health Expenditure and Economic Burden: Evidence from Kerala, South India'. *International Journal for Equity in Health* 10(1): 1–13.

Navaneetham, K., and A. Dharmalingam. 2002. 'Utilization of Maternal Health Care Services in Southern India'. *Social Science and Medicine* 55(10), 1 November: 1849–69.

Nichter, M. 1978. 'Patterns of Resort in the Use of Therapy Systems and their Significance for Health Planning in South Asia'. *Medical Anthropology* 2(2): 29–56.

———. 1980. 'The Layperson's Perception of Medicine as Perspective into the Utilization of Multiple Therapy Systems in the Indian Context'. *Social Science and Medicine* 14(4): 225–33.

———. 1981. 'Idioms of Distress: Alternatives in the Expression of Psychosocial Distress: A Case Study from South India'. *Culture, Medicine and Psychiatry* 5(4): 379–408.

Nichter, M. 1983. 'Paying for What Ails You: Sociocultural Issues Influencing the Ways and Means of Therapy Payment in South India'. *Social Science and Medicine* 17(14): 957–65.

——— (ed.). 1992. 'Introduction'. In *Anthropological Approaches to the Study of Ethnomedicine*, ix–xxii. Montreux, Switzerland: Gordon and Breach Publishers.

———. 1997. 'Project Community Diagnosis: The Role of Participatory Research in Primary Health Care'. In *Anthropology in Public and International Health*, ed. Robert Hahn, 300–24. Oxford: Oxford University Press.

Nichter, M., and C. Nordstrom. 1989. 'A Question of Medicine Answering'. *Culture, Medicine and Psychiatry* 13(4): 367–90.

Nichter, M., and G. Quintero. 1996. 'Pluralistic Therapy Systems: Why Do They Co-exist and How Are They Used'. In *Encyclopedia of Cultural Anthropology*, eds D. Levinson and M. Ember, 1–17. New York: Henry Holt.

Pinto, S. 2004. 'Development without Institutions: Ersatz Medicine and the Politics of Everyday Life in Rural North India'. *Cultural Anthropology* 19(3): 337–64.

Population Centre. 1978. 'Classification of Districts in Karnataka State by Health Status'. *Population Centre Newsletter* 4(3), Bangalore, India.

Ranga, V., and P. Panda. 2016. 'Private Non-degree Practitioners and Spatial Access to Out-patient Care in Rural India'. *GeoJournal* 81(2): 267–80.

Rani, M., and S. Bonu. 2003. 'Rural Indian Women's Care-seeking Behavior and Choice of Provider for Gynecological Symptoms'. *Studies in Family Planning* 34(3): 173–85.

Rao, P. H. 2005. 'Profile and Practice of Private Medical Practitioner in Rural India'. *Health and Population* 28(1): 40–49.

Rohde, J., and H. Viswanathan. 1994. *The Rural Health Practitioner*. New Delhi: Oxford University Press.

Saroha, E., M. Altarac and L. M. Sibley. 2008. 'Caste and Maternal Health Care Service Use Among Rural Hindu Women in Maitha, Uttar Pradesh, India'. *Journal of Midwifery and Women's Health* 53(5): 41–47.

Singh, P., R. J. Yadav and A. Pandey. 2005. 'Utilization of Indigenous Systems of Medicine and Homoeopathy in India'. *Indian Journal of Medical Research* 122(2): 137.

Sudhinaraset, M., M. Ingram, H. K. Lofthouse and D. Montagu. 2013. 'What is the Role of Informal Healthcare Providers in Developing Countries? A Systematic Review'. *PloS One* 8(2): e54978.

Thirthalli, J., L. Zhou, K. Kumar, J. Gao, H. Vaid, H. Liu, A. Hankey, G. Wang, B. N. Gangadhar, J. B. Nie and M. Nichter. 2016. 'Traditional, Complementary, and Alternative Medicine Approaches to Mental

Health Care and Psychological Wellbeing in India and China'. *The Lancet Psychiatry* 3(7): 660–72.

Williams, S. J. 1995. 'Theorising Class, Health and Lifestyles: Can Bourdieu Help Us?'. *Sociology of Health and Illness* 17(5): 577–604.

four

Medical Pluralism and the Political Economy of Obstetric Care among Bangladeshi Women in Britain

Sultana Mustafa Khanum

Deployment of medical pluralism in everyday contexts of seeking care is common in almost every society. The context, process and ways of seeking assorted healing practices vary from culture to culture. This chapter will contextualise Bangladeshi migrant/Briton women's deployment of medical pluralism around obstetric care within their experiences of 'coerced integration' into the host society and maintaining an 'intrinsic link to' the kin network back home in Bangladesh. Drawing on intensive field work over a period of 27 years involving first, second and third generations of Bangladeshi migrant/Briton women in Manchester, UK, the chapter discusses how perceived/experienced institutional racism and their own cultural agencies induce women to blend the use of biomedicine with indigenous medicine (particularly ayurvedic and unani medicine, and the use of medicinal herbs) and healing practices. Such blending goes beyond individual bodily practices. For example, both biomedicine and indigenous medicines become items of gift exchange between the women living in England and their relatives back home, thus enabling them to maintain a sense of belongingness. Yet at the same time, perceived belongingness to two cultures creates ambivalent responses towards medicalisation of pregnancy and imperatives of technological interventions at childbirth. For these women, while biomedicine was perceived as essential to regaining strength or preventing further complications, indigenous medicine was viewed as indispensable to expel the side effects of such medicine. Finally, while such hybrid medicine is desired, availability of both biomedicine and indigenous medicine depended on the position of the woman in her family as well as in the wider society, where the power of both the family elders and medical personnel are decisive factors.

This chapter draws on ethnographic fieldwork spanning three generations of Bangladeshi migrants in the UK. Data are collected through oral testimonies, 'using self as informant' (Keyes 1987) and focusing on 'body gesture' from the epistemological point of view (Bourdieu 1984). Almost all my respondents were from the Sylhet district of Bangladesh and use the Sylheti dialect, very different from the Bengali language. My great advantage was that I am from the same district, speak the same dialect and lived with them as a member of the community in the UK. In addition to in-depth interviews, the emphasis was given to 'chatting' (Keyes 1987) and storytelling. Kirkham (1997) rightly pointed out that a story tells more than a tale; it also demonstrates context and values. During the first spell of my fieldwork, I adopted snowball sampling procedures but later it was evident that the number restricts the conceptualisation of the themes and takes away the essence of the diverse nature of data. The first spell of formal data collection was between 1990 and 1994. The second spell was in 2001–04, while the third started from 2010 and is continuing now with an interval of a few months almost each year. Besides formal fieldwork, I maintain everyday contact with my respondents through letters, mail, email, phone and Skype. This enables me to remain informed of any changes that occur in the community and the trajectory of the changes relating to obstetric care. This longitudinal study is being carried out in a small part of Manchester, UK, for which I used the pseudonym 'Ochingram'.

'Sojourner to Settlers': Bangladeshis in Britain

Popular impressions portray Bangladeshi women in the UK as being unreceptive, isolated and a 'mute group'. This is true to a certain extent, especially in the case of the first generation of women having rural backgrounds, but the second- and third-generation/Briton demonstrate a higher level of achievement in terms of education, employment and participation in the social and political spheres (Ahmed, et al. 2001; Dale, et al. 2002). A few of them have even been elected as Members of Parliament in the UK. Moreover, women who entered Britain with a Tier 1 or Tier 2 visa have engaged themselves in corporate as well as 'high-skilled job' sectors. Despite showing remarkable enthusiasm and good performance in education, a large section of them 'experience disproportionate rate of employment and other socio-economic deprivation' (Eade and Garbin 2003; Khanum 1994, 2000a, 2000b).

The Bangladeshis in Britain are heterogeneous in terms of education, employment, background, span of migration and demographic set-up in Britain as well as back home. In order to understand these differences, it is essential to shed some light on the background and process of migration of this group. There was a great influx of male migrants to the UK after the promulgation of the British Nationality Act of 1948. Most of them were from the least privileged class in Bangladesh, with very little education, who came to Britain as *khalasees* (galley hands) and started off in the UK as factory workers. After the collapse of a huge number of textile industries, most of them engaged themselves in the restaurant business, either as workers or owners. By the early 1970s, they started bringing their families to Britain and earned the status of settlers, transforming, as described by Ballard (1994: 11), 'from sojourners to settlers'. This group encapsulated themselves within their own community, inclined to preserve their own cultural norms and practices. In the late 1960s, a few educated/professional groups began to enter Britain. In order to keep pace with others in this competitive society, they more or less integrated themselves into White culture. This group prefers to keep a deliberate distance from the working/less educated groups. When they themselves fell victim to British institutional racism, they held the lifestyle, that is, cultural practices, of the first immigrants responsible for it. Hence, the Bangladeshi migrants/settlers are polarised into two groups on the issue of their reluctance or inclination to be assimilated into White culture. In course of time, a large number of second-generation migrants coming from the so-called uneducated/less educated families have been able to place themselves in the higher strata of the society in Britain in terms of education, employment, business, politics, etc. Despite their everyday contact with mainstream culture, they retain their own cultural norms and practices with dignity. Hence, neither income, nor education, nor even occupation, is an effective criteria of distinction.

Based on their cultural practices rather than on class or status, Bangladeshis in Britain have gradually come to form two categories: the integrationist group (referred to here as Culture A) and the people who prefer to retain their own cultural ideals (Culture B), as categorised in Khanum (1994). Although the first-generation members belonging to

Culture B maintain a 'myth of return' to their homeland, the second/third-generation of this group perceives Britain as their homeland. At the same time, like their parents, they also maintain connections with their relatives residing in Bangladesh, and these 'connections remain to be the political, economic, familial or even imagined' (Gardner and Ahmed 2006: 1). For them, 'home' is often located in two places—in the UK and Bangladesh, because close family members live in both the locations (Gardner 1993). Hence, these families make frequent visits to Bangladesh and they view 'such visits ... as a way of reinforcing family bonds for their children and exposing them to Bangladeshi ways to doing things' (Gardner and Mand 2012: 2).

'Doing things in Bangladeshi way' makes them a distinct community, subject to the effect of racial stereotype and action. A large body of research revealed that Bangladeshis faced discrimination in terms of employment, wages, housing and health services (Eade and Garbin 2003; Husband 1982; Mares, Henley and Baxter 1985; Khanum 1994, 2000a; Townsend and Davidson 1982). It is evident that ethnic people also suffer an 'ethnic penalty' (Stubbs 2008), for example, 'service providers usually make assumptions based on stereotypes and prejudice about the needs of these users without trying to know their true needs' (Chahal 2004). With regards to obstetric health care, Bangladeshi women in the UK were able to meet their midwives according to their need/desire, only 50.65 per cent compared to 78.1 per cent of White women (Miller 2008). Some studies claimed that the mass media attempts to construct an image of 'Asian criminality' (Webster 1997). After September 2001, Islamophobia was expressed in many ways (Werbner 2004), including physical attacks, verbal abuse, institutional racism, etc. The second/third-generation Bangladeshis/Britons are reluctant to accept second-class status like their ancestors did. When they face racist attacks, they fight back. In such a situation of perceived and institutionalised racism, 'community cohesion' becomes a means of collective strength to retain a distinct identity and respond to practices of racism where required. Such cohesion is sought to be established through frequent visits to Bangladesh. Through these visits, the Bangladeshi cultural agency is also transmitted to the UK. One such cultural practice relates to traditional/indigenous knowledge and practices, including more tangible matter like the herbs. In the subsequent section, I describe the extent, nature and process of employment of indigenous healing practices in this community.

Medicalisation and Politics of Obstetric Health

Obstetric care has been covered by medical jurisdiction since the beginning of the twentieth century, but the process of medically separating a woman's body from herself and gaining control over her life had started in the seventeenth century, as Oakley (1984: 2) indicated: 'Antenatal care may be equated with other forms of social control over women on the basis of what is said by the clinicians.' She added, 'A pregnant woman is encouraged to hand over responsibility for the management of her condition to others (the medical professionals)' (Oakley 1979: 46). A large group of feminists viewed the intervention of technology in pregnancy as a way for others to exercise the power to control women's bodies (Carden 1973). The medicalisation of childbirth literature is well established. In the Western context, this is the starting point of the politics of pregnancy/childbirth. While on the one hand, the State exerts control over reproductive bodies through medicalising childbirth, on the other hand in Bangladesh, there exists a different form of politics of pregnancy where the elderly women in the community exercise their power over the pregnant women through a series of prescriptions and proscriptions. These are related to their cultural practices concerning food, movement, remedial measures, etc. I will describe the nature, context and seeking out of such practices in the subsequent sections.

In the UK, the pregnant Bangladeshi women have to abide by the instructions concerning indigenous health practices mainly for two reasons: (a) In Bangladeshi culture, the daughter-in-law usually remains under the control of her in-laws, especially elderly members of the family. She has very little decision-making power relating to the uptake of health services. (b) Medical assistance in childbirth is still quite sparse in some areas of rural Bangladesh, especially in the areas from where most of the Bangladeshis have migrated. Moreover, first-generation migrants hardly had any opportunity to receive such facilities in Bangladesh. Despite the Bangladeshi government's sincere efforts and provision of institutional delivery at the root-level health centres in some areas, only 26.5 per cent women received a medically trained attendant at delivery (Government of Bangladesh 2012) due to several sociocultural constraints. Taufikuzzaman (2015) reported that women tried their best to avail themselves of institutional delivery if they found a facility nearer to their place, and that 44 per cent of the births were attended by medically trained providers. In such a situation, what would the attitude and practices of those women who have migrated to the UK, where medical assistance is easily available, be? What about the indigenous cultural practices relating to health, which are supposed to have disappeared in Britain because of access to institutional delivery? Interestingly, Bangladeshi settlers/Britons are caught between these two systems and worldviews. Some of them adopt medicalisation of obstetric care without any demur but also actively use their own traditional healing practices. They simultaneously take up hospital services and traditional remedial measures, which they regard as 'essential' and 'desirable', respectively, as Sharma, et al. (2013) termed while discussing the issue in the context of India. With regard to food taboos or following a special diet during pregnancy, previous research found that these do not depend on the women's age, education or duration of migration. Women living with their mothers-in-law or nearer to their mothers' houses sometimes observe these practices to please them. On the other hand, some of the mothers-in-law are against such taboos/practices; some women observe these through their own initiative (Khanum 1994).

Medical Pluralism among the Bangladeshis/Britons in Britain

Uses of remedial measures, either biomedical or traditional or a dual system, differ from family to family within the same Bangladeshi community in Britain, depending on a series of factors such as demographic set-up, duration of residency in the UK, educational and occupational status of the household members, linkages with people back at home, status/presence of elderly in the family, nature of kin support, attitude towards authoritative knowledge in the community, experience of racism, etc. Interestingly, age does not play a significant role in this regard. Availability of such measures and the presence of people holding authoritative knowledge have a great bearing on women's healing practices. Authoritative knowledge is socially endorsed, which demands that 'people actively engage in (its) production and reproduction ... thus continuously reinforcing its validity' (Floyd and Sargent 1997: 183). In the present study, I relate the authoritative knowledge among Bangladeshis to the practices concerning obstetric care. This knowledge relates to indigenous health practices during pregnancy, childbirth and the post-natal period.

Migrant parents prefer to get their children married to Bangladeshi relatives to keep their kinship network strong. Irrespective of geographical distance, the parents-in-law have control over the nuclear household as well (Khanum 2001). After getting married to a British Bangladeshi groom, when a Bangladeshi woman arrives in the UK, she either finds herself isolated due to her unfamiliarity with the surroundings or is placed under the control of her in-laws, which restricts her mobility and suppresses her decision-making power in terms of health seeking behaviour. In spite of that, some of these women can adopt their desirable remedial measures by exercising their own agency while some have to succumb to the desire of seniors in the family. Nevertheless, it was revealed that women prefer medicalisation of pregnancy relating to antenatal care, but they are against technological intervention in childbirth (Khanum 2003). They prefer hospital delivery but without any artificial intervention. In their opinion, introduction of a monitor at the time of labour hampers the normal movement, thus delaying delivery. Most of them have a negative attitude towards drip or oxytocin, which is used during the second stage of labour to amplify the labour and speed up delivery. This injection is also used to prevent post-partum hemorrhage. The senior/elderly women have maintained that this injection prevents the expulsion of *dushito rakto* (impure/filthy blood), resulting in the thickening of the abdomen, leaves the uterus delicate and leads to long-term complications. On the other hand, young educated women/Britons feel that overdoses of oxytocin may lead to hasty delivery, leaving perineal tears, uterine rupture, etc.

In rural Bangladesh, the delivery takes place with the women lying, kneeling or in a squatting position. Women are supported by a number of female relatives/neighbours during labour and a series of rituals are associated with childbirth (Blanchet 1984; Islam 1985; Khanum 1994). These practices relating to childbirth and food taboos are very common throughout South Asian societies and widely documented in India in general (Jeffery, et al. 1989) and Tamil Nadu in particular (Ferro-Luzzi 1973); Malaysia (McElroy and Townsend 1989); and rural Bangladesh (Blanchet 1984; Islam 1985; Khanum 1994, 2000; Walton and Schbley 2013). Even Choudhury, et al. (2012) found some beliefs and practices relating to childbirth and post-natal periods in the urban slum areas in contemporary Bangladesh. It was also found that when a rural woman was taken to the health centre for delivery, she was accompanied by a *dai* (traditional birth attendant) because the household members believed that she would help lessen the pregnant mother's labour pain by introducing indigenous techniques like moving her fingers (soaked with mustard oil) around the navel, lower abdomen and cervix of the pregnant woman; help her exert pressure down by massaging the lower part of the back; soothe her by chatting/story telling; etc. The dai claimed that when the ejection of placenta was delayed, she induced vomiting in the mother by giving her some water mixed with *neem* (a herbal plant). That helped the expulsion of the placenta. She did that in the presence of the health staff and none of them prevented her from doing so (Khanum and Anwar 2017).

During labour pain, drinking hot water, tea or hot milk prevents reverse motion of the foetus. A piece of consecrated jute or the flower of the *hatisuri* tree (another herbal plant) is tied around her waist or thigh. Sometimes the birth attendant places a *kula* (a winnowing platter, used to separate the grain from the husk) below the mother's birth passage, inviting the unborn baby to come (a gesture of separating a new born from its mother's womb). In case of delayed ejection of placenta, some rituals are performed, such as unlocking the padlocks, unhinging the doors of the room, cutting off the tying ropes of thatched roofs, or cutting off the bamboo nodes (Blanchet 1984; Khanum 2003). Some of these practices are still in operation in Bangladesh, but none of these exist in Ochingram. The women who gave birth to their children in Bangladesh or attended others' deliveries informed me that they miss these practices in the UK, which they would like to have. However, some of them use homeopathy medicine to quicken delivery. Sanctified water brought from Mecca is also given to the woman to drink. Some of this water is sprinkled over her body. This is done in the presence of the birth attendants in the labour room.

It is thought that the more excessive the bleeding, the more the possibility of an earlier recovery. In order to expel the dushito rakto after delivery, a *shek* (hot compress) is important. A lump of dried soil is heated in the fire bowl inside the room. This hot lump is wrapped properly in a piece of cloth and pressed gently on the lower abdomen and external genital parts of the mother. This heat helps her uterus to retract and heals the injury of the womb. Sometimes the mother is asked to take her meal from an earthen plate. After finishing the meal, the plate is heated in the fire and a hot compress is made with this plate. It serves a dual purpose:

First, radiating the abdomen in this way clears out clotted blood from the uterus, and second, it helps the woman get rid of any evil spell which might have invaded the body with the food.

The earthen plate or the lump of soil epitomises the gift from the earth, while burning represents the fire. Besides, a hole is made in the ground where *baro bakhor* (12 types of spices such as cumin, black cumin, cloves, coriander seeds, cassia, cinnamon, comfit, nutmeg, cardamom, black pepper, ginger and garlic) are placed and a fire is lit. When the flame comes up, the woman squats over the hole. Sometimes the mother is asked to sit on a hot brick. The reference to soil, earth, fire, water or later, the cold, hot and fluid substances stems from the syncretic forms of ayurveda and unani in Bangladesh. In Bangladesh, Shadhona and Shakti are two popular brands of ayurvedic medicine, while Hamdard represents the unani system to a certain extent.

It is thought that the entire health status of a mother depends on the nature of the treatment she receives and her food intake during the post-natal period. Since she is internally *kancha* (bruised), her body needs warmth for healing. She cannot get warmth through taking hot food as her digestive system remains weak because of the vulnerable state of her health. At the same time, for regaining strength she needs nutritious food that is easy to digest. Moreover, through pregnancy/delivery she accumulated excess fluid in the body. Dry food is required to absorb the fluid. Thus, the food should be selected very cautiously in order to provide her with the necessary warmth and strength, to absorb the excess fluid without disturbing the digestive system. Taking all these factors into account, food is divided into five main categories, namely *thanda* (cold), *gorom* (hot), *rosal* (fluid based), *shukhna* (dry) and *badi* (excluded). Cold food contains fruit, milk, yogurt, etc., while the hot foods are meat, eggs, oily fish, etc. Milk, soup, juice and pulses are fluid based. Dry and excluded foods are puffed rice, *ghee* (purified butter), bread, grounded rice, nuts, baro bakhor (the combination of the 12 types of spices, mentioned earlier), molasses, honey, etc., and small fish, chili, sour, pumpkin, etc., respectively. The morning after delivery, the mother is served ginger juice and the sap of *tuni mankuni* (a kind of herb) leaves with honey. This relieves acidity and indigestion. A bowl containing a mixture of roasted ground rice, honey, molasses and baro bakhor are kept near the mother's bed. At intervals, she eats this mixture throughout the day. After three days, she is served soft, over-boiled rice with a special soup. The soup is prepared with the leaves of *rujat*, neem, *dhan kolash*, *amtal*, *bashak*, tuni mankuni, *rashmanik* (all wild herbs), etc. These are made into a paste. This paste is then mixed with baro bakhor. The mixture is fried in ghee and two pints of water are added to it, and it is brought to boil. Afterwards, one or two small *shing maach* (cat fish) or a pigeon chick are added to the boiling soup and boiled for a few minutes (Khanum 1994, 2000). From the eighth day of delivery, the new mother can start taking other restricted foods in small quantities.

Although meat is prohibited from the very beginning, she is provided with specially prepared chick/pigeon soup. A processed chick/pigeon is added to a jar with cinnamon, clove, cardamom, garlic and ginger in it. Water is boiled in a pot and the jar containing the chick/pigeon is placed in the boiling water. Half an hour after it has been cooked, the chick/pigeon is taken out and is squeezed properly to extract the juice. Though this yields very little juice, it is rich in protein and vitamins. It does not have any meat or bulk of the fluid, thus it does not add any extra fluid in the body or affect the digestive organs.

There are also some traditional homemade specific herbal preparations which can prevent obstetric complication and help speedy recovery. These include powdered dried leaves of neem and jute, powered black cumin, roasted rice mixed with honey and ghee. Small balls are made out of that. The mother eats these balls frequently. It may prevent the swelling of legs, cervical pain, anorexia, indigestion, dizziness and helps drying of the *kancha nari* (weak and bruised fallopian tube). *Tri fala* (combination of three types of dried fruits, namely *amla*, *bohera* and *haritaki*) are soaked in water. The water is drunk to purify blood. *Shutika* (post-natal diarrhoea) could be prevented by massaging a paste of the leaves of *chalta* (a kind of fruit) to the middle of the scalp and washing it off after half an hour. Massaging the scalp with warm oil smoked with freshly ground ginger and garlic protects against *bela otha* (continuous headache and burning skull).

Although many of their everyday remedies are prepared with medicinal plants and herbs that are easily available in rural Bangladesh and require little processing, none of them are available in the market in the UK. People collect these from Bangladesh while they or their friends/neighbours visit Bangladesh or a relative/friend visits Britain from Bangladesh. In such cases, these remedial measures become items of gift exchange (Khanum 1994, 2000). They also bring Shadhona, Shakti and Hamdard medicine from Bangladesh. On the other hand, biomedicine such as Nurofen, vitamins and food supplements, namely Berocca, Vitabiotics, etc., are taken to Bangladesh as gift items.

It also happens that women manage to take preferred food items prepared with herbs and baro bakhor, even when their family members prohibit this. Bina's neighbours were a good source of the desired food. During my fieldwork she gave birth and stayed in hospital for three days. It is customary among Bangladeshi women to visit a patient/new mother in the hospital in a group. But in Bina's case, they came separately so that each could bring at least one dish secretly, without Bina's husband and the health staff noticing. In fact, it is very difficult to ascertain which women from which specific generation will adopt indigenous food or cultural practices. It may happen that a first-generation mother-in-law got her son married to a Bangladeshi bride; when she arrived in the UK, the bride was also regarded as first-generation Bangladeshi. Despite being members of the first generation, both mother-in-law and daughter-in-law may hold completely different worldviews and attitude towards indigenous health practices. In some such cases, the elderly mother-in-law may try to impose these practices on the daughter-in-law, who might dislike them. On the other hand, it may also happen that the first-generation daughter-in-law takes the indigenous preferred food/medicine secretly, without the knowledge of her mother-in-law, who perhaps migrated more than 30 years previously and holds negative views towards such food/medicine. It appears from the field data that the case of each woman is unique and that each of them represents a part of their cultural heritage. It is also apparent that a significant number of Britons are more enthusiastic in embracing indigenous health practices than the young first-generation Bangladeshi migrants.

A number of first-generation women mentioned that they had followed these healing practices and observed food taboos in Bangladesh, but no longer did so in Britain. Around 12 per cent of the Bangladeshi women surveyed did not wish to practise them but were obliged to do so in deference to their mothers-in-law or other senior women (Khanum 2000a, 2000b). It is worthwhile to note that the first-generation elderly women usually compelled or encouraged their daughters-in-law to use indigenous healing practices, while the first-generation young women overwhelmingly preferred and used biomedicine and hospital services. Most of them tried to avoid traditional remedial measures. There might be two reasons for such a state of affairs. First, most of them migrated from the least privileged rural areas, where modern medical treatment is still sparse. Despite their willingness, they were not able to avail themselves of the same due to financial as well as sociocultural constraints. When they found an opportunity to do so, they accepted it as a blessing of living in a modern society. Second, in order to compensate for their deficiency in other sectors (in employment, education, status, language), these women tried to present an image of modernity through using hospital treatment. A good number of them viewed using traditional healing practices as a sign of being 'backward' and 'uncivilised'. Even then, most of them used traditional healing practices to comply with their mothers-in-law's demand or desire, as Shumi states:

> I do not have any faith in these *gachamo oshudh* (medicine made with medicinal plants/herbs) but I have to take these to please my mother-in-law. Otherwise she would make a fuss. Furthermore, I must show some respect to her by obeying her order. (Shumi, age 23, first-generation settler, living with mother-in-law)

Some of them use a mix of biomedicine and traditional medicine, and Rehana identifies the reasons for that:

> What is the benefit of living in a modern society if you cannot reap the benefit of modern treatment? While I was in Bangladesh I used to crave for hospital delivery and modern medicine but could not avail that due to our inability to bear the expenses. Now I take antenatal check-ups, hospital delivery but also use gachamo oshudh because it helps me to purify my blood and expel the bad elements of the biomedicine that I have taken. (Rehana, age 38, first-generation settler, living in a nuclear household)

Rehana used to collect herbal medicine from Bangladesh through relatives and friends who visited their homeland. Her case depicts that social capital plays an important role in availing of and using indigenous remedial measures. On the other hand, an antagonistic relationship and mistrust between mother-in-law and daughter-in-law prevent a woman from using traditional medicine in spite of wanting it. Shafina's case can illustrate the situation:

> I never take these preparations ... I always throw these away secretly, without the knowledge of my mother-in-law. Because I guess she mixes some *pora pani/pora tel* (sanctified water/oil) to this herbal preparation to deteriorate my relationship with my husband so that he will divorce me and marry his mother's niece, Shapla. My mother-in-law wanted to get my husband married to Shapla so that she can bring her to the UK

> and help her brother, that is, Shapla's father. Subsequently Shapla will bring her father and brothers as well. It would have been nice if any of my natal relatives could visit me; I would ask them to bring gachamo oshudh prepared/procured by my mother or sister. (Shafina, age 21, first-generation settler, living with mother-in-law)

Perceived racism also tempted some of the women to use indigenous medicine, which is apparent from the following case:

> I have changed my general practitioner several times; I even rushed to Royal Hospital. When none of these worked I went to the private practitioner ... I spent nearly 1,000 pounds. But there was no difference. Do you know why? None of them even heed to me because I am not an *engraje* (White). Then my husband's aunt brought me some medicine prepared with herbs. Would you believe that it worked tremendously? Now I do not have any cervical pain. (Rini, age 24, second-generation Briton, working in a bank and living in a nuclear household)

It is interesting to note that while first-generation women, especially young women, have a negative attitude towards indigenous medicine, a large number of second/third-generation/Briton women have high regard for such medicines and use these. One of the reasons might be that they are educated and share the increasing global concern about the iatrogenic effects of biomedicine and, hence, they demand alternative medicine and healing practices, especially ayurvedic/herbal medicine, which is part of their heritage. A similar phenomenon of using herbal preparations to cure not only diabetes but also address social ills is noted among South Asian migrants in Edinburgh (Porqueddu 2013, 2017). Moreover, despite their acquisition of British citizenship/residency, Bangladeshi migrants are still subject to the effects of racist stereotyping and actions, which inspired them to use and restore their traditional remedial measures, as Nabila mentions:

> I am as British as John. If he can uphold his cultural symbols why should I not? I was born and bred here, earned higher education and a decent job, pay handsome tax to the British government but still they, that is, Whites, treat me as a trespasser to their land and blame me for not doing things like them. Why should I? They also call us 'uncivilised'. You know we ... I mean Bangladeshi British, have an age-old cultural heritage as well as sound remedial measures that date back to 5000 BC. I want to let them know that we have our own healing practices, which are more beneficial than biomedicine. I want to restore these measures and try to diffuse them

> throughout the world. We are not rootless, we did not come to the earth out of the blue ... we have a long-lasting legacy. (Nabila, age 24, third-generation Briton, working as a lawyer and living in a nuclear household, near her natal family)

These discussions with the women interviewed show that a series of interrelated factors have contributed to the transmission of indigenous remedial measures from Bangladesh to Britain and *vice versa*, which has enabled the Bangladeshis living in the two countries to deploy medical pluralism.

Conclusion

A myriad of interrelated factors have contributed to resorting to indigenous remedial measures in Britain, such as thrust for maintaining kinship ties, quest for identity maintenance, restoring cultural heritage, deference to the norms and practices of descendants, self-esteem, desire to uphold one's own cultural endowment, pride in one's own cultural resources, perceived as well as experienced institutional racism, health benefit, etc. It is evident that despite the availability of modern treatment, a large number of migrant Bangladeshi/Briton women continue to value traditional lore and practices relating to obstetric care, but they do not do so as blind followers or cultural dupes. Their deployment of medical pluralism is a product of many intermingled factors. First-generation Bangladeshis belonging to the Culture B group had not been able to enter mainstream British society because of their lack of institutional education, language difficulties and accompanying hesitation and lack of confidence. Finding themselves excluded and powerless in every sphere of life, they tried to compensate their disadvantage through employing the 'authoritative knowledge' in the community. On the contrary, institutional racism induced a section of Britons with Bangladeshi origins to use and restore their traditional healing measures. For them, their 'cognitive contours' and experiences of perceived institutional racism encouraged them to reinstate their cultural practices relating to health. But none of the groups escapes biomedicine. They use it according to their perceived need and blend it with their indigenous medicine that helps continue the deployment of medical pluralism within the Bangladeshi community in Britain.

References

Ahmed, N., C. Phillipson and J. Latimer. 2001. 'Transformations of Womanhood through Migration'. Working paper no. 8, Centre for Social Gerontology, Keele University.

Azmat, J., and O. Razum. 2014. *Medical Sociology in Africa*. Switzerland: Springer International Publishing.

Ballard, Roger. 1994. 'Introduction: The Emergence of DeshPardesh'. In *DeshPardesh: The South Asian Presence in Britain*, ed. Roger Ballard, 1–34. London: Hurst.

Basham, A. L. 1976. 'The Practice of Medicine in Ancient and Medieval India'. In *Asian Medical Systems: A Comparative Study*, ed. C. Leslie, 18–34. California: University of California Press.

Blanchet, T. 1984. *Women, Pollution and Marginality: Meaning and Rituals of Birth in Rural Bangladesh*. Dhaka: University Press Limited.

Bourdieu, P. 1984. *The Habitus and the Space of Life Style in Distinction: A Social Critic of Judgement and Taste*. London: Routledge.

Carden, M. L. 1973. *The New Feminist Movement*. New York: Russell Sage.

Chahal, K. 2004. 'Experiencing Ethnicity: Discrimination and Service Provision'. Joseph Rowntree Foundation. Available at https://www.jrf.org.uk/report/experiencing-ethnicity-discrimination-and-service-provision (accessed 2 December 2016).

Choudhury, N., A. Moron, M. A. Alam, K. Z. Ahsan, S. F. Rashid and P. K. Streatfield. 2012. 'Beliefs and Practices during Pregnancy and Childbirth in Urban Slums of Dhaka'. *BMC Public Health* 12(1): 790.

Dale, A., N. Shaheen and V. Kalra. 2002. 'Routes into Education and Employment for Young Pakistani and Bangladeshi Women in the UK'. *Ethnic and Racial Studies* 25(6): 942–68.

Eade, J., and D. Garbin. 2003. 'Bangladeshi Diaspora: Community Dynamics Transnational Politics and Islamic Activities'. Report for the Foreign and Commonwealth Office, UK.

Ferro-Luzzi, G. E. 1973. 'Food Avoidances of Pregnant Women in Tamilnad'. *Ecology of Food and Nutrition* 2: 259–66.

Floyd, R. D., and C. Sargent. 1997. *Childbirth and Authoritative Knowledge: Cross Cultural Perspectives*. California: University of California Press.

Gardner, K. 1993. 'Desh-Bidesh: Sylheti Image of Home and Away'. *Man* 28(1): 1–15.

_____. 2002. *Age, Narrative and Migration: The Life Course and Life Histories of Bengali Elders in London*. Oxford: Berg.

Gardner, K., and K. Mand. 2012. 'My Away is Here: Place, Emplacement and Mobility amongst British Bengali Children'. *Journal of Ethnic and Migration Studies* 38(6): 969–86.

Gardner, K., and K. Mand. n.d.'Transgender Childhoods: Diasporic Children in East London'. University of Sussex.

Gardner, K., and Z. Ahmed. 2006. 'Place, Protection and Migration in Bangladesh: A Londoni Village in Baiswanath'. Working paper no. T18, Development Centre on Migration, Globalisation and Poverty, University of Sussex, Sussex.

Government of Bangladesh. 2012. 'Bangladesh Health Bulletin'. Ministry of Health and Family Welfare, Dhaka.

Husband, C. 1982. *Race in Britain: Continuity and Change*. London: Hutchinson Company Limited.

Islam, M. 1985. *Women, Health and Culture*. Dhaka: Women for Women Study Group.

Jefferey, P., R. Jefferey and A. Lyon. 1989. *Labour Pains and Labour Power: Women and Child Bearing in India*. London: Zed Books.

Keyes, S. M. 1987. 'The Native Anthropologists: Constraints and Strategies in Research'. In *Anthropology at Home* (ASA monograph no. 25), ed. A. Jackson. London: Tavistock Publications Limited.

Khanum, S. M. 1994.'We Just Buy Illness in Exchange for Hunger: Experiences of Health Care, Health and Illness among Bangladeshi Women in Britain'. PhD dissertation, Keele University, UK.

———. 2000a. 'Habitus and its Implication in Constructing Kinship Ties: Data From a Bangladeshi Settlement in Britain'. In *Culture, Creation and Procreation: Concept of Kinship in South Asia Practice*, eds Aparna Rao and Monika Böck, 199–218. New York and Oxford: Berghahn.

———. 2000b. 'The Role of Kinship in Perpetuating the Politics of Pregnancy among the Bangladeshi Women in England'. *Man and Life* 26: 5–30.

———. 2001.'Household Patterns of a Bangladeshi Village in England'. *Journal of Ethnic and Migration Studies* 27(3): 489–504.

———. 2003. 'Child Birth Practices in Bangladesh'. Banglapedia, National Encyclopaedia of Bangladesh, Asiatic Society of Bangladesh.

Khanum, S. M., and A. K. Anwar. 2017.'The Status of Health Service Utilization by the Fistutla Patients: Data from Northern Bangladesh'. Research report, funded by Social Science Research Council, Dhaka.

Khanum, S. M., and U. Sharma. 2003. 'Penetrating Roots and Encountering Barriers: The Politics of Pregnancy for the Bangladeshi Women in England'. Paper presented at the ASA Decennial Conference on Anthropology and Science, University of Manchester, UK, 14–18 July.

Kirkham, M. 1997. 'Reflection in Midwifery: Professional Narcissism or Seeing with Women'. *British Journal of Midwifery* 5(5): 167–82.

Maloney, C., K. M. A. Aziz and P. C. Sarker. 1981. *Belief and Fertility in Bangladesh, Rajshahi*. IBS, University of Rajshahi.

Mares, P., A. Henley and C. Baxter. 1985. *Health Care in Multiracial Britain*. Cambridge: National Extension College.

McElroy, A., and P. K. Townsend. 1989. *Medical Anthropology in Ecological Perspective*. Boulder, Colorado: Westview Press.

Miller, T. 2008. *Making Sense of Motherhood*. Cambridge: Cambridge University Press.

Oakley, A. 1979. *Becoming Mother*. Oxford: Martin Robertson.

———. 1984. *The Captured Womb: A History of the Medical Care of Pregnant Women*. Oxford: Basil Blackwell.

Porqueddu, T. 2013. 'Living with Diabetes: Accounts of South Asian Migrants in UK'. In *Multiple Voices and Stories: Narratives of Health and Illness*, eds A. Mishra and S. Chatterjee, 193–217. New Delhi: Orient BlackSwan.

———. 2017. 'Herbal Medicine for Diabetes Control among Indian and Pakistani Migrants with Diabetes'. *Anthropology and Medicine* 24(1): 17–31.

Sharma, B., G. Giri, K. Christensson, K. V. Ramani and E. Johansson. 2013. 'The Transition of Childbirth Practices among the Rural Women in Gujarat'. *BMC International Health and Human Rights* 13(1): 41.

Stubbs, S. 2008. 'In Place of Drums and Samosas'. *The Guardian*, 14 May.

Taufikuzzaman, M. D. 2015. 'The Nature of Receiving Obstetric Care among Rural Women in Northern Bangladesh'. Unpublished PhD thesis, University of Rajshahi, Bangladesh.

Townsend, P., and N. Davidson. 1982. *Inequalities in Health: The Black Report*. DHSS, Harmondsworth: Penguin.

Walton, L. M., and B. Schbley. 2013. 'Cultural Barriers to Maternal Health Care in Rural Bangladesh'. *On line Journal of Health Ethics* 9(1): 1–12.

Webster, C. 1997. 'The Construction of British Asian Criminality'. *International Journal of the Sociology of Law* 25(1): 65–86.

Werbner, P. 2004. 'The Predicament of Diaspora and Millennial Islam'. *Ethnicities* 4(4): 451–76.

II

Documentation and Systematisation of Traditional Knowledge

five

From Siddha Corpus to Siddha Medicine

Reflection on the Reduction of Siddha Knowledge through Exploration of Manuscripts

Brigitte Sébastia

When I decided to conduct anthropological research on siddha medicine in 2005, one of the sites I chose was the district of Kanniyakumari in the southern state of Tamil Nadu, India, well known for its numerous traditional practitioners. Compared to institutional siddha doctors[1]—those trained in siddha colleges—siddha traditional practitioners acquire their medical knowledge from their relatives, parents and quite often grandparents, and for some, notably in this region, from *ācāṉ(kaḷ)*, a local term referring to teacher(s) or person(s) regarded as being highly proficient and knowledgeable in a specialty that defines the siddha tradition. Traditional practitioners possess siddha-related items they inherited from their family, and sometimes from their ācāṉ(kaḷ). These items include ancestors' photographs, diplomas, grinders and apparatus used to prepare medicines, surgical instruments, medicinal components (regarded as 'precious' because of their unaltered state considered as belonging to categories of medicines whose preparation required high skill) and manuscripts. During visits to these practitioners with my husband, it was rare that we were not exposed to these items. My husband, who documented the fieldwork in terms of photographs and video recordings, was on most occasions invited to take pictures of such almost unobtainable medical artefacts. Several practitioners, concerned with the preservation of manuscripts they inherited from their forefathers, consulted my husband regarding the process of cleaning and maintaining them and, occasionally, requested him to conduct the work.

The large quantity of manuscripts we discovered in the Kanniyakumari district led, seven years later, to the submission of a project on the digitisation and cataloguing of siddha manuscripts and items to the Endangered Archives Programmes of the British Library, sponsored by the philanthropic foundation, Arcadia. The two-year project, referenced EAP810, and entitled Conservation, Documentation and Preservation of the Knowledge of Siddha Medicine, began in July 2015.[2] The digital manuscripts, according to the British Library policy, will be accessible online. My objective in conducting this project was not only to preserve siddha knowledge, but also to encourage research on siddha medicine and on its allied subjects (philosophy, alchemy, yoga, etc.). This field is still neglected in India and hardly known outside the country, compared to ayurveda and its allied subjects developed in Sanskrit literature. Therefore, such research may offer keys to comprehending mutual influences between these Tamil and Sanskrit traditions, and to identifying the specificities of the siddha corpus in a comparative perspective with Asian traditions.

This chapter aims at sharing my reflections on this project. Based on the growing interest in siddha manuscripts I have been observing through encounters with individuals who have constituted manuscript collections they obtained from practitioners, I will discuss the motivations of such collectors as well as their openness or reluctance to participate in the project. The second discussion will be on the content of the manuscripts, some of which illustrate the complexity of siddha knowledge as well as the lack of clarity on the subjects they refer to. Although the project as it was formulated targeted medical manuscripts, the descriptive catalogue testifies that in many texts the medical matter is inextricably enmeshed with other subjects, namely alchemy and magic, philosophy and spirituality, ascetic practices and astrology, and forms that I would call the 'siddha corpus'. This corpus differs from the content of what is today called siddha medicine, whose institutionalisation in schools modelled on the British educational system at the time of colonisation led to a clear separation between subjects defined as medical and those considered as falling under philosophy and history of sciences or of religions.[3] Given that the syllabus in siddha colleges is increasingly being infiltrated by subjects related to biomedical practice and concepts, this raises questions about how this corpus, taught to the students of siddha colleges, is relevant in clarifying the transformations of traditional knowledge resulting from its institutionalisation, and in documenting its reception by the students. This subject, analysing the encounters between tradition and modernity, and between beliefs and rational and scientific thought, has been widely debated since the pioneering work of Leslie (1976). Quite often these encounters have been discussed by researchers in terms of the transformations of medical practice, such as diagnostic methods, medication and terminology (Alter 2005; Langford 1995, 2004; Leslie 1992). This chapter proposes another area of observation: the comparison between the knowledge contained in manuscripts and that imparted in the colleges.

Definition of the Project to Preserve Siddha Knowledge in Manuscripts

The project, once finished, will comprise around 400 siddha manuscripts. The manuscripts are composed of a variable number of texts going from 1 to 65, attributed to a *cittar* (class of yogis; explained later) or written by an anonymous pactitioner.[4] The texts, composed in verse or prose, are written on palm leaves collected from palm trees (*Borassus flabellifer*) and talipot palm trees (*Corypha umbraculifera*), the latter being rarer (Image 5.1).

The palm leaves, prepared by being buried for a few days to darken them and make them flexible, or being soaked in water to make them flexible, were then cut out, and holes pierced in one or two places for receiving the thread that bound them between two boards constituted of hardwood or palm leaves. The scripts were then engraved on the leaves with a sharp stylus. Their size is variable; those engraved on talipot palm leaves, characterised by fine texture and great flexibility, are quite often minuscule, indicating the high skill of the writer. The writers were siddha practitioners or copyists they hired to duplicate a manuscript they possessed or borrowed from peers. The manuscripts have almost disappeared since paper replaced palm leaves and printing replaced copyists in the first decades of the twentieth century. The important production of siddha manuscripts, still in the hands of practitioners and collectors or kept in diverse libraries in Tamil Nadu,[5] contradicts the common idea that the knowledge of traditional practitioners was based strictly on practice and ignored siddha concepts; an idea that endures today in the milieu of siddha doctors who claim the superiority of their knowledge received in college over that of traditional practitioners. This shows that in the past, siddha practitioners were well-educated and able

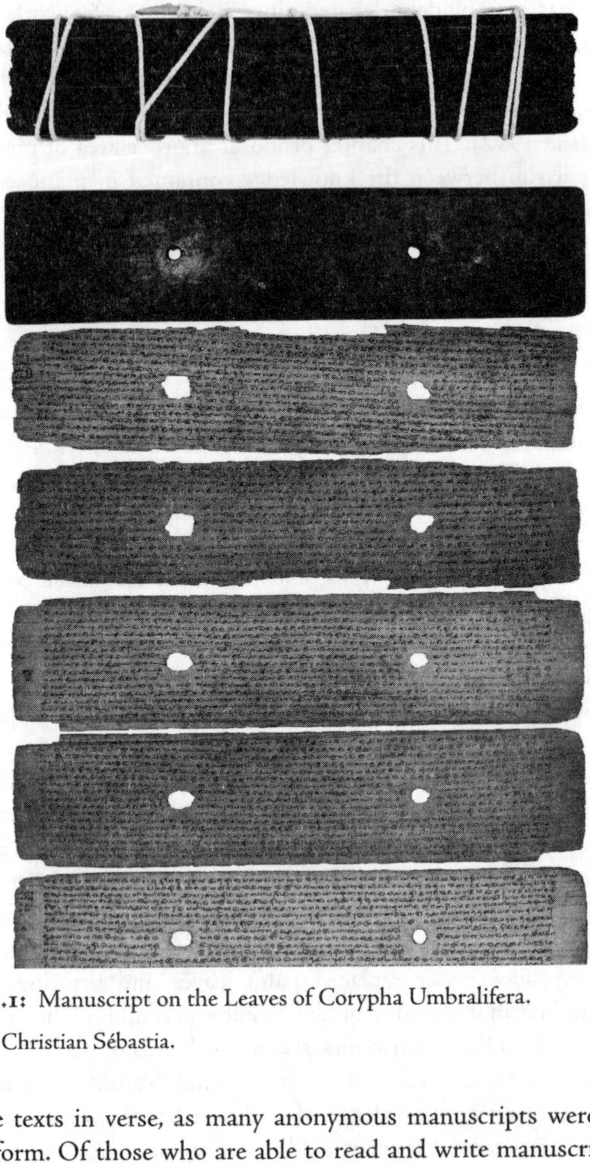

Image 5.1: Manuscript on the Leaves of Corypha Umbralifera.
Photo © Christian Sébastia.

to write texts in verse, as many anonymous manuscripts were written in this form. Of those who are able to read and write manuscripts (rare due to the lack of transmission of this practice), some continue to record information on their medical practice in notebooks (Image 5.2) and consult published books too.[6]

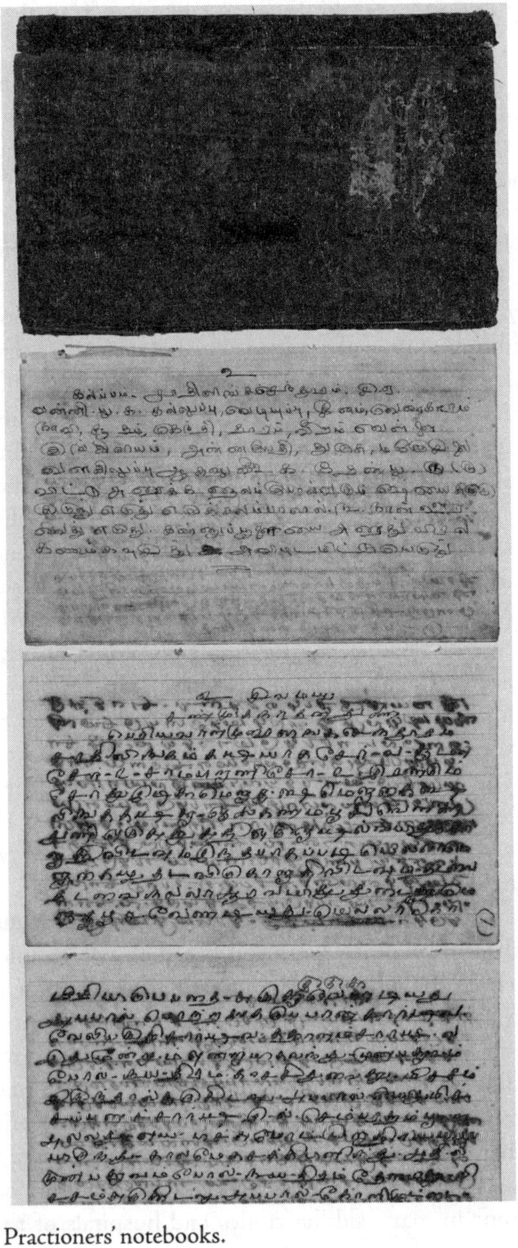

Image 5.2: Practioners' notebooks.
Photo © Christian Sébastia.

In most manuscripts, the leaves are numbered on the left part of the recto, a process conducted either once the leaves were ready to be inscribed or during the writing of texts. This numbering, and according to the texts, that of verses, offers the possibility to reorder the leaves when they are mixed up, or to reconstruct texts when leaves have been removed from the manuscripts. The displacement of leaves from a manuscript may be due to neglect, notably when the thread binding the manuscript has broken. It might result from the medical practice as, before going to the patient's bedside, traditional practitioners selected leaves from texts on astrology, nosology, diagnosis and treatment, corresponding to the patient's condition. A type of medicine box belonging to a practitioner of the Kanniyakumari district who inherited it from his grandfather attests to this practice—among its 23 compartments for storing remedies and instruments, the box has a long central case for receiving palm leaves.

The project was drawn up in order to digitise and catalogue manuscripts collected from Kanniyakumari and other districts. The digitisation is conducted at the residence of Akila Thiruvithancore Siddha Vaidhya Sangam (ATSVS) or 'Association of Siddha Practitioners of Travancore', Munchirai, for the collection of Kanniyakumari, and at the French Institute of Pondicherry for the manuscripts of other districts. The descriptive catalogue is prepared by two experts on manuscripts; the one from Tanjavur is in charge of manuscripts of all the districts except for those of the Kanniyakumari district, which are catalogued by the president of the ATSVS, a siddha practitioner. The descriptive catalogues are translated in a comprehensive manner into English and, to maximise access to texts, are presented in the database in two versions, Tamil and English.

The distinction between manuscripts coming from Kanniyakumari district and those from other districts is based on two grounds. The first is that numerous manuscripts, comprising the collection of ATSVS and manuscripts of traditional practitioners, were identified in the Kanniyakumari district, and the owners were willing to digitalise. Second, the difference in the manuscripts' origins allows for assessing the specificities commonly credited to the medical practice of Kanniyakumari district—a therapy based predominantly on plants; and a practice of acupressure and manipulation called *varmam*. During my observations on consultations in many siddha clinics and hospitals of this region, I noticed that practitioners prescribed complex medicaments, made up of metals and minerals prepared by iatrochemical processes only when the disease resisted treatments based on medicinal plants. Practitioners justify their extensive usage of plants by the availability and diversity of species, favoured by climatic conditions and by the varied topography of this region, which offer the means to treat almost all ailments. However, the manuscripts of the region do not reflect this therapeutic practice. The recurrence of medicaments based on metals, minerals or metallic salts such as *centūram*, *pa<u>r</u>pam*, *cuṇṇam* or *kaṭṭu*,[7] as well as of iatrochemical processes for purifying metals, metallic salts and minerals, and of alchemy-related products such as *muppu*, *racamaṇi*,[8] *some kaṭṭu*, *cuṇṇam* and *centūram* is as significant as in manuscripts coming from other districts. The discrepancy between formulations described in manuscripts, dating from the early nineteenth to early twentieth century CE, and those prepared and prescribed in the Kanniyakumari region today is the result of at least four factors.

The first is the influence from the neighbouring state of Kerala, well-known for its practice of ayurveda that gives primacy to herbal formulations. The second is the cost of raw materials, time of preparation and level of skill, which must be much greater to produce metal/mineral-based medicines. The lack of skill in preparing complex medicaments is pointed out by some practitioners who denounce the decline of siddha knowledge (Sébastia 2013); others complain about the present mentality of practitioners, especially those trained in colleges who, in quest of 'easy money', are not eager to throw themselves into the preparation of elaborate products. The third factor is awareness of intoxication risks due to the utilisation of poisonous substances (Sébastia 2015). As in the West, medicinal plants, even though they are not always free of risks due to environmental contamination or toxic components, are rarely seen as harmful in India.[9] Lastly, current practice may have been influenced by Maruttuva Āciriyam, a book written in the mid-nineteenth century by Po<u>n</u> Mikēl Ñā<u>n</u>iyār of Kāriyāviḷai (Kanniyakumari district), very popular in this region. In this text dealing with preparations of medicines, some formulas of *centūram*, *pa<u>r</u>pam*, pills and *kaṭṭu* are described but compared to the numerous formulations based on medicinal plants, they are under-represented.

On the other hand, manuscripts on varmam (vital spots; treatment of injured vital spots) are numerous in Kanniyakumari district, while none comes from other districts. Practitioners of the Kanniyakumari region attribute the practice of varmam to the Nāṭār community. The Nāṭārs form a caste partly constituted of ex-Cānārs[10] who held the traditional occupation of climbing coconut and palm trees (*Borassus flabellifer*) to collect the fruits and sap, which they converted into alcohol and sugar (*karupaṭṭi*). This labour, realised by rudimentary means and still practised today, led to severe injuries resulting from falls for which a medical field, called varmam, was developed by the Nāṭār community. Varmam is practised conjointly with bone-setting and siddha medicine.[11] The deciphering of texts on varmam requires an expert to clarify the meaning of the term itself, which varied according to context.[12] Varmam refers to *varma kalai* or art of vital spots, which comprises two arts: that of neutralising or killing enemies by injuring vital spots (martial art) and that of reviving unconscious people and of healing injured vital spots (therapy). These two arts, relying on the common knowledge of the exact location of vital spots in the body, are performed together by some practitioners. The vital spot is a location where the breath of life circulates (*piraṇam*). Varmam refers to a category of pressure; it is necessary to apply this on specific spots to release the circulation of piraṇam (Sankrit, *praṇa* or life energy), which causes the injury. Varmam is a deep and sustained pressure for treating serious injuries.[13] The texts of varmam present a description of the number of vital spots located in diverse parts of the body, explanations of the types of acupressure according to the injured varmam, and preparations of internal and external medicines to treat injuries. They rarely mention the cause of injuries, but a text we have digitised specifies those resulting from fighting and occurring during the practice of the martial art called *varma aṭi* (literally, hitting the vital spot) or *cilampam*.

Varma kalai is, nevertheless, not unique to Kanniyakumari; it has been developed in Kerala through the martial art called *kaḷari payaṭṭu* and the therapy called marma (Alter 2005; Zarrilli 1998). The differences in terminology are not so much substantive as an expression of regional identity politics (Alter 2005). The similarity between these two traditions has to be understood by the fact that the district of Kanniyakumari was associated with the southern part of present-day Kerala to form the Travancore kingdom before the creation of Tamil Nadu and Kerala in 1956. As pointed out by Immanuel (2002), just as the practice of varmam was developed by the Nāṭārs, in the same way, marma was in the hands of the E̱lavas, a caste assimilated to that of the Cānārs of Tamil Nadu from the sociocultural viewpoint. This therapeutic technique seems to be spread more through Kerala than through Tamil Nadu, thanks to oil massages, which constitute a part of the therapy *pañcakarma* (meaning 'five actions'; these are therapies that aim at purifying the body) that has become the emblem of ayurveda.

The comparative content of manuscripts between those coming from the Kanniyakumari district and those from the other districts testifies clearly that the varma (marma) practice is specific to the ex-Travancore region. This specificity is well-illustrated by the authorship of texts such as Varma Kaṇāti, Varma Muṟivu Cāri 1200 or Varma Vil Vicai Cūttiram, attributed to Akattiyar. In the Kanniyakumari region, the number of manuscripts under the name of Akattiyar is much more significant than in other districts; this is a reflection of his status as 'father of medicine' that the siddha practitioners of Kanniyakumari region attribute to him. Lastly, while from the point of view of the utilisation of organic and inorganic components in formulas it is difficult to assert a difference between Kanniyakumari district and other districts, it is worth mentioning that many manuscripts of Kanniyakumari refer to a medical specialty such as treatment of child and mother, skin diseases, eye diseases, mental illnesses and poisoning, in addition to varmam. These specialties are learned in siddha colleges, but they are integrated into general medical practice, rarely as specialties. However, the increasing popularity of varmam has been leading siddha doctors to set up a varmam clinic after having improved their practice with ācāṅkaḷ from the Kanniyakumari district (Sébastia 2010, 2016; Sieler 2015).

Private Manuscript Collections: Multiple Motivations

The rearrangement of palm leaves in manuscripts is a complex task when the material given for digitisation is badly maintained, as in the case of a collection of bundles and leaves we obtained from an ayurvedic doctor[14] of Karaikuti (Sivagangai district), who was unable to reconstruct the texts (Image 5.3). The classification of leaves based on physical criteria, notably size of leaves, number of holes for receiving the thread and their location and type of writing, then checked by the expert in manuscript reading, led to obtaining 98 manuscripts of diverse numbers of palm leaves, which belong to the siddha corpus.

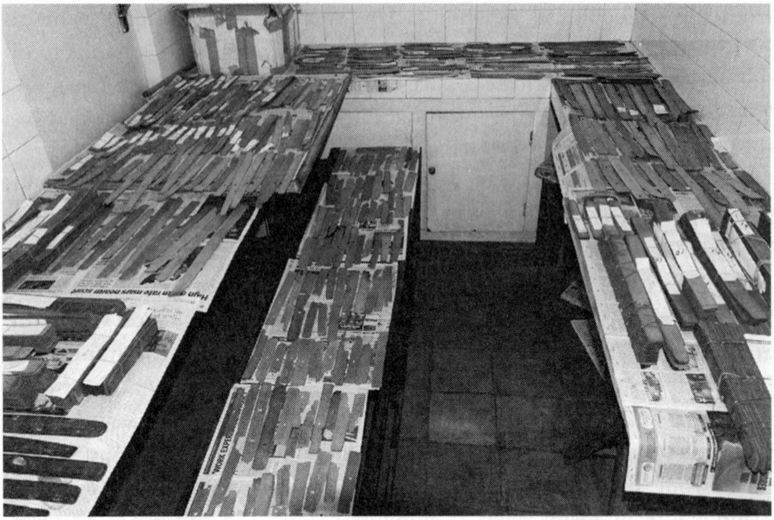

Image 5.3: Classification of Manuscripts

Photo © Christian Sébastia.

The necessity for an expert in siddha knowledge for reconstructing manuscripts is due to the poor maintenance of collections, in some cases by individuals who have created an association to constitute collections.[15] They justify this work by recurrently arguing: 'Practitioners have no interest in manuscripts, and thus, we requested them to give them to us in order to preserve the siddha knowledge for the future generations'. It is a fact, as I have observed several times, that the manuscripts are discarded by their owners, notably when they are in bad condition or when descendants are not interested in siddha medicine. However, the adequacy of the verb 'to preserve' is questionable as these collectors simply store the manuscripts without providing the necessary care to stop deterioration by insect larvae and eggs, and fungus, or even to protect healthy manuscripts from contamination caused by affected ones. Among the collectors I met, some are siddha doctors or traditional practitioners. Siddha doctors give their manuscripts for digitisation easily as their objective is not driven by a study of their content, and they see the project as an opportunity to reorder and clean them. The underlying motivation to collect this material seems to go along with my observations of the milieu: to gain the credibility of their clients by exhibiting manuscripts or other iconic objects in their clinics. Indeed, when patients have recourse to a private siddha clinic, they quite often turn to traditional practitioners who have acquired a solid reputation because of their family, rather than to siddha doctors who have no link with siddha tradition.

In contrast, traditional siddha practitioners who have collected manuscripts from their peers are not inclined to share them. Their goal is neither to preserve the knowledge contained in texts nor to obtain legitimacy as they are already recognised. Their intention is to study texts in order to improve their medical practice or knowledge, to write books, develop new medicinal formulas or seek information on *materia medica*, remedies and occult techniques to increase longevity, or on processes to produce highly iconic substances of the siddha tradition, especially the *mūppu*, a combination of three salts. Although numerous manuscripts provide formulas to prepare mūppu, it seems that the veritable and authentic recipe needs to be discovered (Venkatraman 1990). This quest, relying on the esoteric and alchemical aspects of siddha knowledge, underwent a growing interest from promoters of siddha medicine and also from practitioners willing to increase their reputation and to be recognised as ācān. They use strategies to hide their secrets from their disciples and reveal them, parsimoniously, only when they have acquired enough confidence in those disciples. The question of secrecy is sometimes mentioned in manuscripts, either to emphasise the importance of maintaining it, especially when the texts describe the vulnerable vital spots and alchemical processes, or to disclose alchemical secrets. A few traditional practitioners denounce their peers' lack of openness. Particularly aware of the loss of siddha knowledge, they are ready to share anything which may serve the purpose of its preservation and promotion. It is with this intention that the owner of a large collection of manuscripts of Kanniyakumari agreed to participate in the project. His objectives were in line with those of his grandfather and father, who were presidents of the ATSVS before him—that of disseminating siddha knowledge.

ATSVS was created in 1937 by Netiyananda Samikal on donated land located on a small hill in the village of Muncirai.[16] The grandfather of the current president participated in the establishment of a small college to supplement the clinical knowledge of siddha traditional practitioners by providing theoretical insights. The college was then developed into a college-cum-hospital which received recognition from the Department of Health and Family Welfare of Tamil Nadu in 1996 for training students and delivering the BSMS degree (Sébastia 2010).[17] A large part of the collection of manuscripts of ATSVS is the work of the first president, who hired copyists to copy manuscripts he collected from his peers in order to establish a library in the college and to develop a range of remedies, some of which are still prepared and prescribed in the hospital. The rest of the collection (around one tier) was undertaken by the father of the present president of ATSVS and by the president himself. His tenacity in obtaining manuscripts from his peers is in accordance with his objectives to improve and make known certain parts of siddha medical knowledge, by publishing books from manuscripts and by participating in the revision of textbooks for students of siddha medicine. In the past, he has written many books on the practice of varmam; his present focus is to write books on the preparation of siddha medicines.

The willingness or reticence to share manuscripts, which is largely dependent on the identity of the collectors, as I attempt to show, demonstrates that this material is highly valued as a resource of authentic knowledge on the siddha corpus. Although many books have been printed from manuscripts, notably those attributed to the major *cittarkaḷ*, the common idea shared by all the collectors is that the manuscripts contain precious information, especially on medical and alchemical formulas, which needs to be discovered.

From Siddha Corpus to Siddha Medicine: A Reductionist Knowledge

Syllabus in Siddha College: Are Students Eager to Learn the Siddha Corpus?

The periods of digitisation conducted at the ATSVS, Muncirai, offered me the opportunity to complement my knowledge and observations on the siddha therapeutic milieu, traditional as well as institutional. On the one hand, I was exposed to traditional practitioners who regularly visited the ATSVS's president for friendship and/or advice related to medical practice (formulas, patient's symptoms, etc.), and on the other hand, I was free to move around in the out-patient wards, the pharmacy where medicaments are given free to patients, and the laboratory where the students learn to prepare medicines. Additionally, I interacted with students during all my fieldwork periods. One of the points of conversations had been to evaluate the interest of students in siddha medicine and to discuss what drove them to join this medical specialty. On a similar point, I learnt, through discussions with students of the government siddha colleges at Chennai and Palaiyamkottai and doctors trained in these institutions, that siddha medicine was rarely the first choice. The students had turned to it because the marks they had obtained to pursue their education were insufficient to gain a seat in government biomedical colleges. The responses of the students of the ATSVS college of Muncirai were similar: they expected to enter a biomedical college, but their marks were insufficient to get a seat not only in a biomedical college, but also in the government siddha colleges of Chennai and Palaiyamkottai. However, they decided to enter this medical field because their focus was to become a doctor, a highly valued profession in India, more attractive from the point of view of prestige and money than from a humanitarian perspective. However, a category of students stands apart: they are those who belong to a family of siddha practitioners.[18] For these students who have already acquired a solid medical knowledge and practice in the family, turning to siddha college is the means to continue their family profession. Since the registration of traditional practitioners was stopped in 1972, an institutional degree is required to practise medicine legally (Sébastia 2010).

As the college of Muncirai was recognised by the government in 1996, its syllabus was changed to comply with that defined by the Central Council of Indian Medicine. Consequently, while in the past the traditional knowledge (siddha corpus) was privileged, the syllabus has progressively integrated more disciplines drawn from biomedical sciences, notably anatomy, physiology, biochemistry, microbiology and pharmacognosy. As I have discussed elsewhere on the institutionalisation of siddha medicine (ibid.), the introduction of biomedical disciplines and concepts into Indian medical colleges results from the repeated strikes organised by students who have attempted to mimic the biomedical model. It offers students the possibility to conduct their internship in biomedical hospitals and, possibly, to reorient their career towards this medical field which offers valorised jobs with better remuneration. The disciplines related to siddha knowledge still have their place, but their importance in the syllabus is dependent on their ability to fit into 'modern' subjects commonly offered in other colleges. While *materia medica* including botany and pharmacopeia (*kuṇapāṭam*), pathology/etiology of diseases (*nōy nāṭal*), physiology and anatomy (*uṭal tattuvaṅkaḷ*) and diagnostic techniques are taught in the whole curriculum, a set of subjects very specific to the siddha corpus called *tōki*, the short form of *tōṟṟa kirama arāycci*,[19] are in the syllabus of the first year and, to a lesser extent, of the second year of BSMS only.[20]

Tōki, which is also translated as history and fundamental principles of siddha medicine, includes the study of 96 *tattuvaṅkaḷ* that comprise physiological and anatomical concepts such as the three humours (*tiridoṣam* or *muppiṇi*), five elements (*aim pūtam*), seven bodily constituents (*eḻu tātu*), five organs of actions (*karumēntiriyam*) and of senses (*ñāṉēntiriyam*) and 10 nerves (*taca nāṭi*), etc., and other concepts difficult to categorise, as they concern the subtle and sensible parts of the body, such as the five states of soul (*pañca cāvastai*), the five cases of sheaths of soul (*pañca kōcam*), the three cosmic qualities (*mukkuṇam*), the three regions (*mūṉṟu maṇṭalam*), the eight passions (*eṇ vikāram*), etc. (Pillai 1931, 1993; Madhavan 1984). Tōki approaches occult aspects of the siddha corpus related to the second category of tattuvaṅkaḷ, such as philosophical concepts of the creation of the universe, conceptions of the body in relation with spirituality (almighty, soul and bondages), ethics and morality, as well as mysticism of cittarkaḷ, alchemy, principles of rejuvenation (*kayakaṟpam*) and yoga. However, tōki is never mentioned when students are questioned on their disciplinary preference; they regard it as odd, irrational and outdated. The president of the ATSVS attributes the lack of interest of students in tōki to the complexity of its intertwining subjects which requires to be taught by an expert, almost impossible to find today because of the change of syllabus in colleges and preferences for disciplines that are more 'modern' and 'scientific'.

Exploration of Manuscripts: The Complexity of the Siddha Corpus

The catalogue presenting the digitised manuscripts describes their physical aspects and the content of text(s), which is based on the information indexed on the left part of the palm leaves or, when it is insufficient or absent, on an exploration of text(s) to identify the subject(s). A catalogue is certainly frustrating for researchers like me who do not have the ability to read the manuscripts, but it provides information on the recurrence of subjects, the enmeshment of subjects in certain texts, and on the identity of certain manuscripts' owners.

A large majority of manuscripts, as they belong(ed) to medical practitioners, concerns medicine-related subjects. Some deal with astrology, quite often in relation to health prediction and astral influences on the body, alchemy, meditative techniques, religious rituals and cults, *mantiram* (mantras used for magic), veterinary medicine, and Tamil literature and epics. The medical matters presented in texts that I would categorise as simple predominantly concern descriptions of nosological categories in terms of aetiology, symptomatoly, diagnostic and treatment, medicinal formulations, sometimes with indications on the diseases for which they are recommended, on their posology, appropriate time of their consumption and dietary regimen, diagnostic methods focusing mostly on pulse reading (*nāṭi kuṟi*) and diseases resulting from their derangement and, as mentioned earlier, of the practice of varmam in terms of anatomical description, pathology and/or therapeutic methods.

The content of texts on nosology and medicinal formulations informs about the prevalence of diseases and disorders at the beginning of the twentieth century and earlier. The most frequently mentioned diseases or troubles result from precarious living conditions, lack of hygiene, excessive hard work and malnutrition or undernourishment. These are fevers of which numerous types, varying according to their aetiology, are described—the dictionary of T. V. Sambasivam Pillai (1931) mentions 77 types—diseases of the urinary tract, digestive disorders such as peptic ulcer, diarrhoea, dysentery or flatus, skin diseases and infections, diseases of the head region especially those of eyes, infectious diseases such as tuberculosis, leprosies, jaundice and disorders of reproductive organs. A disease, recurrently mentioned in the texts, drew my attention as it concerns the psychiatric field on which I conducted anthropological research 15 years ago (Sébastia 2007, 2009). This 'disease' is *caṉṉi*, translated as delirium. Its recurrence is reflected in the dictionary of Pillai (1931), who describes 50 types of delirium defined in siddha medicine, to which he adds more. Caṉṉi, as he mentions accurately, is a symptom occurring in many diseases such as typhoid, tetanus, syphilis, neurological disorders, alcoholism and poisoning, which are caused by lack of adequate health policy, unhygienic conditions of life (anaemia and undernourishment, premature pregnancy, hard work, crowded habitat, etc.) and consumption of toxic substances.

Compared to these simple texts, others are much more obscure and ambiguous as they approach multiple subjects belonging to the siddha corpus, but in an extremely tangled way. Books and articles introducing siddha medicine have not neglected to present the diverse aspects of the siddha corpus referred to previously as tōki (Kandaswamy Pillai 1998; Kannan 2000; Narayanswami 1975; T. V. Sambasivam Pillai 1931, 1993; Subbarayappa 1997; Subramanian and Madhavan 1984; Thirunarayanan n.d.; Uthamaroyan 2005). However, they treat these aspects separately and briefly, so the feeling of confusion reflected in the manuscripts is hardly perceptible. Except for the introduction to siddha medicine by T. V. Sambasivam Pillai (1931, 1993),[21] these works not only simplify the siddha corpus, but also reduce it to its medical dimension. The best example is the use of products such as *centūram, cuṉṉam, ceyanīr* or *kaṭṭu* obtained by iatrochemical processes which are presented as remedies, while in certain manuscripts it is not possible to distinguish if they are used in the domain of alchemy or of esotericism, to obtain the ability to perform magical acts (*aṣṭakarmam*) or to increase the potentiality of meditation during the practice of the *kuṇṭaliṉi yōkam*. This process of reduction, which precludes disciplines and concepts deemed irrational, has enabled traditional medicine to be recognised as one of the Indian systems of medicines as it fits the requirement of scientificity extolled by supporters of Western medicine since the nineteenth century.

A specificity of texts which has been conserved and has served to define this medicine is the authorship of texts. Even though a large majority of texts confined in manuscripts are anonymous, siddha medicine is attributed to cittarkaḷ. Cittar refers to a category of accomplished yogis who would have acquired supernatural powers (*citti* from Sanskrit *siddhi*) through stringent meditative practices whose ultimate goal is to transcend the materiality of the sensory world in order to attain liberation, that is, union with the supreme deity (Sébastia 2015; Weiss 2009). According to Tamil tradition, as well as in the manuscripts which mention cittarkaḷ, their number is 18. However, it reaches more than 90 if we consider the lists presented in siddha literature (Ganapathy 1993; Shanmugavelan 1963; Venkatraman 1990; White 2004) and in the catalogues of manuscripts (Madhavan 1984; Palanichamy 1973; Samuel 1998). Historians have pointed out that many siddha texts were written under the name of famous cittarkaḷ such as Agattiyar, Tēraiyar, Irāmatāvar or Pōkar (Kutumbiah 1973; Venkatraman 1990).

Venkatraman (1990) and Meenakshi (2001) have pointed to the anti-conformist character of cittarkaḷ which is expressed by their opposition to brahmanical ritualism, casteism and orthodoxism, and by their tantric orientation favouring the cult of Śiva-Śakti.[22] The cittarkaḷ were in line with the siddha groups which emerged in the north of India from the middle of the first millennium CE and initiated heterodox practices and concepts, which were defined thereafter under the denomination of tantrism (Gray 2016; White 2004). Tantrism or tantric traditions, as Gray proposes, represent the plurality of practices and thought of the siddha sectarians (ibid.). The adherence to tantrism is perceptible in the manuscripts mixing medicine, alchemy, religion, magic, yoga, etc., and it is this affiliation that makes the siddha corpus obscure and, for students, hardly credible.

The high value attributed to cittarkaḷ is due to its association with the development of medical knowledge under the name of siddha medicine. No study, to my knowledge, has tried to explore when this association occurred. It seems, however, that it emerged in the first decade of the twentieth century during the period of Tamil revivalism, which fought against the cultural and linguistic hegemony of north India (Weiss 2009). While the previous committees appointed by the British government to evaluate the pertinence of establishing a School of Indigenous Medicines in their reports mentioned only ayurvedic and unani medicines, that by Hakim Muhammad Usman, appointed secretary in 1923, uses the term siddha for the first time (Usman 1923). Hausman (1996) has pointed out that the previous reports of committees did not overlook the fact that Tamil Nadu had a specific traditional medicine, but it was called 'Tamil medicine' or 'Tamil ayurvedic'. These terms were also used in some records of missionaries and travellers who visited the region, with other words such as 'native medicine' or 'bazaar medicines' with reference to drugs and raw material (Chakrabarti 2006). However, the siddha corpus had induced many debates during the period preceding the opening of the school of Indian medicines in 1924 for determining whether it was scientifically acceptable. If siddha medicine was finally integrated into colleges, this was at the price of a transformation and of a selection of the subjects belonging to its corpus, as reflected in yoga which has been dispossessed of its spiritual and magical qualities to become a therapeutic tool, and in the content of tōki which does not approach magic, while that is very much present in the manuscripts. Magic participates in the construction of the figure of certain cittarkaḷ described as able to perform magical deeds (*cittikkaḷ*), thanks to the supernatural powers acquired through rigorous ascetic practice. It is a therapy for treating diseases diagnosed as resulting from bad influences (*doṣam*), transgressive acts, sorcery (*cuniyam*) and evil spirits (*pēy*). Magic is also related to spirituality as the practitioner uses the supportive intervention of gods and goddesses to heal.

Two collections of manuscripts digitised during the project illustrate the importance of magic as well as of occult practices in the milieu of traditional siddha practitioners. The identity of the owner of the first collection is unfortunately not known, as the siddha doctor who obtained it during a tour to identify manuscripts in the Tirunelveli district did not conduct an interview with the owner on the history of his manuscripts. However, the poor condition of the manuscripts shows clearly that they were frequently used. The palm leaves of those containing *mantiraṅkaḷ* (mantras) and *yantiraṅkaḷ* (letters inscribed in geometrical figures) for performing both black and white magic (around a third of the collection) were stuck by fungus and mould, developed by repeated exposure to sandal water sprinkled during rituals to invoke deities (*pūja*).

The second collection concerns the 98 manuscripts that I mentioned earlier. It is illustrative of the complex enmeshment of subjects which blurs the context for which formulas are detailed. Its history is not only fascinating, but also shows that the practice of magic and alchemy could be destructive if it was not used properly. The present owners (the nephew and his paternal uncle) belong to a Telugu Brahmin family established in Tamil Nadu for several generations. The uncle has identified six generations before him; the practice of medicine was developed by his ancestor belonging to the second one, called in manuscripts Parappuvayal Subbayyan. The collection of manuscripts began with him. He resided in the hamlet of Parappuvayal close to Navalur, in the present Ramanathapuram district.[23] In the past, this hamlet was near a road which went to Ramesvaram (one of the four major Viṣṇu temples in India). Subbayyan, who had learnt the medicine from practitioners of the region, took an interest in all practices allied to medicine, among them alchemy, magic, yoga and astrology that he learnt from ascetics coming from north India who went regularly to Ramesvaram. However, his deep involvement in the practice of alchemy and magic ended up endangering his family. As the uncle shared:

> The manuscripts were collected and copied by Subbayyan. He was very attracted by alchemy and he spent his life and his money to search through texts and to make gold. He did not succeed in preparing pure gold and his fascination with alchemy ruined his family. We learnt that the land where Subbayyan had lived was pervaded by negative waves: no owner has succeeded in keeping the land for long because of misfortunes.[24]

Scared by the detrimental effects of both alchemy and magic, he encouraged his son to quit the region and to set up in a region of the present district of Pudukottai, which was reputed for its richness in medicinal plants. The son set up his practice in the village of Arimalam where, on the recommendations of his father, he held himself back from practising alchemy and magic which had destroyed his family. Although the manuscripts in which his name is mentioned do not differ from those of his father as they deal with medicine, iatrochemistry, alchemy, yoga, astrology and magic, he dedicated his life to medical practice. It seems that he inherited from his father the fascination with ascetics, as his house is close to a shrine which was inhabited by a yogi that he frequented regularly; a gate of the garden attached to this house gives direct access to the shrine. This yogi is still venerated today and the uncle used to visit the shrine. The medical practice of Subbayyan's son continued to flourish through his descendants, as this house became a residence-cum-hospital. Named Mani Iyer Hospital, it is used for family celebrations, and especially every Sunday to treat patients, work that the uncle,[25] who resides in Tiruracchirapalli, has undertaken since his father's death in 2002. He treats patients with the same medicines, notably medicated oils, developed by his ancestors that he learnt to prepare from his father. Emphasising their effectiveness, he relates that in 2008, he received an award from the WHO dedicated to his father for his contribution to treating patients, especially children affected by polio.

Conclusion

The two collections presented in this chapter come from practitioners who are no longer living. However, the practice of magic and alchemy is still alive among a few traditional practitioners, not always old. Their practice is very close to that described in the manuscripts: they prepare medicines, extemporaneously, according to the specific condition of the patient; they use astrology for treating a patient and recite mantiraṅkaḷ over the patient and over the medicines they prepare to increase their efficacy; they expose their medicines in the pūja room in front of the picture of the divine couple Cakti-Śiva; and they conduct experiments in pharmaceutical and alchemical fields to develop components to treat or prevent (*kaṟpam* 'rejuvenation') diseases. Such practices, which manipulate diverse kinds of knowledge, are on the verge of disappearing, and it is not certain that the practice of siddha medicine, as it is taught now in colleges, will be able to maintain the holistic approach contained in the manuscripts. As a practitioner told me when we were discussing changes in medical practice, 'Even us [traditional practitioners], we do not use magic to treat. I learnt some mantiram from my grandfather, I don't use them. They were effective and according to the condition of the patients they give good results. They have psychological effects.'[26] Interestingly, a siddha practitioner I met did not regard the alchemical conversion of metals into gold as a means to become rich. He argued: 'Remedies with gold are essential to fight severe diseases. When we need gold, we require the patients to buy it. For rich patients, this is not an issue. But for poor, it is the duty of the practitioner to make gold in order to prepare these remedies.'[27]

However, a resurgence of interest in siddha medicine and its corpus is discernible among young people, especially among the children of siddha families. Having developed a website on siddha medicine on which, among other things, I present diverse certificates, legal and illegal, and evoke issues on education and registration, I am regularly requested for information on schools which provide courses on siddha medicine or, in case of children belonging to siddha families, on the way to getting a siddha diploma or to be registered as a siddha practitioner. The attraction to the prestige attached to a medical profession, even though it is not biomedicine, seems to be the cornerstone of the interest of the majority of enquirers. However, some justify their requirement by talking about their quest to learn siddha medicine 'authentically'. This recalls the statement made by several students of the Government Siddha College and Hospital at Palaiyamkottai: 'If you want to know what siddha medicine is, don't stay here, go to Kanniyakumari and visit my ācāṉ.' These students, therefore, become the repositories of two kinds of knowledge that they consider as complementary. The college provides for them a composite and modern medicinal knowledge and the degree to practise legally, and their apprenticeship with several ācāṉ(kaḷ) chosen according to the specialty that they seek to develop, enables them to legitimise their practice; the names of ācān(kaḷ) being the proof of the authenticity of their knowledge. In this context, where the siddha corpus faces a significant erosion of its knowledge but where, at the same time, siddha medicine is experiencing a revival movement, the manuscripts have a role to play as a resource of 'authentic' knowledge. Their digitisation with free access is thus pertinent, or will be if means are developed to train people in manuscript reading. This is the dream of the president of ATSVS who requires that this discipline be included in the curriculum of siddha colleges, and that his family collection of manuscripts receives appropriate attention.

Notes

1. I use the term 'doctor' to differentiate practitioners who possess a medical degree, which allows them to append the title of Doctor to their names, from those without formal medical training. Siddha degrees are of two types: Bachelor of Siddha medicine and Surgery (BSMS) obtained after completing five-and-half-year courses, and Doctor of Medicine [MD (siddha)] given after additional three-year courses, including the submission and examination of a PhD dissertation related to one of the six branches of siddha medicine: general medicine (*potu maruttuvam*), *materia medica* and pharmacopeia (*kuṇapāṭam*), child's medicine (*kuḻantai maruttuvam*), nosography and pathology (*nōy nāṭal*), toxicology (*nañcu maruttuvam*) and special medicines (*cirappu maruttuvam*) comprising skin diseases (*tōl nōykaḷ*), mental illnesses (*kirikai nōykaḷ*), yoga, bone and joints disorders (*varmam*) and rejuvenation/prevention of diseases (*kayakarpam*). The Tamil words used in this chapter observe the rules of transliteration defined in the Tamil lexicon (Chennai, University of Chennai). The plural forms follow the Tamil grammar: addition of *kaḷ* after consonants and vowels, except for the plural of words finishing with 'm' which is nasalised (*ṅkaḷ*) and by 'a' and 'ā' which induce a change of sound given by the doubling of 'k' (*kkaḷ*).

2. This project is hosted at the French Institute of Pondicherry (IFP) and conducted in co-partnership with the Centre of Traditional Medicine and Research (CTMR), Chennai. The IFP provides rooms for the cleaning and digitisation of manuscripts and the CTMR gives a space for clerical work. In addition to the supervisor and the co-partner, the team is composed of a photographer, two experts in manuscript reading and a graduate in siddha medicine charged with translating and typing the catalogues. One of the experts, who is the president of the association ATSVS, provides the space for cleaning and digitising the manuscripts of the Kanniyakumari district that include his collection.

3. This separation is well-mirrored in books focusing on a particular part of the siddha corpus, such as those by R. Venkatraman (1990) and Kamil V. Zvelebil (1993) which, while defining the work of *cittarkaḷ*, focuses much more on their philosophy and occult practices (meditation, alchemy, magic) than on medical matters, or that by T. N. Ganapathy (1993), which is strictly concerned with the philosophical school of cittarkaḷ.

4. The length of texts is extremely variable. In manuscripts composed of a large number of texts, their length may go from a half-leaf to 30 leaves; the short texts may be composed of several verses excerpted from an authored text and/or of information provided by the author of the manuscript based on experience, such as medicinal formulas, iatrochemical processes and treatment of diseases.

5. The main places where siddha manuscripts are stored: the Central Research Institute for Siddha (Chennai), Government Oriental Manuscripts Library and Research Centre (Chennai), Sarasvati Mahal Library and Tamil University (Tanjavur), Annamalai University (Chidambaram) and the French Institute of Pondicherry. A large collection of siddha manuscripts is also kept in Kerala at the Oriental Research Institute and Manuscripts Library (Thiruvananthapuram).

6. It is worth mentioning that several practitioners have shown me notebooks in which their parents had copied from their manuscripts important information, notably medicinal formulas.

7. *Centūram* is a red calcined powder (oxidation); *paṟpam* and *cuṇṇam* are alkalin calcined powder, quite often white; and *kaṭṭu* is a stone-like medicine used by rubbing it on a mortar, the fine powder obtained is mixed with milk or honey.

8. *Muppu* is, in principle, a combination of three salts including a salt called *pūnīr* or *vaḻalai* collected in specific places, during the nights of the dark moon in May and June. Muppu, for which multiple formulas are provided in manuscripts, is the most emblematic product of siddha alchemy. *Racamaṇi* is a bead of solidified mercury, also known in Sanskrit alchemy. It is prepared by rubbing quicksilver with minerals and diverse juices of plants. It is sometimes used to treat severe diseases, in amulets as protection from bad influences, or swallowed by the alchemist-cittarkaḻ to obtain supernatural powers.

9. Certain plants used in siddha/ayurveda formulas, as for example *Semicarpus anacardium*, *Datura stramonium*, *Aconitus*, *Strychnos nux-vomica*, *Cannabis sativa*, *Commiphora mukul* or *Plumbago zeylanica*, require a process of purification (*cutti kiramam*) before being used (Maurya et al. 2015; Natarajan 1984).

10. The change of caste name from Cānār to Nāṭār occurred at the end of the nineteenth century. It followed a long political movement and recurrent conflicts conducted by Cānār/Nāṭār demanding a better status and abolition of their untouchability; see Hardgrave (1969), Sébastia (2007), Templeman (1996), and also Immanuel (2002) who, focusing on the Nāṭār of Kanniyakumari, shows the roles that some of them played in the history of this region in terms of politics and social development.

11. The practice of certain practitioners is, however, more centred on varmam and bone-setting, so the medicines they prepare correspond to this medical field. These remedies use mostly plants and animal products such as snails, frogs, hens and peacocks (today forbidden, as they are protected).

12. Two factors validate the recruitment of an expert in manuscripts of Kanniyakumari region: the specific terminology of varmam and the medical terminology which is particular to this region or comes from Malayalam. In fact, it is extremely difficult to differentiate varmam from marma and siddha from ayurveda.

13. The study on the practice of varmam, realised by Roman Sieler (2015) with a few practitioners of Kanniyakumari, is helpful to understand the concept of varmam and the anatomical siddha terminology. As I have noticed, his definitions related to varmam are not always supported by all practitioners; this is because of the lack of homogeneity of this knowledge, each practitioner having their known concepts. The definitions I use here result from discussions with the president of ATSVS, who has written numerous books on varmam from manuscripts.

14. When I ask him why he learned ayurveda while the medical specialty of his paternal family is siddha, he explained that the choice was determined by the examination board, which took into consideration his knowledge of Sanskrit acquired at school.

15. For maintaining anonymity, I will not mention the name of the associations.

16. This land was chosen for its location—close to a Siva temple frequented by siddha practitioners, it dominates the plain covered by coconut trees from where emerge some rocks that local legend assimilates to the petrified tears of Ravana (information of the president of ATSVS).

17. See http://atsvssmc.org/ (accessed 5 March 2017).

18. This college, due to its affiliation with ATSVS and the significant practice of siddha medicine, receives many more children from traditional siddha families than other siddha colleges.

19. *Tōṟṟa* means origin or evolution of life or things; *kirama* order, morality; and *arāycci* investigation.

20. The first year comprises the study of (a) tōki, (b) Tamil language, (c) communicative English, (d) biochemistry, (e) medicinal botany and pharmacognosy, and (f) microbiology. The second year comprises the study of (a) Western anatomy, (b) siddha physiology (a part of tōki), (c) biomedical physiology, and (d) siddha *materia medica*. The third year comprises (a) siddha pathology, (b) Western pathology, (c) forensic medicine and toxicology, and (d) hygiene, community health and health policies. The fourth year comprises (a) siddha and Western nosography, (b) external therapy, including varmam and special medicine, (c) surgery, and (d) siddha and Western gynaecology and paediatrics.

21. Let us mention also the work of A. Shanmugavelan (1992), which extensively presents the diverse aspects of the siddha corpus due to the fact that they participate in the principles of rejuvenation and longevity (theories of the universe and of the body; physiology; yoga; *materia medica*; alchemical products; magical power; etc.).

22. The Śiva-Śakti principle is the union of Śiva with Śakti which, through *kuṇḍalinī yōkam*, allows for the attaining of the state of blissfulness where 'all consciousness of duality and fear of falling again into the bond of *samsara* are removed forever' (Ganapathy 1993: 87). Kuṇḍalinī yōkam is performed to develop the eight supernatural powers (*citti*): *aṇimā* (power of becoming very small), *laghimā* (of becoming very light), *prāpti* (of obtaining everything), *prākāmya* (of having irresistible will), *mahimā* (of increasing one's size), *iśitva* (of becoming superior, great), *vaśitva* (of bringing others under one's control), and *kāmāvasāyitā* (of suppressing passion) (Banerji 1992: 628). The names of the supernatural powers are in Sanskrit.

23. In Tamil, *Vayal* means paddy field. This village belongs to the taluk of Thiruvadanai. In manuscripts, the name of the village of the practitioner precedes his name.

24. Fascinated by this story, I proposed to go to Parappuvayal. The land, unsellable, is now used to extract earth for brickwork. According to neighbours we met, the land would have been affected by the ill-effect of a statue of Kālī which belonged to this land. But we succeeded neither in finding the statue nor in learning more about it.

25. When I asked him about his registration, which he did not previously have due to the fact that he did not take siddha medicine as a profession, he explained that after his retirement, he applied to be registered and his application was accepted. He is registered as a siddha medical practitioner.

26. Information from Rajendran, Kanniyakumari district (July 2008).

27. Information from Rajkumar Vaittiyar, Kanniyakumari district (February 2017). I met this practitioner, who knows how to write on palm-leaf manuscripts, thanks to the president of ATSVS. He arranged the meeting in order to make a documentary on the subject. The documentary is entitled,*A Declining Tradition in Siddha Practice: Writting on Palm-leaf Manuscripts*.

References

Alter, Joseph S. 2005. 'Āyurvedic Acupuncture—Tansnational Nationalism: Ambivalence about the Origin and Authenticity of Medical Knowledge'. In *Asian Medicine and Globalization*, ed. J. S. Alter, 21–44. Pennsylvania: University of Pennsylvania Press.

Banerji, Sures Chandra. 1992. *New Light on Tantra*. Calcutta: Punthi Pustak.

Chakrabarti, Pratik. 2006. '"Neither of Meate nor Drinke, but What the Doctor Alloweth": Medicine amidst War and Commerce in Eighteen Madras'. *Bulletin of the History of Medicine* 80(1): 1–38.

Ganapathy, T. N. 1993. *The Philosophy of the Tamil Siddhas*. New Delhi: Indian Council of Philosophical Research.

Gray, David B. 2016. 'Tantra and the Tantric Traditions of Hinduism and Buddhism'. Oxford Research Encyclopedia of Religion, Oxford University Press. Available at http://religion.oxfordre.com/view/10.1093/acrefore/9780199340378.001.0001/acrefore-9780199340378-e-59 (accessed 12 March 2017).

Hardgrave, Robert L. 1969. *The Nadars of Tamilnad: The Political Culture of a Community in Change*. Berkeley/Los Angeles: University of California Press.

Hausman, Gary. 1996. 'Siddhars, Alchemy and the Abyss of Tradition: "Traditional" Tamil Medical Knowledge in "Modern" Practice'. Unpublished thesis, University of Michigan, Ann Arbor.

Immanuel, M. 2002. *The Dravidian Lineages, a Socio-historical Study: The Nadars through the Ages*. Nagercoil: Historical Research and Publications Trust.

Kandaswamy Pillai. 1998 [1979]. *History of Siddha Medicine*. Chennai: Department of Indian Medicine and Homoeopathy.

Kannan, R. 2000. 'Siddha: A Unique System' (folio). *The Hindu*, 8 October.

Kutumbiah, P. 1973. 'The Siddha and Rasa Siddha Schools of Indian Medicine'. *Indian Journal of History of Medicine* 18: 21–33.

Langford, J. M. 1995. 'Ayurvedic Interiors: Persons, Space, and Episteme in Three Medical Practices'. *Cultural Anthropology* 10(3): 330–66.

———. 2004. *Fluent Bodies: Ayurvedic Remedies for Postcolonial Imbalance*. New Delhi: Oxford University Press.

Leslie, Charles (ed.). 1976. *Asian Medical Systems: A Comparative Study*. Delhi: Motilal Banarsidass Publishers.

———. 1992. 'Interpretations of Illness: Syncretism in Modern Āyurveda'. In *Paths to Asian Medical Knowledge*, eds C. Leslie and A. Young, 177–208. Berkeley: University of California Press.

Madhavan, V. R. 1984. *Siddha Medical Manuscripts in Tamil*. Madras: International Institute of Tamil Studies.

Maurya, Santosh Kumar, Ankit Seth, Damiki Laloo, Narendra Kumar Singh, Dev Nath Singh Gautam and Anil Kumar Singh. 2015. 'Śodhana: An Ayurvedic Process for Detoxification and Modification of Therapeutic Activities of Poisonous Medicinal Plants'. *Ancient Sciences of Life* 34(4): 188–97.

Meenakshi, P. 2001. 'The Siddhas of Tamil Nadu: A Voice of Dissent'. In *Tradition, Dissent and Ideology: Essays in Honour of Romila Thapar*, eds R. Champakalakshmi and S. Gopal, 111–34. New Delhi: Oxford University Press.

Narayanswami, V. 1975. *Introduction to the Siddha System of Medicine*. Madras: Pandit S. S. Anandam Reseach Institute of Siddha Medicine.

Natarajan, Kanchana. 1984. 'Purification Processes in Siddha System'. In *Heritage of the Tamils: Siddha Medicine*, eds S. V. Subramanian and V. R. Madhavan, 117–31. Madras: International Institute of Tamil Studies.

Palanichamy, K. 1973. 'Works on Medicine by Siddhars'. *Bulletin of the Indian Institute of History of Medicine* 3(2): 71–75; 3(3): 132–134.

Samuel, G. John. 1998. *A Descriptive Catalogue of Palm-leaf Manuscripts in Tamil* (Volume 5, Part II). Chennai: Institute of Asian Studies.

Sébastia, Brigitte. 2007. *Les Rondes de Saint Antoine: Culte, Affliction et Possession en Inde du Sud*. Paris: Aux Lieux d'être (sous prétexte de médecines).

_____. 2009. *Restoring Mental Health in India. Pluralistic Approaches, Pluralistic Therapies and Concepts*. New Delhi: Oxford University Press.

_____. 2010. 'Governmental Institution versus Associations: Multifaceted Expression of Siddha in Tamil Nadu'. *Regionalism and Cosmopolitanism South India*. Available at http://rcsi.hypotheses.org/317 (accessed 10 April 2016).

_____. 2013. 'A Medicine in Loss of Identity'. IIAS newsletter no. 65, Autumn.

_____. 2015. 'Preserving Identity or Promoting Safety? The Issue of Mercury in Siddha Medicine: A Brake on the Crossing of Frontiers'. *Medical Mercury: A Global Commodity in Transition* 64(4), Special Volume of Asiatische Studien, ed. D. Wujastyk: 933–69.

Shanmugavelan, A. 1963. *Siddhar's Science of Longevity and Kalpa Medicine of India*. Madras: Sakthi Nilayam.

_____. 1992. *Siddhar's Science of Longevity and Kalpa Medicine of India*. Madras: Directorate of Indian Medicine and Homoeopathy.

Sieler, Roman. 2015. *Lethal Spots, Vital Secrets: Medicine and Martial Arts in South India*. New York: Oxford University Press.

Subbarayappa, B. V. 1997. 'Siddha Medicine: An Overview'. *Lancet* 350: 1841–44.

Subramanian, S. V. and V. R. Madhavan (eds). 1984. *Heritage of the Tamils: Siddha Medicine*. Madras: International Institute of Tamil Studies.

Templeman, Dennis. 1996. *The Northern Nadars of Tamil Nadu: An Indian Caste in the Process of Change*. Delhi: Oxford University Press.

Thirunarayanan, T. n.d. *An Introduction to Siddha Medicine*. Tiruchendur: Thirukumaran Publishers.

T. V. Sambasivam Pillai. 1931. *Tamil–English Dictionary of Medicine, Chemistry, Botany and Allien Sciences (Based on Indian Medical Science)* (Volume 1). Madras: The Research Institute of Siddhar's Science. [Volume 2 (1991), Volume 3 (1931), Volume 4 (1998) and Volume 5 (1994).]

T. V. Sambasivam Pillai. 1993. *Introduction to Siddha Medicine*. Madras: Directorate of Indian Medicine and Homeopathy.

Usman, Khan Bahadur Muhammad. 1923. *The Report of the Committee on the Indigenous Systems of Medicine*. Madras: Government of Madras.

Uthamaroyan, C. S. 2005. *A Compendium of Siddha Doctrine* (trans. Anandan Anaivari R.). Chennai: Department of Indian Medicine and Homeopathy.

Venkatraman, R. 1990. *A History of the Tamil Siddha Cult*. Madurai: N. S. Ennes Publications.

Weiss, Richard S. 2009. *Recipes for Immortality. Medicine, Religion and Community in South India*. New York: Oxford University Press.

White, David Gordon. 2004 [1996]. *The Alchemical Body: Siddha Traditions in Medieval India*. New Delhi: Munshiram Manoharlal Publishers.

Zarrilli, Phillip B. 1998. *When the Body Becomes All Eyes: Paradigms, Discourses and Practices of Power in Kalaripayattu, a South Indian Martial Art*. Delhi: Oxford University Press.

Zvelebil, Kamil V. 1993 [1973]. *The Poets of the Power: Freedom, Magic and Renewal*. Lower Lake, CA: Integral Publishing.

six

Family Repositories to 'Knowledge Commons'

The Discourse of Documenting Local Health Traditions in Contemporary Kerala

Harilal Madhavan and Praveen Lal

The Ambiguity of Pluralism and Discourse of Documentation

This chapter intends to understand the discourse of documenting the knowledge and practice of local health traditions in contemporary Kerala. In this chapter, we use 'local health traditions' as a common terminology to explain the indigenous medical traditions in Kerala (as equivalent to the Malayalam term, namely *nattuvaidyam*), which is largely uncodified. In Kerala, local health traditions have different terms of reference, though they are meant to refer to community-based forms of knowledge. Vishavaidyam, tribal medicines and even the medicines practised by astavaidyas were generally known as vaidyam or medicine prior to the introduction of modern medicine, but some of them partially codified with the arrival of textual ayurveda, and partially, remain as local health traditions. The term 'classical traditions' is used here to refer to the institutionalised and codified form of medical tradition since the turn of the twentieth century, like ayurevda, siddha, etc. We discuss the discourse of the documentation of local health traditions through a close examination of three dominant models in the state of Kerala. The codification of medical knowledge was influenced to a great extent by the discourse of pluralism, which emerged in the state through the support of princely states in Kerala, especially Travancore,[1] the rise of sociopolitical democratic organisations and through the growth of print media and education (Abraham 2013; Girija 2017a). The contemporary codification, either by the State, academia or other stakeholders, owes much directly or indirectly to medical identities and lineages of specific caste groups. In Kerala, it draws particular attention not only to the context of the historical pertinence of local health traditions in public health delivery services, but also to the domination of the different stakeholders and political factors shaping the sphere, leading to varied practices of documentation by different institutional types. The uniqueness of this documentation process in the state is to sustain the role of local healers as an 'indigenous alterity' to the codified systems, reflected both in its historical and contemporary pluralistic therapeutic attitude.

An important question is: How far is the term 'revitalisation' adequate to express the recent documentation efforts of local health traditions in Kerala? These living traditions falling under the broad realm of indigenous medicine captured an ambiguous space in Kerala's health care. They are distinct in the sense that many of them are partially written in the local languages and kept in the old formats like palm leaves within the confinement of families, and a lot of them are still not recorded in any usable format but largely lost in intergenerational transfers. Identifying the extent to which this knowledge is acknowledged in policy documents and utilised at various stages of Kerala's health care development might be necessary to understand whether the new forms of collection and preservation of knowledge, including documentation, indeed constitutes revitalisation of such knowledge and practices.

The Kerala narrative of medical pluralism suggests that the dichotomy of the formally trained 'experts' and informal 'practitioners' (Collins and Evans 2002) is not a truism. Within the informal knowledge domain, there are experts 'licensed' or accredited by various authorities[2] like the regional government councils, royal authorities, etc. (Unnikrishnan and Koike 2010). The exchange of knowledge between the formally trained physicians and traditionally reputed healers is apparent in Kerala (Varier 2002). Two categories of physicians practised in the early half of the twentieth century—'registered practitioners', whose name was entered in the register of practitioners, and 'qualified practitioners', who possessed the recognised qualification as per Section 19 of the Travancore Medical Practitioners Act (Government of Travancore 1946: 50–51). The separation of institutionally and otherwise qualified practitioners (just like not all ayurvedic practitioners in Kerala have the same qualifications or titles) is difficult and in the highly hierarchised plural medical system, this will add more ambiguity regarding the identities of practitioners. There were even diverse practices following the gurukula system with improvisations in Charaka Samhita, Susrutha Samhita, Ashtanga Hridaya or Ashtanga Samgraha. The lineage-based system of gurukula was considered a major component of uniquely variant regional practices. For example, the astavaidya families in Kerala (18 families with highly qualified knowledge that practised eight branches of medicine) acquired their knowledge through oral lineages and later incorporated their experience into the gurukula method, where a more systematised curricula was followed for medical instruction. The differences between the institutionally trained/licensed practitioners and indigenous practitioners became significant not for epistemological but for political reasons when licensed practitioners felt it important to make such a distinction. Both the categories were earlier referred to as nattuvaidyam (local medicine) (Unnikrishnan and Hariramamurthi 2012). Girija (2017b) points out that this need to distanciate from non-institutionally trained practitioners was reinforced by the introduction of educational institutions to teach vaidyam (medicine).

During colonial times, the place of indigenous medicine in the newly emerging system of health services in Kerala was a major point of debate as in other parts of the country. The main challenge was to create an entirely new cultural milieu in the wake of the introduction of Western medicine or find possible ways to retain, preserve and sustain the cultural heritage, which necessitated revisiting the past and present in detail (Panikkar 1992). The public health emergency created by the spread of communicable diseases in the late nineteenth and early twentieth centuries (Madhavan 2011) and predominantly high domestic demand for medicines kept the revitalisation and institutionalisation of the experiential systems in possible loop. A grant-in-aid system was started by the Travancore authority to pool locally experienced physicians and help them start their own *vaidysalas* (hospitals), when there was a cholera and small pox threat in the region (Madhavan 2008). But subsequently, the demands for therapeutic evaluation and efficacy privileged the classical traditions (codified traditions) even while the non-classical traditions were ready to open up their knowledge to serve public health needs.

The state's policies in both education and registration of medical practitioners created hierarchies within the medical system. In early twentieth-century Travancore, with the involvement of the Rockefeller

Foundation, British and American medical imperialism joined hands in shaping health care, and Western knowledge was introduced as scientific truth and its technology as superior and progressive (Menon 2002). As Cleetus (2007) argues:

> The terms of indigenous medicine itself was defined in different ways in colonial times and it oscillated between the large compendiums of health care practices followed locally and regionally, and in caste and ethnic minority contexts and also the dominant health care tradition that traced its lineage from the Samhita texts. Under colonialism the latter form of knowledge was deemed to indicate the entire corpus of indigenous medical knowledge under Ayurveda. (ibid.: 148)

Besides the presence of the dominant biomedicine, hierarchies were constructed within the different indigenous systems itself. Social mobility and caste politics had a major role in redefining the relation between the heterogeneous practices of codified (and institutionalised) and indigenous medical traditions in Kerala. As a highly valued service, the social groups that practised medicine subsequently gained higher social status and class advantage within the non-elite classes like the Ezhavas (considered a lower caste of agricultural labourers, small cultivators, toddy tappers, etc.) in Kerala. This, in a sense, prevented the spread and development of medical knowledge from remaining confined within the brahmanical tradition or astavaidya families. Later, these lineages within the different caste groups are reflected in both the institutionalisation process (by establishing educational institutions) and in gaining economic benefits (through manufacturing outlets). This makes a strong categorisation of the knowledge as codified and folk systems analytically difficult in the state, and hence, the revival of ayurveda in twentieth-century Kerala can also be considered a revitalisation of regionally variant, but submerged strands of local healing traditions.

Within this complex, unequal relationship among pluralistic traditions, the astavaidya tradition has been enriched over centuries through interactions with folk medical practices of Kerala (Menon and Spudich 2010). Each astavaidya family had its own set of special formulations. Many such formulations were gathered, put into verse and written down on palm leaves. Each family also had its own collection of such secret preparations (ibid.). Even though the practices based on vernacular texts like Sahasrayogam and Chikitsamanjari were considered informal, and hence the practitioners were not considered authentic or included in the classical group, some of them have reappeared and been practised as separate entities later as *siddhavaidyan*[3] (siddha medical practitioners). These oral/partially codified traditions remained unorganised in the form of localised health traditions scattered and confined within traditional families, tribes and remote regions in need of State recognition or identity. But many of these practitioners continued their practice, received popularity among the people served and reemerged in the process of revitalisation, through commercialisation. However, the pluralistic space remained ambiguous in Kerala for a long time. When opportunities arose for commercial production, a number of practitioners across castes and communities came forward, made their 'unique' family medical recipes commercially available and marketed them under their family name. Along with medicines from classical texts, formulations from local texts were also produced and marketed as ayurvedic medicines, catering mainly to a local clientele (Abraham 2013).

Efforts at systematic documentation of indigenous medical knowledge is not new in the province as the foremost classical work in botany/medicinal flora in the world, *Hortus Malabaricus* by Hendrik Adriaan Van Rheede, was written in Kerala between 1686 and 1703 in 12 volumes (with illustrations of 794 plant species, out of which 539 are identified as medicinal plants). It is also said that this textbook formed a main reference work for Carl Linnaeus (the father of modern taxonomy) (Rajasekharan, et al. 2016). *Hortus Malabaricus* was published with the help of Itty Achuthan,[4] a renowned Ezhava scholar of traditional and folk practices of Kerala. The medicinal preparations for the ailments of Dutch soldiers in India were imported from Europe and the realisation of possible local substitution was the main cause behind this documentation of knowledge and plants.

In the early nineteenth century, the codification remained within the confines of familial boundaries and many families preserved the secret nature of their practice, and hence had a right-based positive protection. The formation of the LSPSS in 1984 initiated discussions about integrating the local health traditions with institutionalised systems and the need for documentation and training at the national level. This movement also established a network of indigenous health practitioners and scientists (Unnikrishnan and Hariramamurthi 2012). In the meantime, codification efforts were also reinforced as a defensive mechanism against the unsolicited encroachment of knowledge by the corporates and other new forms or expressions of the market. In the national context, obviously there is a larger rationale for the documentation process beyond revitalisation (Hafeel, et al. 2004). The issues of protection of traditional knowledge, bio-piracy and fair and equitable sharing of benefits arising out of the utilisation of traditional knowledge are very important as evidenced in the recent cases of bio-piracy, like the wound-healing properties of *manjal* (turmeric), or patents on hypoglycemic properties of bitter gourd, brinjal, etc. Most of the Kerala codification narratives connect strongly to this national emergency for protecting the legitimate rights of the indigenous population. But even before the official start of the Traditional Knowledge Digital Library (TKDL) at the national level, many regional institutions, especially NGOs, local science movements and academic institutions, with the support of the State or otherwise, have started collating and codifying knowledge with minor or medium funds.

In Kerala, the Kerala Sasthra Sahithya Parishad (KSSP) or Kerala Science-Literature Forum, an NGO working towards making science and technology work for the needs and priorities of the local communities through reorienting science towards their lived experience, was at the forefront in bringing local knowledge together in the second half of the twentieth century. Even though most of the institutions provide the rationale of defensive protection against bio-piracy, any kind of preservation initiatives by the State have impeccable relevance, as many of the traditional healers and the astavaidya practitioners (who are now confined to five main families) are in the latter part of their lives, and hence there is a threat of extinction of knowledge. The intergenerational mobility of knowledge also seems to be at stake, as the new generation is not too enthusiastic about following this lineage. For example, in Payyannur (north Kerala), nearly 70 per cent of the institutionally trained ayurveda doctors in their 50s are from traditional healer families. However, among the children of these doctors, very few have chosen ayurvedic practice as their professions (Unnikrishnan 2004). Many traditional practices are on the peripheries due to either their vernacular forms of codification or no codification, and hence many of these practitioners, after long efforts towards striving for recognition, are now ready to give up the family secrets for codified use. For example, one of the popular physicians from south Kerala practising the closely linked traditions of *marmavidya* (knowledge of vital spots) and *kalaripayattu* (martial art originating in Kerala) mentions:

> I contacted the government multiple times through the association for the recognition of *kalari marma chikitsa* (classical treatment based on vital points of the body). I got this[5] knowledge orally from my grandfather. But now, if I try to share knowledge orally, no one has the ability and patience to learn. So documentation is important, I am interested in and open to documentation and patenting my knowledge if better benefits are possible. I am not confident of my son in this case nor any of my *sishyas* (disciples). If it is documented, it could be even part of the school curriculum.

Intergenerational translation requires dedication and commitment to taking this tradition along, but completely lacks institutional support in the context of increased standardisation of the market-dominated model. This has worsened with the lack of any coherent or cooperative move from traditional practitioners in achieving a space for practice within the pluralistic domain; on the contrary, they have tried to disqualify each other. This unhealthy competition has led to discrediting their own professions and subsequently checked any kind of upward mobility. The disruption of traditional ways of living may also cause younger generations to lose interest in learning about these traditions (Abbot 2014). In the context of existing ambiguity in its translation, most of the valuable knowledge is irrecoverably lost. We now discuss the salient features of some of the recent documentation initiatives in Kerala and examine the problems and possibilities emerging out of various reassuring models.

Major Initiatives of Documentations in Kerala

One of the grave disadvantages of local health traditions is that its information base is fuzzy, incomplete and fragmented. The manuscripts kept in private repositories are dusty, brittle and under daily threat of damage due to lack of knowledge and means for preservation. Apart from the sporadic efforts of practitioners, the sheer existence of amassed knowledge of various kinds (for example, both donated and collected manuscripts kept at the government ayurvedic colleges and other academic institutions) necessitated some coordinated codification efforts from the state and academia.

The state of Kerala has recently taken interesting steps for the protection of traditional community-based medical knowledge through initiatives and polices—it was the first state to attempt state-level intellectual property protection for traditional knowledge in 2008, even though it has not been successful in executing this under the federal law. It was also the first ever state, in 2016, to have a separate policy on Indian systems of medicine. A close analysis brings forth many intriguing attempts to promote and protect indigenous knowledge through the medium of documentation with the involvement of a variety of stakeholders. They protect the local values and autonomy and, therefore, also the legitimacy of the local modes of reasoning (McGonigle 2016) within the same judicial systems and avoid the tensions of 'epistemic subsidiarity' (Jasanoff 2013).

The discourse of documentation, however, has not solely emerged as a mechanism of revitalisation, but is considered important in the context of incentivising innovations and defending bio-piracy both in national and international contexts. Protective mechanisms like intellectual property rights are not designed for the protection of traditional knowledge in its original form (that is, in its oral and non-documentation existence). The intangible features make the knowledge inaccessible for inspection by patent officers and, therefore, 'facilitate' bio-piracy when patents are granted on innovations that were based on existing knowledge. As a consequence, the traditional knowledge documentation (TKD) project has been accepted as an interim tool to overcome the shortcomings of the existing legal framework. Having a state that has expansive medical knowledge users among communities like the Kanikkars in southern Kerala and the Kurichiar tribal communities in the northern parts of the state, being the home of experts in vishavaidyam (poison therapy), manorogachikitsa (mental health) and also being home to a number of families that store such abundant knowledge in their own scriptures and palm leaves, it was natural that the state and other organisations stepped in to document this knowledge, even though it was left to the national discretion in the international legislative frame.

The last decades of the twentieth century have seen a few serious attempts in the case of documentation and policymaking in Kerala. The uniqueness in the relative dominance of the stakeholders in different approaches, the process through which it is executed and the governance systems used for the same warrant a close look at some of the dominant documentation models. For this purpose, we selected three cases, including the community-academia-market linkage model by the

Jawaharlal Nehru Tropical Botanical Garden and Research Institute (JNTBGRI), the open-source, public-domain model by Traditional Knowledge Innovation, Kerala (a project by the directorate of the Medical Education and Health Department, Government of Kerala) and the decentralised management model by the Kerala State Biodiversity Board (Peoples' Biodiversity Register or PBR), from among the various such efforts.[6] Various political, institutional, legal and economic rationales dominate these documentation efforts and offer rich comparative insights and lessons. The translation of knowledge, its ownership patterns, the livelihood of the knowledge holders, public–private partnerships, hierarchical politics, institutional complexities and epistemological debates all figure in the discussion of these approaches. In the following sections, we use the information gathered from various policy documents, institutional brochures and records of the organisations involved in the documentation and the various interviews conducted with the organisation heads and academicians during multiple field visits from October 2014 to July 2015.[7]

JNTBGRI: Community-academia-market linkage as a viable source of protection

The contemporary policy discussions regarding documentation and protection of knowledge date back to the CBD (1992) that introduced an obligation to seek prior informed consent (PIC)[8] for the commercial use of any traditional knowledge, ensuring benefit-sharing with the knowledge holders. However, even before this historical landmark declaration, JNTBGRI[9] (henceforth, TBGRI) had a team of scientists (including botanist, ethnobiologist, taxonomist, institutionally trained ayurvedic physicians) enthusiastic about the collection and preservation of *nattarivu* (local medical knowledge) through ethno-biological expeditions. The research and development activities of TBGRI are integrated and geared to achieve the most tangible results of conservation as well as development of value-added and product-oriented sustainable utilisation of plant genetic resources of the region. Even the department of ethno-medicine and ethno-pharmacology in TBGRI was borne out of the research enthusiasm that the members shared during the early 1990s.

TBGRI's tryst with the local medical knowledge documentation started in 1987 with a major project (All India Coordinated Research Project on Ethno-biology or AICRPE), sponsored by the Ministry of

Environment and Forest (MoEF) for inventorying and documenting the multidimensional perspectives of the life, culture and traditions of the tribes as well as their knowledge system associated with the utilisation of the local biological resources. As part of this larger survey, the former director of TBGRI and his team introduced a benefit-sharing method, namely the Jeevani Model. Jeevani is a restorative, immune-enhancing, anti-stress and anti-fatigue agent, based on the herbal medicinal plant *Arogyapacha* (Trychopus zeylanicus), used by the Kani tribal population in south Kerala in their everyday medicine. The knowledge was divulged by Kani members to the scientists, who isolated 12 active compounds from *Arogyapacha* and developed the drug Jeevani (Gupta 2002). Five process patent applications were filed on the drug (Bijoy 2007). Arya Vaidya Pharmacy Ltd (AVP) of Coimbatore, one of the largest herbal pharmacies in India, was chosen as the primary manufacturer, and in 1995 AVP signed a seven-year licensing agreement with TBGRI and paid a $50,000 licensing fee. Under the terms of the agreement, TBGRI would receive 2 per cent royalties on any sales of the Jeevani drug. The licensing agreement with AVP was primarily to establish a market for Jeevani products, after which TBGRI maintained the right to license its manufacturing technology to other companies if it so desired. Through this benefit-sharing arrangement, TBGRI actually recognised the intellectual property rights of the Kani tribe even before the CBD came into existence. In November 1997, a trust consisting of nine Kani tribal members was formed with the assistance of TBGRI. Named Kerala Kani Samudaya Kshema Trust (the Trust), the two Kani members who imparted the traditional knowledge to TBGRI were appointed as president and vice-president of the Trust (Rajasekharan, et al. 2012). About 60 per cent of the Kani families of Kerala are members of this Trust. From February 1999, the amount due to them has been transferred to the Trust with an understanding that the interest accrued from this amount alone can be used for the welfare activities of the Kani tribe.

However, the forest law permits the Kani to collect only minor forest produce and not the endemic plant, *Arogyapacha*. When they started collecting *Arogyapacha* on a commercial basis, criminal cases were foisted on members of this community. This created an institutional tension in sustaining the model effectively. AVP had written to the Kerala Forest Department and the Tribal Welfare Department proposing a plan for the cultivation of *Arogyapacha*, whereby it would pay the Kani initial seed money for the cultivation of the plant and enter into a buy-back arrangement with them to buy the leaves harvested from the cultivated plants. AVP was prepared to buy five tons of leaves a month. However, the forest department rejected AVP's proposal, explaining that the collection and harvest could not be permitted because they concerned an endemic species. Some stakeholders pointed out that if the forest department had been involved from the beginning in this value chain, perhaps there might have been better institutional support (Gupta 2002).

Even though the Jeevani initiative is known for pioneering the benefit-sharing model of local health traditions in the community-academia-market-based path, it was not successful in sustaining the revitalisation of knowledge and its public health outcome. The disruption in the production of this drug after a few years of technology transfer reminds the stakeholders about the close connection of indigenous knowledge with bio-resources and that sustainability has a broader meaning beyond just the protection of knowledge. In the meantime, it has demonstrated a possibility that traditional communities can be empowered to preserve/protect their knowledge, avail their rights while sharing their resources and taking the knowledge to the market, and bring in more innovations and value additions.

While very few documented knowledge of these surveys are made eligible for further processing, huge information is digitised and kept with the institute. It is partly based on PIC and the permission to reveal for the public or commercialise. The concept of PIC was introduced into international policy initiatives through CBD only in 1999–2000, while the JNTBGRI model is a forerunner in this case, inspiring such an inclusion. During the past few decades, JNTBGRI led a number of documentation initiatives, some of which are shown in Appendix 6.1.

Many of these documentation processes resulted in the enviable collation of regional knowledge. Part of this information is disseminated to the selected people who can make the best use of it, for example, after documenting through video films or other electronic database, it is disseminated to AYUSH doctors through workshops. Such workshops were conducted in 14 districts in Kerala every year for the effective use of these methods in their treatment. Some scientists who worked on these documentation efforts have later started a different institution apart from TBGRI to pursue the possibilities of drug development from this knowledge.[10]

The TBGRI developed a web-based database on traditional knowledge related to the plants used for food and medicine with the technical support of the Centre for Development of Imaging Technology (C-DIT). This database contains details of locations, information related to plants, conditions, treatment, method of preparations, dosage and restrictions, and also the details of the single and poly-herbal formulations. It has facility for different directory, assimilating all types of data, and to store the images, audios and video files. TBGRI has signed an agreement with one of the vaidyas from south Kerala for the preclinical study on his knowledge of diabetes medicine. There are more market linkages in the pipeline, like drugs for hypertension, which needs a proficient institutional coordination to sustain the benefits, unlike the Jeevani Model.

The TBGRI documentation is interesting in many regards: First, the interdisciplinary team managed the entire process—those who are able to understand and discuss the meanings and intricacies of the local health traditions that are documented. Second, they have effectively introduced PIC to protect the legal rights of the knowledge holders. Third, they have taken a professionalised procedural system of documentation and a multi-stakeholder view of its promotion—networking with the community and the market. The flaw in the sustainability of this model was from an institutional failure in terms of coordinating the public-private partnerships[11] and in problematising community ownership.[12] Nevertheless, on the documentation front, it had another important consequence. The effort of TBGRI to trace the plant *Arogyapacha* back to textual ayurveda did not only mean taking the plant away from oral, indigenous, tribal knowledge to bring it into the realm of a written, scholarly, institutionalised Indian system of medicine, but also implied changing its economic status. This is visible in the case of the Jeevani in two steps—one, where the textual reference of *trychopus zyelanicus* was established, linking it to the category of medicines called *varahi* (woody climber found in the Western Ghats) in Sushruta's text, and two, finding an existing combination of ayurvedic enhancers like *ashwagandha* (*withania somnifera*) to pose as ayurvedic medicine. Interestingly, through this connection the formulation could be legally registered as Ayurvedic Proprietary Medicine, even if *trychopus zyelanicus* had never been mentioned within the numerous lists of botanical plants used in classical ayurveda (that is, *shastric* or classical) preparations. While there are claims that knowledge is emerging from the tribal or local populations, the question of its efficacy is always attached to an established tradition than to any alternative ways of promotion. It raises questions about how local health traditions can be documented in their totality, in the context in which they are practised, retaining the multidimensional nature of their knowledge.

People's Biodiversity Register: Decentralised governance and co-management of knowledge

There has been active community-level resource mapping and decentralised planning in Kerala since the late 1980s (Soman 2014). The possibility of having control over local resources is a significant component in decentralised management. The latest initiative in this regard, the Peoples' Biodiversity Register (PBR), was started as a pilot project in 1997 under the aegis of the state planning board and the state government, and was given substantial financial and administrative support for the process of documenting through the Gram Sabhas (local self-government forums) in the Ninth (1997–2002) and Tenth (2002–07) Five-Year Plans. A large part of the methodology for developing the register was conceptualised by KSSP with the help of the teachers, students and members of local bodies (Anuradha, et al. 2001).

The main idea behind this is the intercommunity exchange of knowledge and capacity-building and sustainable monitoring of the resources to keep away from the commercial and private exploitation for extended patented products. This is also the time when the discussions at the national level and state consultations have started to form a biodiversity bill. The 'people's campaign for decentralised planning', launched under the Ninth Five-Year Plan for the state, has made remarkable headway in making the process of administration more participatory. The State Biodiversity Committee comprising a variety of representatives from local self-government institutions, academic and research organisations and KSSP, helped the state to disseminate the capacity-building process with close involvement of the communities. Biodiversity and knowledge mapping of the Ernakulum district by KSSP, and of the Wayand district by M. S. Swaminathan Research Foundation in the late 1990s, has laid the foundation for further knowledge documentation in Kerala. Discussions on the experience of the Kani benefit sharing, and the documentation efforts and consultations for initiating a tribal property rights bill by KIRTADS,[13] have all interestingly guided the decentralised knowledge mapping process. At the international level, the CBD has emphasised that stakeholder participation in the development of biodiversity policy is critical for effective implementation, and that the process by which such policy is developed is as important as the product. To emphasise, the local-level discussions on the protection of local traditions of healing was already initiated at different levels by the NGOs (KSSP) and autonomous institutes (TBGRI) and research collaborators (KIRTADS), where the national and international context of bio-piracy complimented the momentum in the state-level discussions. PBR seeks to document the local knowledge, practices of propagation, sustainable harvests and conservation, as well as economic uses of biodiversity resources that reside with India's local communities.

The PBR process is also developed to enhance the state's attempt to follow the CBD with the focus mainly on three broad ways:

> (1) to respect, preserve and maintain the knowledge, innovations and practices of indigenous and local communities embodying traditional lifestyles relevant for the conservation and sustainable use of biological diversity; (2) to promote the wider application of such knowledge, innovations and practices with approval and involvement of the holders; and (3) to encourage the equitable sharing of the benefits arising from the use of such knowledge, innovations and practices. (Article 8(j) of the CBD)[14]

It is expected to extend the already successful decentralised model of governance in Kerala to the management of natural resources and to create the basis for equitable sharing of benefits. The documents bring together important locational-specific information on biodiversity resources and the ecological processes affecting them (Gadgil 2000). The biodiversity register is only one among the different models, which is direct and efficient in providing a long-term sustainability option.

The Biological Diversity Act of India (Government of India 2002) is being implemented through a three-tier system—the National Biodiversity Authority (NBA) at the Centre, state biodiversity boards at the state level and Biodiversity Management Committee (BMC) at the Gram Panchayat/municipality/corporation level as the third tier or base unit. The Kerala biodiversity rules of 2008, in consequence of the Biodiversity Act of 2002, Section 41, and biodiversity rules 2004, Section 41, required the state to form the BMC within the jurisdiction of the local self-government with eight members[15] representing a cross-section of the society—herbalists, agriculturists, fisherfolk, academicians, community workers, non-timber forest produce collectors/traders, etc. In 2012, the state government had formally declared the constitution of BMCs in all the 978 Gram Panchayats, 60 municipalities and five corporations in the state.[16] From the beginning of 2017, the road map of conservation under PBR entrusted further role to a major stakeholder, Kerala Institute for Local Administration (KILA),[17] for conducting mass contact programmes incorporating the panchayat functionaries with a major role for members of the Mahatma Gandhi National Rural Employment Guarantee Scheme (MGNREGS) in awareness campaigns. There was also further discussion to extend the terms of the BMCs to five years, to make them co-terminus with the panchayat committees (Nandakumar 2015). At present, the BMC coordinates the register compilation with the help of the ward-wise volunteers/study groups through direct observation and discussion with the knowledge holders. The state biodiversity boards train the selected district coordinators and they, in turn, train and provide contact information to the BMC, and facilitate the process of data collection. The cost of protection of medical knowledge is exercised through a local biodiversity fund. It is interesting to note that the institutions created for the protection of knowledge can also help in the conservation of resources. A further plan is to link the local self-government bodies with the BMC to ensure sustainable utilisation of medicinal plants and fair benefit-sharing.[18] Stricter enforcement of biodiversity legislations and mandatory registration for collectors of wild plants and those who sell through herbal shops is recommended with proper inventory, and monitoring of harvesting impacts. The focus is on strengthening the local self-government and BMC for resource management and then formation of a medicinal plants trading society. This would ensure the location and source of collection, and their local names, in order to support traceability to the collection area. A proposal for Good Manufacturing Practices (GMP) certification to be linked with the traceability of resources is part of future plans (Laladhas, et al. 2015).

Encapacitating and empowering the local group of institutions to have the add-on capacity of 'knowledge watch groups' beyond just the 'environmental watch groups' (Mithrambika et al. 2016) would be an additional direction that the institutions can think of in dealing with the state of significant local knowledge. This may also call for different sets of protection strategies simultaneously, as we know that in the case of healing traditions, both these are very closely linked and destruction of one may lead to the loss of the other.

Traditional Knowledge Innovation, Kerala: A project transferring knowledge from families to the public domain

An institution, namely a patent cell under the aegis of the directorate of ayurvedic education in Kerala, was established by the planning board and the government of Kerala, initially to bring awareness about the patenting and intellectual property issues in indigenous medicine, but later was largely focused on entextualisation of old manuscripts and pamphlets from traditional physician families and those collected and kept with the Ayurvedic Medical College library, Thiruvananthapuram. It is an open-source public-domain model of documentation officially started in 2005, with intermittent funding from Ministry of Health, Kerala, and the AYUSH department.

The scientific officer and co-coordinator of this initiative, known as Traditional Knowledge Innovation, Kerala (TKIK), mentioned the main purpose of this documentation process:

> Our institute has sought the help of institutionally trained physicians and litterateurs to read, decode and transliterate the contents in the palm leaves, which are considered as the treasure trove of knowledge system in Kerala. TKDL, an initiative at the central government level, is not adequately covering [sic] the extensive medical knowledge in the state, where largely the knowledge is partially textual or mostly experience based ... we have collected the knowledge through advertisement in the media and medical journals, and hence the large bundles of knowledge scripted within the family traditions (contributed by vaidyas) are yet to be comprehended, collated and publicised for common use.[19]

As the collected scripts are kept in the medical college library, doctors and medical students have had access to it, but many of the institutionally trained allopathic/ayurveda doctors are not able to read and understand this knowledge, as a large portion of it is written in old scripts and sometimes in verse form. The knowledge is accumulated from those families and groups that are willing to contribute to the larger welfare and promotion of the knowledge with no expectation of rewards. The coordinator of the TKIK programme also added:

> We have gathered more than 2,000 bundles of palm leaf manuscripts from various sources such as indigenous practitioners, gurukulas, houses of old

> vaidyas and *aacharyas* (most senior and experienced traditional medical practitioners). The number of leaves comes around more than 45,000. Till now we documented five volumes both in English and Malayalam that could cover only 4–5 bundles and the rest is still waiting to be documented ... and we continue to receive much more from the traditional practitioners. However, the real problem is sustainable funding. These leaves have to be properly preserved; otherwise, they will be completely ruined, because the maximum life span of the dried leaves is 300 years.

This throws light on the expanse of knowledge that is confined within vaidya families which could be put to public health use for further exploration, validation and drug development, but the financial support for it remains a major hurdle. This initiative was not primarily intended to validate the knowledge, but recently, TKIK has signed a memorandum of understanding (MoU) with the first public-private consortium of ayurvedic manufactures in Kerala, namely the Confederation of Ayurvedic Renaissance, Keralam (CARe Keralam),[20] for the preparation of a dossier, drug master file (DMF) and further substantiation of this knowledge. The first one in the series has just been initiated—a DMF for a newer preparation for diabetes. The cluster innovation centre, CARe Keralam, stands as an excellent example for public-private partnership in the promotion of grassroots innovations in the field of ayurveda in Kerala (Madhavan 2013), and now it also facilitates the validation process and incubates local medical traditions.

The Integrity and Governance of Translation in the Three Models

The institutional initiatives for protecting and reviving local health traditions and related resources are evident in the various policy steps that the state has undertaken at various points. The dialogues for an intellectual property act for traditional knowledge (initiated in 2008) and state policy on Indian systems of medicine and local health traditions (draft in 2016) were formulated after various levels of political confrontations, resource mapping process and ample experiences from the earlier models.

The summary of the three models discussed are presented in Appendix 6.1. The discussed approaches raise a number of systemic concerns on the nature of codification and process of validation within the revitalisation discourse. One is the element of path-dependency of the non-codified systems to ultimately validate themselves (the TBGRI model). This model raises larger questions about the local knowledge and its revitalisation through documentation, connected to the market for herbal products and the implications it has on the agency of local health traditions in the revitalisation process. While TBGRI has been successful in establishing the connection of local knowledge of the community with the market and providing a legal framework for the protection of knowledge through PIC, it has failed to protect the agency of these traditions owing to the regulations of the modern market. By drawing references from established ayurvedic texts (to be certified as an ayurvedic drug that satisfies the Drugs and Cosmetic Acts of India and hence the permission for market entry), the new form of this documentation reinforces that local health traditions are peripheral, and hence, the validation requires the lens of an institutionalised system. As in the case of Jeevani or TKIK documentation, it either requires the institutional patronage of ayurveda or adequate references from ayurveda to seek its legitimacy.

It is argued that the codified Indian traditional medicines offer a similar worldview as that of the folk traditions and, hence, they are better tools of assessment for the folk health traditions (Unnikrishnan and Shankar 2004). This criterion has been used for a while now. For example, in the case of ethno-veterinary practices, FRLHT, Bangalore, used the rapid-assessment method through dialogue and consensus with a group of experts including local healers, veterinary doctors, researchers, community members and other ethno-veterinary experts (Nair and Unnikrishnan 2010). TBGRI has also used the same method of consensus in the case of Jeevani validation, but it cannot be called a rapid assessment as it involved clinical and laboratory studies at a later stage. Here, a comparative assessment is used only in finding the source or reference of the folk knowledge in the ayurvedic text. Two, it also raises concerns about the suitability of the commodification process—the challenge of reducing the plural practice of a community or family to position as a product (pharmaceutical) in the herbal drug market through modern reformulative regimes and scientific validations (TBGRI, TKIK, and perhaps the PBR).

The subjugation and disappearance of a section of the local health traditions in Kerala is usually justified through the closely woven development and enviable exchanges between the locally practised forms and the codified systems of knowledge, often referred to as mutually shaped cultural traditions. It is a known fact that contrary to other states, Kerala stayed different from the usual commercialisation path in ayurveda, offering a 'medical alterity' (Kudlu 2016) dominated by traditional therapies and shastric medicines than other derivatives of herbal formulations. Being a tradition that is very closely knit in everyday cultural practices, local health traditions in the state contribute to the public health needs of a large section of the population, which may require a different paradigm of revitalisation altogether. This paradigm of indigenous alterity works complementary to the medical alterity that already prevails in the codified medical sector in Kerala. The idea of 'creative (knowledge) commons' in the Intellectual Property Bill of Kerala (2008), sustainable options from *within* like participatory protection and possibilities of social entrepreneurships (Torri and Herrmann 2011) in the promotion of revitalisation efforts sufficiently feed the image of indigenous alterity. Local practitioners share a common ethos with their patients and they are equipped to deliver socio-cultural sensitive health care (see, for example, Nichter and Nordstrom 1989; Sujatha 2009). The local traditions are enriched with the health care techniques of many ethnic communities such as those of the Vannan and Malayan in Kerala. Most of the ritual procedures of healing are related to sacred groves and Theyyam worship.[21] Some of the devotional procedures that have become extinct, such as *thachumanthram* (traditional curative practice for the evil eye), resemble, to some extent, the new streams of alternative medicines such as *reiki* (traditional energy healing technique) (Unnikrishnan 2004). This necessitates protecting not only the knowledge, but also the communities and rituals associated with it in one or the other form. The knowledge of healing, hence, also remains inseparable from the plurality within—cultural, traditional, habituations and ethos—and ultimately what the documentation efforts may be representing is the skeletons of these traditions, which is not realistic for any kind of revitalisation.

The extent to which the existing codified mechanisms like TKDL provide incentive for the knowledge communities to share knowledge remains a concern. The digitisation process that confines itself to the codified traditions raises a number of questions: (a) About the possible decontextualisation of practice and, hence, the capture of intangible properties (ritualistic aspects, customary protections, etc.) in the new digital formats, derivatives or products (Peekay 2016); (b) How do we establish legitimacy? Is there a way to filter the legitimate practice through documentation?; and (c) And if legitimacy is the second stage of documentation, what kind of validation system is in existence? Or is it necessary to validate at all? These questions need to be confronted in the context of validation efforts in the explained models.

Apart from the aforementioned systemic concerns, the models raise many political, economic and financial questions at its implementation level. The local healers under the existing regulations of medical practice in Kerala have no legal security, but the state follows the policy of non-interference in their practice within the confinement of the community and tribe, but the responsibility for any implications lies with the practitioners in this case. Any kind of practice outside the community calls for immediate regulative systems in place. Many of the documentation efforts like TBGRI's have attempted to provide legitimacy through documentation and further validation. One of the pioneers of documentation from TBGRI mentions:

> These healers can treat within their communities as the government has allowed that freedom, and hence the knowledge is utilised within them. But due to the popularity and effectiveness of their treatment, many people approach them from outside. I suggested these healers to have pretreatment consent mentioning that they are treated upon the request made by them and they will solely be responsible for negative implications, if any! More scientific validation of the folk system is important and relevant, and hence they can treat within the regulative structure and under the support of the State.[22]

Many attempts were made by various traditional healers' associations at different intervals to obtain legal validity for their practice but they remained unsuccessful, leaving many such healers to either practice within their community or adopt promotional instruments such as videos and public speeches to attract patients from outside the community. The state needs to make sure that it does not curtail the communities' and tribal healers' right to access the resources while trying to provide defensive protection. As a senior official in the Kerala Biodiversity Board states,

> Strong regulations are already in place; now the main issue is the coordination of various departments like agriculture, forestry and animal husbandry. We have instances that the fertilizer developed to protect agriculture has killed the biodiversity in that geographical region.

The decentralised power structure may be effectively utilised in nurturing medical pluralism through the existing governance system to translate BMCs into biodiversity sustaining committees with an additional mandate to implement mechanisms to refurbish the local ecosystem in addition to the role of protecting existing resources and knowledge. The documentation in Kerala, as we have seen from different approaches, is not an end in itself, but a first step towards the revitalisation objective. This also means that these steps need to survive various internal political challenges too. One such issue is the prevalence of caste politics, where the knowledge has tended to alienate the original knowledge holders and formed a new social milieu, which erodes the original intent of family health care. This is a huge shift from the situation in Kerala, where the vaidyam is being practised not only by the elite, but also within many lower castes. With the promotion of Sanskrit texts and universalisation of English education, many bundles of lower-caste medical inscriptions are either neglected or lost (Chandran 2016).

The second is dealing with the political governance structure, especially in the case of the BMC, where the party-based political set-up may keep changing the structure of the local bodies and corruption can creep in at various levels of management. This is pertinent while dealing with corporate capital entry into the indigenous medical sector, where the new wave of herbalism is being cashed upon and exploitation of resources is closely linked to attaining permission through loopholes in the existing local political monitoring groups. The lack of awareness regarding the value of traditions and related resources among the local politicians may be easily hijacked for economic gains. The PIC, which was informally executed (only through oral consent between the informants and the ethno-botanists) in the case of Jeevani, was developed later as an official tool for protection in further documentation by TBGRI. This stands as a major instrument for creating the trust of knowledge holders and other stakeholders in the execution of bioprospection. One of the Kani physicians mentioned that he had to withdraw the knowledge from further validation when he felt that the knowledge may be hijacked by other members in the chain of commercialisation. In his words:

> They had done research on my combination. It was a medicine for treating diabetes. After checking, the doctor said that it is a fantastic medicine. For the verification, they sent it again to regional laboratory and they confirmed that it is a successful combination. After the first session, the

> public lab demanded my medicine sample again and again for validation. That time I felt that they will misuse my knowledge. So I didn't give sample again. I have marketing rights for three medicines of blood cancer, sugar and psoriasis, but somehow in this case, I was deliberately being drawn into an unfair process.

The state policies in Kerala have to essentially deal with the local issues of governance, legitimacy and trust enhancement among the knowledge holders in the process of documentation, which in a way may complement the national and international policy efforts. The nitty-gritty and complexity of the documentation process can at times easily lead to a situation where the knowledge holders are exploited due to their weak bargaining power. What these documentations recently matured into is a concept of 'knowledge commons', which was put forward by the state intellectual property bill discussions in the previous decade. The state proposed a new *sui generis* framework to revitalise local health traditions by creating 'knowledge commons'.[23] This is a pool that consists of all the documented local medical knowledge from various tribes and physicians, and the members outside the knowledge-holding communities are free to utilise this knowledge for strictly non-commercial purposes, and are required to deposit whatever improvements and refinements they make to this knowledge into the 'knowledge commons'. That means the value-added knowledge needs to be reinvested into the knowledge pool. But this calls for concrete provisions for safeguarding the knowledge that would be invested in the 'knowledge commons' and also regulations to curtail the misuse of the knowledge taken from the repository. While this does not stop the viable knowledge from commercialisation with due permission through a well-defined agreement with the real owners, this strategy claims to utilise the amassed wealth of knowledge lying idle on the shelves and in digital repositories through various documentations. The policy also calls for the knowledge holders' cooperatives to help the right holders commercialise the knowledge with the help of academic institutions and private manufacturing entities.

Even though the state holds the ownership of such knowledge, all the actual practitioners of this knowledge will have an autonomous license for right of commercial use from the state. However, these licensees are not empowered to sub-license (sublet) this right of commercial use, and the right of transferring licenses will solely rest with the state. Therefore, the ultimate aim of the legislation is not to protect the financial interests of the knowledge holders but the benefit of the society at large. The documentation attempts attain further meaning with the close involvement of traditional healers in state-facilitated development and public health programmes. This is part of the state strategy to facilitate local knowledge, as a major component of development strategy, through incentives for livelihood and improving access to local public health facilities. The Kerala Biodiversity Board has started such initiatives at the local level, incorporating tribal physicians in conducting health camps and forming tribal cooperatives. Within the Kani tribal region, the state government, with the help of local practitioners, is funding many public health camps. The major attempts now are to make knowledge holders aware about the possibilities and potentials of the knowledge. The historical linkages of different caste and social groups in practising medicine and exchanging knowledge in Kerala were reaffirmed and reproduced when the AVP (the firm started by an upper-caste vaidya) readily came forward to commercialise the tribal knowledge-based product, Jeevani, within the ambit of the TBGRI documentation procedure.

Conclusion

The contribution and role of local health practices in Kerala's development experience (known for its high social and health status coexisting with low economic development) cannot be ignored as it offers access to cost-effective and quality health care and results in higher utilisation in public health services (Priya and Shweta 2010). Local health traditions occupy a large share of the health care choices of millions with their presence as home remedies, poison therapists, traditional bone-setters and birth attendants and, hence, provide an indigenous alterity to the mainstream systems. Though their expertise and services are in demand, these health care providers are under severe pressure due to their semi-legal status, the aggressive marketing of biomedical drugs and biomedicine's social prestige (Bode and Hariramamurthi 2014).

Documentation is important and useful; it depends on specific contexts and objectives pursued by local communities and the interest of the actors involved in the process. The purpose of any documentation is to protect the knowledge with its heterogeneity, possibility for further improvement and citation of its original holders. We saw that not all documentations serve all the purposes, for example, the Jeevani model offered some benefits to its knowledge holders despite the limitations, while that of the TKIK has not offered the benefits yet as many aspects of the knowledge are brought into the public domain, but surely offers avenues of further innovations through print forms. While the Kerala narrative of documentation of local health traditions attempts to place the rationale within the national effort for the protection of indigenous knowledge (as claimed by most of the cases), it is clear that the present effort has much to do with the historical pluralistic ambiguity within the state and is probably a continuation of the partial effort of many communities and elite groups for continuous codification and innovations. It is not surprising that some of the cases referred to here attempt to complete the codification that is partially done within the communities and families.

When the legal structure and market realisation require a material artefact for revitalisation, which often manifests as pharmaceuticals or food supplements or a cosmetic product in the modern world, the knowledge, which is often owned by the community or groups and realised as intangible capital before the commoditisation, usually get obscured or suppressed. The various models of documentation practices in Kerala cannot be accepted uncritically in this regard, but surely offer possibilities and directions of inclusive mechanisms. The challenges are of a varied nature—epistemological, cultural, political, economic, legal, social and policy level. The experiences gained in the various stakeholder models may initiate interstate and national dialogues of revitalisation, which has shown a clear impetus in the recent past through the institutionalisation and integration process. The discussions to initiate the 'creative commons' or 'knowledge commons' strategises to coordinate the documentation approaches of various institutions in Kerala, where both the purpose of revitalisation and protection of local healing traditions may be connected. Unlike the TKDL that works as a defensive mechanism,[24] 'creative commons' may offer the possibility of institutional networking for commercialisation and hence the revitalisation of knowledge through creativity, circulation of knowledge and value additions through innovations. As Wolfgram (2012) rightly pointed out, the documentation provides us with a methodological and analytical tool through which we see how the complexity and political economy plays out both in the circulation of the existing knowledge and in the production of new knowledge.

Appendix

Appendix 6.1: Three Major Models of Documentation in Kerala

Model	*Project Aims*	*Nature of Revitalisation*	*Funding*	*Who Owns the Documentation*	*What is the Result of Documentation*
TBGRI	• All-India coordinated research project on ethno-biology (AICRPE), 1987–95, 200 panchayats covered. • Three districts project: planning board, 2004–06. • Kerala state for science and technology, 2005–09. • Coastal ethno-botany: 2012. • 5. Tribal knowledge documentation: recent project.	• Documentation, validation and product development	• Kerala State Planning Board • Kerala State for Science and Technology	• Knowledge is with the institute as a digital database.	• Digital database (not public domain). • Product development. • Benefit-sharing model.
PBR	• Collection and protection of knowledge in various panchayats.	• Collection of knowledge from individual communities at panchayat, municipality and corporation level (LSG), and with help of local people (BMC). • Validation and product development in plan.	• National Biodiversity Board. • Government of India • Rs 125,000 for Gram Panchayats. • Rs 250,000 for municipalities. • Rs 500,000 for corporation.	• BMC • (not public domain).	• Biodiversity Register. • Participatory projects with panchayats.

(Contd)

Appendix 6.1 (Contd)

Model	*Project Aims*	*Nature of Revitalisation*	*Funding*	*Who Owns the Documentation*	*What is the Result of Documentation*
TKIK	• Pamphlet reading. • Reuse of old manuscripts, partially codified, kept in the oldest ayurveda college (Thiruvananthapuram).	• Collection of pamphlets. • Reading and conversion into readable format.	• Government of Kerala and AYUSH. • Rs 40 lakh per year (initial three-and-a-half-years: health department). • Rs 71 lakh per year given by AYSUH. • Rs 50 lakh per year (health department).	• Public domain.	• Six volumes have been published so far, from 4–5 bundles of pamphlets kept with the Ayurveda Medical College in Thiruvananthapuram. • 150 more bundles—40,000 pamphlets—have been scanned, which have around 7,000 formulations. • Digital database. • Contracts with the ayurveda cluster for product development.

Source: Compiled by the authors.

Notes

1. Colonial Kerala consisted of the British-ruled Malabar in the north and two princely states: Cochin in central Kerala and Travancore in contemporary south Kerala.

2. Madras Medical Practitioners' Act 1914, Travancore Medical Practitioners Act 1119 (Malayalam Era), etc., are examples of the various acts under which the practitioners received recognitions or qualifications.

3. There were individual and group efforts for the recognition of traditional vaidyas at different points of time in Kerala. In the process, some formed siddha vaidya associations in both Kerala and neighbouring districts in Tamil Nadu like in Kanyakumari (ATSVS), and many have received certificates and permission of practices as siddha vaidyas in consultation with government functionaries (Interview with a vaidya from Thiruvananthapuram, 12 May 2015).

4. An Ezhava *vaidyan* (physician) named Itty Achuthan was at the time forbidden from using the official written form of Malayalam, *vattezhuthu*, because he was not from the upper caste. His certificate in *kolezhuthu*, published in *Hortus*, is a testament to this though, ironically, he was the chief protagonist in the documentation.

5. Personal interview with Kalidasan Gurukkal at Thiruvananthapuram on 28 June 2015.

6. One such attempt of the documentation projects in Kerala is by Dr Sudha Gopalakrishnan as a part of the endangered archives project of the British Library, namely 'Preserving Memory II: Documentation and Digitization of Palm Leaf Manuscripts from Kerala, India'. See the online resource available at https://eap.bl.uk/project/EAP584 (accessed 10 April 2019).

7. This is done as a part of the larger project on the revitalisation of local health traditions (2014–16), funded by APU, for which research was conducted in three south Indian states, Kerala, Tamil Nadu and Karnataka.

8. Since the tribal or indigenous people contribute to both the knowledge and conservation of biodiversity, Article 8(j) states that their contributions must be 'respected' and consent must be sought before such knowledge can be disseminated or used, as well as 'encouraging' the equitable sharing of the benefits. The provision calls upon the states to include such communities in negotiation for benefit-sharing and the PIC mechanism. Even though a state is not obligated to unilaterally dictate how benefits should be shared in private transactions, it has an obligation to facilitate the equitable sharing.

9. TBGRI is an autonomous research body established by the Government of Kerala in 1979. It has been accorded the status of a Centre of Excellence in Conservation and Sustainable Utilisation of tropical plant diversity by the Ministry of Environment and Forests, Government of India.

10. The contribution of the Amity Institute for Herbal and Biotech Product Development can be seen as an extension of the market-led commercialisation process of TBGRI. This is an institution based in Thiruvananthapuram led by Dr Pushpangadan, the former director of National Botanical Research Institution and JNTBGRI. The institute was efficient in linking the knowledge from the community with the lab and market (the institute was mainly involved in taking the cue from the ethno-botanical project) and producing other documentations to file 28 patent applications on the developed formulations (personal conversation with Dr Pushpangadan).

11. The main criticisms raised in media reports were regarding the involvement of the private firm in the commercialisation purpose, even when there was a presence of reasonably better-performing public firms in the state. In a multi-stakeholder model where the private parties are involved, the chances of conflict cannot be undermined due to the political dimensions of networking. The issues of not-so-transparent and incomplete contracts came forward when the forest department was non-cooperative on the entire process of documentation and commercialisation.

12. The ownership of the community knowledge was contested by some institutions, as the Kani tribe extends beyond the location of the actual collection of knowledge, and there were disputes about the confinement of ownership and benefit-sharing to some sections of the tribe. Hence, KIRTADS, the Scheduled Caste and tribal organisation in Kerala, raised concerns about the scope of benefits to the entire community. This led to some tensions between TBGRI and KIRTADS in the process of benefit-sharing.

13. KIRTADS is purely a governmental organisation under the Scheduled Castes (SCs) and Scheduled Tribes (STs) development ministry and functions as a separate directorate. Its main objective is to carry out research that helps promote development among the scheduled communities in Kerala. It also attempts to identify the needs and problems confronting the marginalised section of the population and suggest recommendations to the government.

14. See https://www.cbd.int/convention/wg8j.shtml (accessed 10 April 2019).

15. The BMC of a local self-government institution is comprised of eight persons: the chairperson, member secretary and six nominated members. As per the Kerala Biological Diversity Rules 2008, Section 22, Sub-section 4, the chairperson of the BMC shall be chairperson of the local body and the secretary of the local body shall be member secretary of the BMC, who shall maintain the records. Besides, six persons are nominated as members by the local body to the committee, of which two should be women (33 per cent) and one member (18 per cent) should belong to the Scheduled Caste or Scheduled Tribe categories. All the six members nominated should be permanent residents of the jurisdiction of the local self-government.

16. The funding for the preparation of PBR during 2010–15 by the National Biodiversity Board was around Rs 125,000 for each Gram Panchayat, Rs 250,000 for each municipality and Rs 500,000 for each corporation.

17. KILA, established in 1990, is an autonomous organisation constituted under the ministry of local self-government, Government of Kerala. The mandate includes conducting research, organising training for the functionaries of the panchayat department and the local bodies, non-officials such as members of legislative assembly, members of Parliament, panchayat presidents and other non-officials concerned with the administration of the local bodies and also advising the government on issues of local administration and Panchayat Raj.

18. Discussion with the member secretary of Kerala Biodiversity Board, 14 June 2015.

19. Discussion with the coordinator of TKIK at the Directorate of Ayurvedic Medical Education, Thiruvananthapuram, 1 January 2016.

20. CARe Keralam Ltd is established as a cluster of ayurveda industries with the support of the AYUSH department of the Government of India and equity partnership from the Government of Kerala through the Kerala State Industrial Infrastructure Development Corporation (KINFRA). Infrastructure facilities are available for the use of ayurvedic product manufacturers and service providers for the standardisation of ayurvedic medicines.

21. Theyyam is a ritual form of worship in north Malabar, Kerala, and some parts of Karnataka. The performers of Theyyam belong to the lower-caste community. People consider Theyyam itself a god and seek blessings. The Peruvannan community has the inherent right to perform Theyyam along with very few others. When epidemics like small pox devastated the world, this community was given the responsibility of cleansing the land. The main duties of this community also included *alakk* (laundry), vaidyam (medicine) and *mantravatham* (black magic), among many others. Since all these jobs were associated with the hygiene and cleanliness of the community, the right to cleanse the society spiritually by performing Theyyam also became their responsibility.

22. Excerpt from a personal interview with a leading scientist of the TBGRI team for documentation, 13 June 2015.

23. The intellectual property policy of Kerala, 2008, available at http://www.wipo.int/edocs/lexdocs/laws/en/in/in048en.pdf (accessed 2 November 2016).

24. TKDL is available with the major patent offices around the world. Patents are denied if the applications establish any connection with digitised knowledge. There are claims that while indigenous knowledge is denied patents on the basis of prior art and when the entire related knowledge has to be disclosed to the applicants for the reasons for rejecting their claim, this can also lead to bio-piracy on a larger scale.

References

Abbot, R. 2014. 'Documenting Traditional Medical Knowledge'. World Intellectual Property Organisation, Geneva. Available at http://www.wipo.int/export/sites/www/tk/en/resources/pdf/medical_tk.pdf (accessed 12 July 2016).

Abraham, L. 2013. 'From Vaidyam to Kerala Ayurveda'. *International Institute for Asian Studies* (The Newsletter) 65: 32–25.

Anuradha, R. V., B. Taneja and A. Kothari. 2001. 'Experience with Biodiversity Policy Making and Community Registers in India: Participation in Access and Benefit Sharing Policy'. Case study no. 3, International Institute for Environment and Development, London.

Bijoy, C. R. 2007. 'Access and Benefit Sharing from the Indigenous Peoples' Perspective: The TBGRI-Kani "Model"'. *Law, Environment and Development Journal* 3(1): 1–19. Available at http://www.lead-journal.org/content/07001.pdf (accessed 15 November 2015).

Bode, M., and G. Hariramamurthi. 2014. 'Integrating Folk Healers in India's Public Health: Acceptance, Legitimacy and Emancipation'. *eJournal of Indian Medicine* 7(1): 1–20.

Chandran, M. D. S. 2016. 'From the Shadows of Legitimacy: The Problems and Prospects of Folk Healing in India'. *Journal of Traditional and Folk Practices* 2–4(1): 74–95.

Cleetus, B. 2007. 'Subaltern Medicine and Social Mobility: The Experience of Ezhava in Kerala'. *Indian Anthropologist* 37(1), special issue on the ethnography of healing, January–June: 147–72.

Collins, H. M., and R. Evans. 2002. 'The Third Wave of Science Studies: Studies of Expertise and Experience'. *Social Studies of Science* 32(2): 235–96.

Gadgil, M. 2000. 'People's Biodiversity Registers: Lessons Learnt'. *Environment, Development and Sustainability* 2(3): 323–32.

Girija, K. P. 2017a. 'Interface with Media and Institutions: The Reordering of Indigenous Medical Practitioners in Twentieth Century Kerala'. *History and Sociology of South Asia* 11(1): 1–18.

———. 2017b. 'Esoteric *vs* Exoteric: Situating Indigenous Medical Practices of Twentieth Century Kerala'. *Journal of Alternative Perspectives in the Social Sciences* 8(3): 357–70.

Government of India. 2002. 'The Biological Diversity Act'. Ministry of Law and Justice, New Delhi. Available at http://nbaindia.org/uploaded/Biodiversityindia/Legal/31.%20Biological%20Diversity%20%20Act,%202002.pdf (accessed 10 April 2019).

Government of Travancore. 1946. 'The Acts and Proclamations of Travancore, 1119-20ME' (Volume 14, Part 1). Trivandrum.

Gupta, A. 2002. 'Value Addition to Local Kani Tribal Knowledge: Patenting, Licensing and Benefit-sharing'. Case study no. 2, WIPO Traditional Knowledge and Intellectual Property Rights. Available at http://www.iimahd.ernet.in/publications/data/2002-08-02AnilKGupta.pdf (accessed 7 August 2016).

Hafeel, A., T. S. Suma and P. M. Unnikrishnan. 2004. 'Documenting and Revitalising Local Health Traditions'. In *Challenging the Indian Medical Heritage*, eds D. Shankar and P. M. Unnikrishnan, 114–27. New Delhi: Centre for Environment Education.

Jasanoff, S. 2013. 'Epistemic Subsidiarity: Coexistence, Cosmopolitanism, Constitutionalism'. *European Journal of Risk Regulation* 2(4): 133–41.

Kudlu, C. 2016. 'Keeping the Doctor in the Loop: Ayurvedic Pharmaceuticals in Kerala'. *Anthropology and Medicine* 23(3): 275–94.

Laladhas, K. P., N. Preetha, B. Baijulal and V. O. Oommen. 2015. 'Conservation of Medicinal Plant Resources through Community Born Biodiversity Management Committee, Kerala, India'. In *Biodiversity Conservation: Challenges for the Future*, eds K. P. Laladhas, V. O. Oommen and P. R. Sudhakaran, 27–39. Chennai: Bentham Books.

Madhavan, H. 2008. 'Home to Market: Responses, Resurgence and Transformation of Ayurveda from 1830s to 1920'. Working paper no. 408, Centre for Development Studies, Thiruvananthapuram.

______. 2011. 'Growth, Transition and Globalization of Traditional Medicine: Case of Ayurvedic Pharmaceuticals in Kerala'. Unpublished PhD thesis, Centre for Development Studies (Jawaharlal Nehru University), Thiruvananthapuram.

______. 2013. 'Towards a "Pharmaceutical Vicious Circle": Revisiting Kerala Ayurvedic Sector' (Special Focus). Research newsletter no. 65 (autumn), International Institute of Asian Studies, 32–35.

McGonigle, I. V. 2016. 'Patenting Nature or Protecting Culture? Ethnopharmacology and Indigenous Intellectual Property Rights'. *Journal of Law and Biosciences* 3(1): 217–26.

Menon, I., and A. Spudich. 2010. 'The *Ashtavaidya* Physicians of Kerala: A Tradition in Transition'. *Journal of Ayurveda and Integrative Medicine* 1(4), October–December: 245–50.

Menon, V. 2002. 'Contesting Healing Power and Knowledge: Health Care in Kerala's Plural Medical System'. *Samyukta* 2(2): 88–101.

Mithrambika, N. B., K. P. Laladhas, N. Preetha and V. O. Oommen. 2016. 'Decentralized Governance for Sustainable Development'. In *Biodiversity for Sustainable Development*, eds K. P. Laladhas, N. Preetha and V. O. Oommen, 165–76. New Delhi: Springer India.

Nair, M. N. B., and P. M. Unnikrishnan. 2010. 'Revitalizing Ethno-veterinary Medical Traditions: A Perspective from India'. In *Ethno-veterinary*

Botanical Medicine: Herbal Medicines for Animal Health, eds D. R. Katerere and D. Luseba, 95–124. New York: CRC Press.

Nandakumar, T. 2015. 'Decentralized Biodiversity Management on the Cards'. *The Hindu*, 10 August. Available at http://www.thehindu.com/news/national/kerala/decentralised-biodiversity-management-on-the-cards/article7520959.ece (accessed 23 November 2016).

Nichter, Mark, and Caroline Nordstrom. 1989. 'A Question of Medicine Answering: Health Commodification and Social Relations of Healing in Sri Lanka'. *Culture, Medicine and Psychiatry* 13(4): 367–90.

Panikkar, K. N. 1992. 'Indigenous Medicine and Cultural Hegemony: A Study of the Revitalization Movement in Keralam'. *Studies in History* 8(2): 283–308.

Peekay, Anoop. 2016. 'Documentation and Indigenous Healers from Kerala'. Talk delivered during the workshop, Dialogue on Revitalization of Local Health Traditions, Azim Premji University, 20 January.

Priya, Ritu, and A. S. Shweta. 2010. 'Status and Role of AYUSH and Local Health Traditions under the National Rural Health Mission'. National Health Systems Resource Centre, National Rural Health Mission, Ministry of Health and Family Welfare, Government of India, New Delhi.

Rajasekharan, S., P. Pushpangadan, P. G. Latha and T. G. V. Nair. 2012. 'Learning from Traditional Knowledge: Intellectual Property, Traditional Knowledge: Community Perspective on Access and Benefit Sharing'. Jawaharlal Nehru Tropical Botanical Garden and Research Institute, Thiruvananthapuram.

Rajasekharan, S., T. G. Vinod Kumar, M. Navas and P. G. Latha. 2016. 'Traditional/Folk Practices of Kerala: Case Studies (Part 2)'. *Journal of Traditional and Folk Practices* 2–4(1): 54–64.

Rautaray, O. P., R. N. Pradhan, P. Behara and H. K. Sahu. 2014. 'People's Biodiversity Register [PBR]: A Community Based New Venture in Odisha to Document Natural Resources'. *Environment and Ecology Research* 2(8): 285–90.

Soman, B. 2014. 'Participatory GIS in Action: A Public Health Initiative from Kerala, India'. *The International Archives of the Photogrammetry, Remote Sensing and Spatial Information Sciences* 40(8). ISPRS Technical Commission VIII Symposium, 9–12 December 2014, Hyderabad, India.

Sujatha, V. 2009. 'The Patient as a Knower: Principle and Practice in Siddha Medicine'. *Economic and Political Weekly* 44(16): 76–83.

Torri, M. C., and T. M. Herrmann. 2011. 'Gram Mooligai Limited Company (GMCL)—An Alternative Bioprospecting and Development Model: Constitution, Structure and its Functioning'. In *Bridges Between Tradition and Innovation in Ethnomedicine Fostering Local Development*

Through Community-Based Enterprises in India, eds M. C. Torri and T. M. Herrmann, 85–120. The Netherlands: Springer.

Unnikrishnan, E. 2004. 'Materia Medica of the Local Health Traditions of Payyannur'. Discussion paper no. 80, Kerala Research Programme on Local Level Development, Centre for Development Studies, Thiruvananthapuram.

Unnikrishnan, P. M., and D. Shankar (eds). 2004. *Challenging the Indian Medical Heritage*. New Delhi: Foundation Books.

Unnikrishnan, P. M., and G. Hariramamurthi. 2012.'Local Health Practitioners in India: Resilience, Revitalization and Reintegration'. In *Medical Pluralism in Contemporary India*, eds Leena Abraham and V. Sujatha, 279–304. New Delhi: Orient BlackSwan.

Unnikrishnan, P. M., and O. Koike. 2010.'Traditional Knowledge for Sustainable Development: A Case from the Health Sector in Kerala, India'. *Global Environmental Research* 14(2): 167–75.

Varier, Raghava M. R. 2002. *The Rediscovery of Ayurveda: The Story of Arya Vaidya Sala Kottakkal*. New Delhi: Viking.

Wolfgram, M. 2012.'The Entextualization of Ayurveda as Intellectual Property'. *International Journal of Cultural Property* 19(3): 313–43.

seven

Documenting 'Folk' Ayurvedic Knowledge in Uttarakhand

Insights from Critical Medical Anthropology

Moe Nakazora

The study of medical pluralism has a rich body of scholarship. Represented by Charles Leslie's work in 1976, which had a great influence on the foundation of medical anthropology in India (Joshi 2016). Initially the literature on medical pluralism shed light on the colonial and postcolonial situations in the Third World, where, despite the spread of biomedical knowledge, 'traditional medicines' remain powerful medial paradigms for local people (Sujatha and Abraham 2012). In the 1990s, several studies started to focus on (post)-modern societies in the West, in which complementary and alternative medicine (CAM) has become one of the major therapeutic options, due to State-sponsored medical pluralism (Cant and Sharma 1999; Scambler 2002; Turner 2004). Although since then, divergent streams have emerged within the field of medical pluralism, overall it has successfully 'relativised' biomedicine by analysing the complexity and dynamism of pluralistic medical traditions or health seeking behaviours of patients, demonstrating how they move across different medical systems in a particular society (Bhardwaj 2010; Young 1981).

Yet, as is argued in the Introduction to this volume, the literature on medical pluralism focuses relatively more on the different 'systems of medicine'. Non-systems of medical knowledge and practice tend to be discussed in isolation or as peripheral to the discussion on the systems of medicine. Indeed, from the early stage (see Leslie 1980), quite a few medical anthropologists have emphasised the importance and efficacy of such overlooked indigenous medical traditions as informal, unsystematic and situated practice (Lambert 1992; Nichter 1992; Trawick 1992). Although medical anthropology as such has produced thick ethnographic studies regarding marginal/subaltern treatments by 'folk' ayurvedic practitioners, traditional midwives, bone-setters and others (Chawla 2013; Jeeva 2010; Lambert 2012; Langford 2003; Sadgopal 2013; Sujatha 2007; Trawick 1992), there is a need to situate these studies in the context of recent policy developments with regard to such therapeutic practices.

Considering this, the recent policy initiatives towards such informal health practice need to be actively pursued in medical anthropology. Since 2000, many of the governmental institutions and NGOs in 'resource-rich nations' (nations enriched in biodiversity and related traditional medical wisdom) have started codification and formalisation of 'valuable' folk medicines. As we will see later, there are several purposes for these documentation projects, including the prevention of misappropriation of knowledge of local health traditions by multinational pharmaceutical companies, as well as its preservation and development to cater to emerging public health needs including strengthening of primary health care. Combining insights from medical anthropology with those of science and technology studies, I propose a new critical approach to examine the socio-material process of documentation of local health traditions. Specifically, I will analyse the particular documentation project in a regional state of India, to show the inclusion/exclusion embedded in the process of documentation and its implications.

Ethnographic Studies of Documenting Local Health Tradition: Insights from Science and Technology Studies

Science and technology studies is a relatively new interdisciplinary field,[1] which a few medical anthropologists have had dialogue with (Martin 2012;[2] Mol 2003; Rajan 2006; Zhan 2009). Though there are different theoretical strands and schools of thought,[3] most of the literature in the field of science and technology studies point out that while modern science claims its universality and neutrality, scientific knowledge is culturally constructed and socially situated (Haraway 1997; Harding 1993). Bruno Latour's (1987, 2007) methodological contribution in this context bears added significance. Criticising the idea of scientific knowledge as a rigid objective truth, Latour paid attention to the *process* of making particular knowledge, by observing what scientists actually do in laboratories or outside laboratories. By this 'following scientists' approach, Latour found out that scientists enrol and *translate* various actors' interests outside laboratories, and thereby that scientific knowledge is a network of humans and non-humans mobilised by such translating activities by scientists. These translations are mediated by various material devices which Latour called 'inscriptions', such as graphs, statistics, diagrams and photographs. For example, Louis Pasteur, in his discovery of microbes, had first of all gained knowledge on anthrax-related diseases from local farmers and veterinarians, and then translated such various 'local' diseases into one possible cause, that is, anthracnose, which was made visible by graphs, diagrams and concrete numbers at his laboratory.

It should be noted that this ethnographic approach of Latour, following the socio-material process of making of scientific knowledge, discloses the *implicit politics* embedded in such a process. The approach of exploring the network that scientists mobilise to make scientific knowledge necessarily articulates who/what are included/excluded in it. For this reason, the influence of this methodology has gone far beyond science and technology studies, and been adopted to critically examine various knowledge practices by other fields such as development studies (Riles 2001).

I argue that this approach has useful insights for the documentation of local health knowledge. Here, I draw on a project undertaken by one NGO documenting the knowledge of *vaidyas* (folk Ayurvedic practitioners) in Uttarakhand, India. I discuss how this project translates the various actors' interests in the *process* of documentation. This chapter draws on data collected through participant observation in various project activities including project meetings, collection of data and documentation process, as well as interviews with various traditional medical practitioners, government officials and NGO members in 2010–11.

Codification of Local Health Traditions in India: Biodiversity and Intellectual Property Right

Among 'resource nations', the Indian government has played a pioneering role in initiating documentation projects. Though in India these projects have had several different purposes, including 'revitalisation' of such traditions for fulfilling the needs of the nation's primary health care, these were also triggered by global market trends and politics for natural and herbal products (Saxena, et al. 2002: 340–43). In the late 1980s, many life-science corporations showed renewed interest in natural resources and indigenous knowledge in the hope of finding leads for developing new drugs. Since then, there has been greater interest in the intellectual property rights of indigenous people and farmers. The 1992 United Nations Convention of Biological Diversity mandated that drug companies accessing indigenous resources and knowledge must share with the source nations and communities any economic benefits that accrue. Although it is in many ways a fragile mandate, the CBD's idiom and institutional framework have had noteworthy effects on the practice of the parties involved. In line with the tenets of the CBD, approval of bioprospecting by scientists has required benefit-sharing agreements with the resource owners and, as a consequence, numerous NGOs and indigenous activists aiming to prevent illegitimate exchange, which they call 'bio-piracy', have emerged.

Following this global trend, since 2000, State actors of 'resource nations' have launched documentation and digitalisation projects to catalogue 'valuable' indigenous knowledge. In India, in the late 1990s, the government and NGOs succeeded in overturning several patents granted by the European Union patent office and the US patent office for neem, turmeric and basmati rice, which were recognised as having originated in India. Since the revocation of granted patents involves huge costs and takes time, to give patent examiners improved access to background information (prior art) of Indian traditional knowledge, it was thought prudent to make a database of traditional knowledge that would make it easier to spot misappropriation during the initial phases of patent examinations (Saxena, et al. 2002: 340–43).

According to the Indian National Biodiversity Act 2002, the national legislation enacted in line with the CBD, in India the traditional knowledge to be databased includes codified (documented) as well as uncodified (not documented, but may be orally transmitted) information, the assumption being that the knowledge-holders for each category are different, namely ayurvedic practitioners and traditional folk healers (vaidya).[4] The Act also specified that the central government is responsible for the databasing of already-documented knowledge such as classical ayurvedic texts and the state governments for recording, collecting, eliciting and databasing what we have called 'local health traditions'.

The People's Biodiversity Register in Uttarakhand

Although the central government's project, TKDL, had a limited purpose, that is, negative protection (prevention of misappropriation of traditional medical knowledge), the state-level project, PBR, included appropriate access and future benefit-sharing in its scope. Consequently, to ensure future legitimate exchanges, PBR projects emphasised the need for registration of not only knowledge but also its 'knowledge holders' and 'their intentions for benefit-sharing' (Brahmi, et al. 2004; Saxena, et al. 2002).[5] The Act obligated each state government to set up a state biodiversity board and BMCs at district, block and panchayat levels, for documenting local health traditions and their 'knowledge holders' in allocated communities with the 'consultation of local people' (Utkarsh 1999).[6] Here, I mainly deal with the case in Uttarakhand in north India, where I did fieldwork in 2010 and 2011 as part of my doctoral research.[7]

Created on 9 November 2000, Uttarakhand is the 27th state of India. Located in the northwestern Himalayas, the environment is rich in important medicinal and aromatic plants, prompting the state government to take steps to develop and project the new state as a 'herbal state' (*jaḍibuti prades*). Drawing on extensive efforts by the state government to attract international and national donors for herbal plant projects, various plans have been formulated to protect medicinal plants and to aid farmers, with support for commercial cultivation, processing and marketing of medicinal plants (Alam, et al. 2006; Mishra and Dutta 2003; Singh, et al. 2005). The PBR is regarded as part of this herbal state policy in Uttarakhand.

The project was officially initiated in 2010 with the formation of the Uttarakhand State Biodiversity Board, consisting of a chair (the head of the forest department), five official members from several state government departments and five specialist members elected from nodal state research institutes and NGOs in the herbal sector. Here, I focus on the documentation activities of one NGO that joined the project as a specialist member in 2013 but had conducted documentation of local health traditions since 2008 as part of their own initiative. This NGO is a 'local NGO', conducting activities only in Uttarakhand, dealing with a wide range of issues including development of ecotourism and disaster management. By using the methodology of science and technology studies, which I explained in the previous section, I will explore the inclusion and exclusion in the process of documentation and registration of subject ('proper' vaidyas) and object ('valuable' folk medicine) in the project.

Inclusion/Exclusion in the Process of Documentation

Subject-making: Registration of 'Proper' Vaidyas

I discuss here the subject-making process of the project, that is, identification and certification of the vaidyas as proper/legitimate knowledge holders. To reiterate, in the PBR project, not only documentation of knowledge but also registration of subjects (and their intentions for benefit-sharing) is considered a crucial part of the project. As I have noted elsewhere (Nakazora 2009a), the global discourse of indigenous intellectual property, especially the CBD, had a particular assumption about indigenous knowledge and its rightful ownership—knowledge has discrete and identifiable subjects who have 'rights' to knowledge, which is itself regarded as a fixed and corporeal object. In other words, there assumed the existence of a 'bounded community' where people, plants and knowledge are bundled together.

As was discussed at the second annual meeting of the National Biodiversity Board (National Biodiversity Authority 2010), how to identify vaidyas caused problems due to the informal nature of their treatment for many states, including Uttarakhand. Unlike in several other states in southern India, where ayurveda and medical tourism have recently become a main source of the states' revenue, and where various occupational groups have come to standardise treatments provided by vaidyas,[8] in Uttarakhand there is no professional organisation that brings together the vaidyas.

Under such ambiguous conditions, how did the project team gather a group of vaidyas for the project? A project coordinator of the NGO explained the method for identifying vaidyas as follows:

> We have to rely on the networks or experiences of the project board members. For example, our NGO organised a cultivation project of medicinal plants in Chamoli last year, and in some cases we happened to know those who approached us for their own benefits or those who had superior knowledge of medicinal plants among participants were vaidyas![9]

Here, we can clearly see that the presence of collective subjects constituting 'Uttarakhand vaidyas' was not an essential precondition for the project. Rather, they were temporally assembled through the contingent networks of the project participants, and through the medium of 'medicinal plants'. Regarding this subject-making process, one should pay attention to two things.

First, the resultant category of 'Uttarakhand vaidyas' includes a variety of subjects (Kala 2005).[10] For example, Table 7.1 includes the project list of vaidyas and their backgrounds in a village in Chamoli district. As one can see, the collected group of vaidyas in this village ranges from hereditary vaidyas (*jāti*) to those who gained knowledge of medicinal plants through interaction with *sādhūs* (wandering Hindi renunciates).

TABLE 7.1: Project List of Vaidyas in Chamoli District, Uttarakhand

	Gender	*Caste*	*Age*	*Qualification*	*How to learn herbal knowledge*
1	Female	Scheduled Caste	70	None	Learning knowledge by living as a *sadhu* (wandering Hindu renunciate)
2	Female	Rajput	29	12th standard	Learning from her friend's grandmother
3	Male	Rajput	45	Matric	Hereditary vaidya
4	Male	Rajput	38	Intermediate	Learning knowledge from a sadhu

Source: Compiled by a local NGO in Uttarakhand (14 September 2010).

Second, the project members were content to regard those who actively participated in other herbal projects as vaidyas. As mentioned above, in Uttarakhand, under the 'herbal state' policy, a number of projects to support farmers with commercial cultivation of medicinal plants have been conducted by governmental institutes and NGOs. To be recognised, that is, made visible as a vaidya, it was necessary to have explicitly shown interest in and knowledge of medicinal plants. Those who did not demonstrate interest or knowledge in medicinal plants did not qualify.

As for this type of subject-making through the medium of 'medicinal plants', Mishra and Nambiar (in Chapter 8, this volume) caution against the exclusion of those vaidyas whose primary mode of healing may not be herbs (bone-setters or traditional midwives, for example). In addition to such exclusion, my field data in Uttarakhand exemplify the possibility of such projects to include those who have not had enough experiences of treatment, only based on their knowledge of and interests in medicinal plants or their participations in other herbal projects. The focus on medicinal plants is partly based on the shared assumption of 'scientific' projects that medicinal plants are the common denominator to translate between scientific and folk knowledge, but more, it reflects the recent global market trend towards herbal treatment, showing how the neoliberal logic of intellectual property permeates the technical details of the project. We can see this permeation in the following stage of the project to interview vaidyas about their *intention* for benefit-sharing. I report a project interview of vaidyas, ostensibly to elicit opinions on the appropriation of their knowledge and on how benefits should be shared.

Subject-making: Vaidyas' Intention for Benefit-sharing

In October and November 2011, I could observe the project team's documentation targeting 32 vaidyas in the Chamoli district. Vaidyas were called to the office of the NGO and interviewed based on the following standard questionnaire form, certified by the State Biodiversity Board:

1. Do you agree with the commercial/scientific application of your knowledge?
2. If you agree, to whom should benefits be given? (individual vaidyas/community [villages]/researchers who added value to knowledge/research institutes/should be used for environmental protection)?
3. What kind of benefits should be shared?
   (a) Monetary benefits.
   (b) Non-monetary benefits (public recognition at national, state and local levels/advertisement through media/support for connection with other traditional knowledge holders/construction of connection with research institutes which attempt to confirm values of traditional knowledge/provision of scientific knowledge about traditional knowledge/trainings of preservation of natural resources used in traditional knowledge).

Here, what I would like to focus on is not the *result* of these interviews. Rather, for the purpose of this chapter, we should pay attention to what happened in the *process* of documentation, and what kind of particular inclusion and exclusion were seen at interviews. I particularly examine the following conversation, seen as the typical interaction between NGO staff and the vaidyas, which was repeated during the course of the interviews.

> **Interviewer 1:** What kind of benefits (*phayada*) do you want in return for sharing your knowledge? Please choose from these options. No. 1 ...
>
> **Old female vaidya:** What?
>
> **Interviewer 2:** Auntie, you are helping someone for his research with your knowledge. He would like to return you something. So, tell me what you want.
>
> **Old female vaidya:** It is our duty (*kartavya*) to help you. As much as we can, we try to help people.
>
> **Middle-aged male vaidya:** Are you from the government? Is it a survey?
>
> **Interviewer 1:** Yes, we are from the government, but it is not survey; it is research, I mean, for a study.
>
> **Old female vaidya:** It is nice to help people who are doing a study for the nation (*bharat ke liye*). Also, we have to show special kindness to the guest from a foreign country.[11]
>
> **Interviewer 2:** By the way, what kind of help do you want from the government?
>
> **Old female vaidya:** It would be a great help for us if they had mercy (*daya*) to organise cultivation projects of medicinal plants.
>
> [After repeating this kind of conversation with other vaidyas several times over, the interviewers changed the question from 'what kind of benefits do you want in return for sharing your knowledge?' to 'what kind of help do you want from the government?').[12]

Here, we can recognise that vaidyas actually express very different ideas of their practice from the project assumption of benefit-sharing. Notably, they legitimised sharing of their knowledge *without any benefits* by using such terms as *seva* (service) or *dana* (gift),[13] instead of *phayada* (benefit). Also, it should be noted that while there was no answer when the interviewers asked the vaidyas what they wanted in return for sharing their knowledge, when they were asked what kind of help or mercy they wanted from the government, they were willing to answer 'cultivation projects'.

We cannot simply ascribe this 'apolitical' attitude (Reddy 2007)[14] to their ignorance of the issue of bio-piracy and global politics regarding bio-resources and related traditional wisdom. According to my interviews with these vaidyas, most of them were well 'aware' of the issue, related to the fact that Navdanya, the NGO leading the international campaign against 'bio-piracy', has its headquarters in Uttarakhand (Shiva 1997). Also, considering that in their daily practices about two-thirds of vaidyas do not accept payments for their treatment, doing it as community service, or sometimes service which is not group-specific but far more general and decontextualised. It could be said that in these interviews excerpted earlier, the responses of the vaidyas suggested an alternative way of thinking about knowledge exchange, rather than simply accepting the global benefit-sharing model as possibly the only one signifying ethical conduct.

However, not all of this kind of complicated interaction and negotiation at interviews was included in the completed form of the project documents. From the above conversation, for example, only the remark of the vaidyas' request that the government conduct cultivation projects for them was recorded and documented. Then, such a remark was decontextualised from its original conversation and recontextualised as an answer to the third question of the form, that is, what kind of benefits should be shared—namely that the values of herbal treatment and knowledge sharing as seva or dana, expressed by vaidyas at the moment of interviews, were excluded in the course of documentation, as they were not fitted into the questionnaire form following the neoliberal logic of intellectual property. As a result of such inclusion and exclusion, in the completed form of the project, vaidyas were represented as the subjects expecting cultivation projects of medicinal plants *in return for* sharing their knowledge.

Object-making: Registration of 'Folk Ayurveda'

In this section, I discuss the object-making process, that is, the process of documenting 'valuable' local knowledge. Regarding such process, there have already been several social scientific works that critically examined the projects in India. As for the project of the central government called TKDL targeting codified ayurveda, Gaudillier (2014) observed that the project decomposed complex compositions in ayurveda and developed the database based not on treatments or recipes, but on medicinal plants. From the Foucauldian viewpoint of 'bio-capitalism', he criticised that such decomposition and reorganisation are in parallel with the recent movement towards approval of patents on living entities or technical manipulation of DNA and genes. Mishra and Nambiar (in Chapter 8, this volume), focusing on state-level projects, also emphasise that documentation includes only tangible aspects of knowledge, more specifically, the knowledge on medicinal plants (name, usage and ailments), systematically excluding other aspects of the knowledge or the social context in which such knowledge is produced and practised (timing, space of collection of plants, prescriptions and proscriptions regarding diet, other aspects of lifestyle or chanting of hymns that are believed to add effectiveness to the therapeutic process). Notably, such findings fall in line with social scientific studies of other indigenous databasing projects, which point out how databasing might transform indigenous knowledge by severing it from the practices that have sustained it (Agrawal 2002).

In addition to such important points, here, from my own ethnographic study that followed the *process* of documentation, I would like to highlight another layer of exclusion. I describe how the project team's assumption to register 'folk ayurveda' as a consistent system that is *different* from biomedicine and formal (codified) ayurveda, excluded the important aspect of the vaidyas' everyday treatment, namely their engagement with multiple medical ontologies such as classical ayurvedic texts, biomedical concepts and knowledge generated through new herbal projects.

As mentioned earlier, the National Biodiversity Act was based on the distinction between codified ayurveda and uncodified (folk) ayurveda, the latter being a target of the PBR project. This policy of categorisation of folk medicine assumes local health traditions as *uniquely* bounded and consistent systems, which are distinctive from formal ayurveda. In the process of documentation, as long as I have observed, this assumption of local health traditions has forced the project team to find out 'what is really unique and original in particular tradition or community', despite negative reaction from vaidyas and other local people.

Notably, the project coordinator of the NGO said that among the herbs used by vaidyas, he especially paid attention to the ones that are not being used in other medical traditions. For example, for making paste for stomachache due to indigestion, many vaidyas mix the herbs of *duna, bahera* (*terminalia bellerica*) and *harad* (*terminalia chebula*). Among these herbs, he said that they focus on duna and should further interview about other usages of this plant, as it does not have any scientific names yet, meaning that it has not been scientifically explored yet and is not used in formal ayurvedic medicine. Regarding this choice, he explained to me that only if plants and related local health traditions are proved to be the unique knowledge of a particular community could they be a source of income for that community when scientifically valued.[15] Also, a senior official in the State Biodiversity Board shared that even for a common plant like neem, there should be unique local tradition in its usage and recognised effects in each community, which should be property documented.[16]

However, at the BMC meetings at the panchayat level, which I attended, most of the local people insisted that except for a few specialists, they lacked any specialised knowledge, as knowledge in the Garhwali villages is basically general knowledge involving the use of common plants such as turmeric in India. Then, as for one kind of such specialists, vaidyas, as I have written elsewhere in detail (Nakazora 2017), even hereditary vaidyas in Uttarakhand gain knowledge from multiple sources, not limited to 'local' oral traditions; for example, one vaidya said that he learned pulse treatment from a vaidya from Bengal, while another learnt treatment of medicinal plants (*jadi buti*) from his friend's father, who acquired such knowledge from a sadhu.

Furthermore, vaidyas often mention written texts as their knowledge source. The knowledge sources include classical ayurvedic texts such as Vaidastha and Sārandhar, as well as contemporary popular ayurvedic books such as *Ghar ka Vaidya* (Vaidya at Home), published for 'doctors, *vaidyas*, and *hakims* who are interested in indigenous medicine'. As for the former, they express their desire for 'authentic' ayurveda, while the latter say that through the pictures in the books, they can learn which medicinal plants are good and what kind of effect they have.

Moreover, the following example of *kiḍe* (bug) shows how their knowledge crosses not only the boundary between codified and uncodified ayurveda, but also that between ayurveda and biomedicine. Joshi (1995) discussed how in Jaunpur, Uttarakhand, the local community believes that there is a bug (kide) which digests food in stomach. However, Langford (2003) reported that the concept of kiḍe has gained far broader meanings than such original context and included the invisible in biomedicine such as cells and bacillus. In my own research in the Garhwali villages, too, some vaidyas mentioned red and white kiḍe, which are considered to be referring to the red and white blood corpuscles in biomedicine.

Such multiplicities of vaidyas' knowledge sources *contradict* the assumption of local health traditions as uniquely bounded oral traditions, or that they do not evolve/respond/adapt to changing times and needs. Raje's (2012) recent account of the Shivarimal *bhagat* (traditional healer) shows how the practice of local health traditions defies any notion of rigidity, timelessness and bounds. Importantly, the object-making process of the project excludes the vaidyas' own idea of revitalising their knowledge. As I have argued elsewhere (Nakazora 2017) and many medical anthropologists have similarly pointed out, for vaidyas the most important thing is the *effect* of their treatment rather than preserving their unique knowledge system, and in their search for *effect* they tend to adopt knowledge from multiple medical sources.

This attitude can be vividly seen at the workshop that I organised with the help of a local NGO in Chamoli (separately from the PBR project), where 16 vaidyas, mainly folk ayurvedic practitioners, got together to discuss the way to enhance their knowledge to solve health problems in the community. At the workshop, they mentioned a variety of ideas and knowledge sources for improving their treatments, from getting proper knowledge on classical texts like Charaka Samhita to scientific cultivation of medicinal plants that they use for their medical practice (Nakazora 2017). The desire for cultivation of medicinal plants is quite strong among the vaidyas in Uttarakhand. This is mainly because after the Chipko Movement, the state forest department strictly restricted the people from collecting forest resources (including non-timber resources), so vaidyas found it difficult to legally collect the medicinal plants that they needed. The cultivation of medicinal plants is seen as the best solution to this impasse.

Thus, in sum, the project model of local health tradition, as rigid and bounded folk medicine, excludes the vaidyas' everyday knowledge-making activities, their engagement with multiple sources of medicine for gaining more *effective* knowledge and, further, their various ideas for improving their medical practices, which cannot be reduced to a single solution of codifying rigid 'local' traditions. It should be noted that as well as the subject-making process, which I have already examined, this object-making process and its particular form of inclusion and exclusion represents how the neoliberal idea of intellectual property is permeated into the project.

This chapter sought to examine the politics embedded in the documentation of local health traditions through following the *process* of documentation, that is, the process in which subjects ('proper' vaidyas) as well as objects ('folk' ayurveda in Uttarakhand) are formulated and reformulated in this new project. The ethnographic explorations have revealed particular inclusion/exclusion and assumed notions about the category called local health traditions. Unlike other studies dealing with the *results* (outcomes of documentation) of projects, this approach examines the technical details of knowledge-making (Latour 2007) to reveal exactly in which parts of the project inclusion and exclusion happen. Only through such detailed analysis of the *process* could we make both practical and useful suggestions for improvement regarding *which parts should be changed for the project to be more inclusive*, rather than denying the whole local effort involved in such a project of documentation. My intention in this chapter is not to critique the activities of the particular NGO or underplay the objectives of documentation, but to show how the neoliberal ideology of intellectual property underlies the project, creating particular forms of inclusion and exclusion. The explicit engagement of critical medical anthropology with recent policy efforts on the documentation and codification of local/folk health traditions is an imperative, as much for the specific projects and initiatives as for the study of medical pluralism.

Notes

1. This field was initiated by Robert Merton, who analysed the *ethos* that a community of scientists (as a social group) shares, followed by Thomas Kuhn, who claimed that scientific fields undergo periodic 'paradigm shifts' rather than solely progressing in a linear and continuous way.

2. Emily Martin (2012) traces the history of the intersection between feminist medical anthropology and science and technology studies. Here, from a rather different angle, I introduce the work of science and technology studies, which could be useful for analysing the documentation process of local health traditions in medical anthropology.

3. India has its unique trajectory of science and technology studies, intermingled with various social activism. First of all, the New Social Movements of the 1970s and 1980s contributed to the emergence of the discipline, as these movements and activist groups influenced by Marxist, Gandhian and deep ecological perspectives could not avoid engaging with modern science and the

modernisation project in the post-colony. In the 1990s, the field became vibrant with the intervention of a group of social historians of science, inspired by postcolonial studies.

4. It should be noted that this distinction itself is an arbitrary construction of postcolonial medical history. Around the turn of the twentieth century, prominent ayurvedic practitioners established professional associations, colleges and pharmaceutical firms, and wrote textbooks organised according to a modern medical division of subjects. Inspired by the thought of British Orientalists, they followed a revivalist ideology, calling for a return to the 'scientific' ayurveda of the classical age through the adoption of institutional practices of biomedicine, while lamenting the descent of ayurveda into magical practices during the colonial era. In the 1920s, this revivalist reform expanded, and received official support from the Indian National Congress that regarded ayurveda as a manifestation of Indian culture. Over time, the gap between 'professional' ayurveda and a host of indigenous practices with which it had once been closely associated has been widened and essentialised into the gap between the professional and folk sectors (a newly separated category) of Indian medicine (Brass 1972; Leslie 1992).

5. This legislation further certifies that the central government regulates bioprospecting by foreign residents, the state governments being responsible for bioprospecting by Indians.

6. The emphasis on 'consultation of local people' is partly because the project format of the PBR is an adoption from the project of an NGO in south Karnataka, FRLHT (Foundation for Revitalisation of Local Health Traditions). FRLHT was set up in 1991, aiming at the construction of a database for preservation of medicinal plants and sustainable development of Indian medical traditions. In the process of documentation, FRLHT attempted to develop the design and methodology for participatory documentation. This emphasis on participation reflects the global transformation of developmental discourses from top-down to participatory development, as well as economic liberalisation and subsequent decentralisation in the 1990s in India.

7. My doctoral work was on an 'Ethnography of Making of Property-owning Subjects: Biodiversity-related Knowledge, Property and Personhood in Contemporary India', University of Tokyo, Japan.

8. For example, in Kerala, there is such an organisation as the Kerala Sidha Marma Chikitsa Sangham (KSMCS), binding vaidyas for knowledge-sharing and standardisation of their treatment.

9. Quoted from my field notes (5 November 2010).

10. C. P. Kala, the ethno-botanist who conducted interviews with 60 vaidyas in eight districts in Uttarakhand, noted, 'In Uttarakhand, there are two routes to become *vaidyas*. Traditional *vaidyas* mean that those who have gained herbal knowledge through hereditary traditions or through other trained *vaidyas*' (Kala 2005: 257).

11. The reference to 'a foreign country' comes from the presence of myself, as a Japanese anthropologist.

12. Quoted from my field notes (30 October 2011).

13. Though we cannot cover it here in detail for the domain of pure or unreciprocated giving in Hinduism, please refer to Parry (1986) and Raheja (1988).

14. Deepa Reddy (2007) analysed a story similar to what we have seen here. The community consultation project of the National Institutes of Health (NIH) in an Indian community in Houston, for which Reddy worked as a consultant, along with requests for blood donations for genomic research, aiming to avoid accusations of biopiracy, also asked about the meaning of the donation. Contrary to scientists' assumptions, however, the Indian donors' attitude was notably apolitical—they themselves legitimised blood donation as a form of community service (seva), or something done for 'the good of humanity', 'the greater good' and, even more generally, 'a good cause'.

15. Quoted from my field notes (30 January 2011).

16. Quoted from my field notes (4 October 2010).

References

Agrawal, Arun. 2002. 'Indigneous Knowledge and the Politics of Classification'. *International Social Science Journal* 54(173): 287–97.

Alam, G., P. V. de Kop and B. de Steenhuusen. 2006. 'Developing a Sustainable Medicinal Plant Chain in India: Linking People, Markets, and Values'. In *Agro-food Chains and Networks for Development*, eds R. Ruben, M. Slingerl and H. Nijhoff, 191–202. New York: Springer.

Bhardwaj, Ruby. 2010. 'Medical Pluralism in India: The Interface Complementary and Alternative Therapies with Allopathy. In *Health, Illness and Medicine: Ethnographic Readings*, ed. Arima Mishra, 30–60. New Delhi: Orient BlackSwan.

Bode, Maarten, and G. Hariramamurthi. 2014. 'Integrating Folk Healers in India's Public Health: Acceptance, Legitimacy, and Emancipation'. *Journal of Indian Medicine* 7: 1–20.

Brahmi, P., R. P. Dua and B. S. Dhillon. 2004. 'The Biological Diversity Act of India and Agro-Biodiversity Management'. *Current Science* 86(5): 659–64.

Brass, P. 1972. 'The Politics of Ayurvedic Education: A Case Study of Revivalism and Modernization in India'. In *Education and Politics in India: Studies in Organization, Society, and Policy*, eds S. H. Rudolph and L. I. Rudolph, 342–71. New York: Harvard University Press.

Cant, Sarah, and Ursula Sharma. 1999. *New Medical Pluralism?: Alternative Medicine, Doctors, Patients and the State*. London: UCL Press.

Chawla, J. 2013. 'Outcaste women, cast-out birth knowledge'. In *Multiple Voices and Stories: Narratives of Health and Illness*, eds A. Mishra and S. Chopra Chatterjee, 75-93. New Delhi: Orient BlackSwan.

Gaudilliere, Jean-Paul. 2014. 'An Indian Path to Biocapital?: The Traditional Knowledge Digital Library, Drug Patents, and the Reformulation Regime of Contemporary Ayurveda'. *East Asian Science, Technology, and Society* 8(4): 391–415.

Haraway, Donna. 1997. *Modest_Witness@Second_Millennium.FemaleMan©Meets_OncoMouse™: Feminism and Technoscience*. New York: Routledge.

Harding, Sandra (ed.). 1993. *The "Racial" Economy of Science: Toward a Democratic Future*. Bloomington: Indiana University Press.

Jeeva. 2010. 'Entering the Dai's World'. Report of Jeeva pilot project. Available at http://www.jeevaresearch.org/pilot-project.php (accessed 16 January 2016).

Joshi, P. C. 1995. 'Don't let me down: Place of worms in culture and reflections on ethno-physiology in a central Himalayan tribe'. *Journal of Indian Anthropological Society* 30: 253–58.

_____. 2016. 'Emergence of Medical Anthropology in India'. *The Eastern Anthropologist* 69: 1–11.

Kala, Chandra Prakash. 2005. 'Current Status of Medicinal Plants Used by Traditional Vaidyas in Uttaranchal State of India'. *Ethnobotany Research and Applications* 3: 267–78.

Lambert, H. 1992. 'The Cultural Logic of Indian Medicine: Prognosis and Etiology in Rajasthani Popular Therapeutics'. *Social Science and Medicine* 34: 1069–76.

_____. 2012. 'Medical Pluralism and Medical Marginality: Bone Doctors and the Selective Legitimation of Therapeutic Expertise in India'. *Social Science and Medicine* 74(7): 1029–36.

Langford, Jean. 2003. 'Traces of Folk Medicine in Jaunpur'. *Cultural Anthropology* 18(3): 271–303.

Latour, Bruno. 1987. *Science in Action: How to Follow Scientists and Engineers through Society*. New York: Harvard University Press.

_____. 2007. *Reassembling the Social: An Introduction to Actor-network-theory*. Oxford: Oxford University Press.

Leslie, Charles (ed.). 1976. *Asian Medical Systems*. Berkeley: University of California Press.

_____. 1980. 'Medical Pluralism in World Perspective'. *Social Science and Medicine* 148: 191–95.

_____. 1992. 'Interpretations of Illness: Syncretism in Modern Ayurveda'. In *Paths to Asian Medical Knowledge*, eds Charles Leslie and Allan Young, 177–208. Berkeley: University of California Press.

Martin, Emily. 2012. 'Grafting Together Medical Anthropology, Feminism, and Technoscience'. In *Medical Anthropology at the Intersections: Histories, Activisms, and Futures*, eds Marcia C. Inhorn and Emily A. Wentzell, 23–40. Durham and London: Duke University Press.

Minocha, Aneeta. 1980. 'Medical Pluralism and Health Services in India'. *Social Science and Medicine* 14(4): 217–23.

Mishra, M. K., and R. Dutta (eds). 2003. 'Base Line Information on Medicinal Plants Conservation and Sustainable Utilization: Uttaranchal'. Sponsored by UNDP/GEF, MoEF, Government of India and coordinated by FRLHT.

Mol, Annemarie. 2003. *The Body Multiple: Ontology in Medical Practice*. Durham, NC: Duke University Press.

Nakazora, Moe. 2009a. 'An Anthropological Approach to the Making of Property-owning Subjects: From Rights to Relations [Shoyu no shutai seisei no purosesu o meguru jinruigakuteki shiron: kenri kara kankeisei]'. *Bunkajinruigaku* [Japanese Journal of Cultural Anthropology] 74(1): 73–85.

———. 2009b. 'Cultural Anthropological Analysis on Subject Formation in "Herbal State" Policy of Uttarkhand: Based on Field Research in the Project Sites of Centre for Aromatic Plants (CAP)'. Research report submitted to Centre for Aromatic Plants (CAP), Herbal Research Development Institute (HRDI), Uttarakhand.

———. 2015. 'Pure Gifts for Future Benefit?: Giving Form to the Subject in a Biodiversity Databasing Project in India'. *NatureCulture* 3: 106–21.

———. 2016. 'Infrastructural Inversion and Reflexivity: A "Postcolonial" Biodiversity Databasing Project in India'. In *Infrastructures and Social Complexity*, eds Penny Harvey, Casper Bruun Jensen and Atsuro Morita, 309–23. New York: Routledge.

———. 2017. 'Temporalities in Translation: The Making and Unmaking of "Folk" Ayurveda and Bio-cultural Diversity in India'. In *The World Multiple*, eds Keiichi Omura, Shiho Satsuka, Atsuro Morita and Grant Jun Otsuki, 140–54. New York: Routledge.

National Biodiversity Authority. 2008. 'People's Biodiversity Register: Simplified Methodology'. Government of India.

———. 2010. 'Report for Minutes of the State Biodiversity Board Interactive and Review Meeting (28 and 29 April 2010)'. Government of India.

Nichter, Mark (ed). 1992. *Anthropological Approaches to the Study of Ethnomedicine*. Philadelphia: Gordon and Breach Science Publishers.

Parry, J. 1986. 'The Gift, the Indian Gift and the "Indian Gift"'. *Man, New Series* 21(3): 453–73.

Priya, Ritu. 2013. 'The Status and Role of AYUSH and Local Health Traditions in Public Health'. Newsletter of the International Institute of Asian Studies no. 65, Focus Traditional Indian Medicine, 24–25.

Raheja, G. 1988. *The Poison in the Gift: Ritual, Prestation, and the Dominant Caste in a North Indian Village*. Chicago: University of Chicago Press.

Rajan, Kaushik. 2006. *Biocapital: The Constitution of Post-Genomic Life*. Durham, NC: Duke University Press.

Raje, Gauri. 2012. 'The Modernizing Bhagat'. In *Medical Marginality in South Asia*, eds D. Hariman and P. Mukharji, 152–70. London: Routledge.

Reddy, D. 2007. 'Good Gifts for the Common Good: Blood and Bioethics in the Market of Genetic Research'. *Cultural Anthropology* 22(3): 429–72.

Riles, Annelise. 2001. *The Network Inside Out*. Ann Arbor: University of Michigan Press.

Sadgopal, Mira. 2013. 'Towards Recognition of Traditional Midwives (Dias): The Jeeva Study'. Newsletter of the International Institute of Asian Studies no. 65, Focus Traditional Indian Medicine, 26.

Saxena, A., S. Roy and K. P. Tripathi. 2002. 'Indian Traditional Knowledge: New Attempts for Fortification and Globalization'. *Journal of Medicinal and Aromatic Plant Sciences* 30: 340–43.

Scambler, Graham. 2002. *Health and Social Change: A Critical Theory*. Buckingham: Open University Press.

Shiva, Vandana. 1997. *Biopiracy: The Plunder of Nature and Knowledge*. Brooklyn: South End Press.

Singh, D., R. K. Srivastava and V. P. Khanduri. 2005. 'Marketing Strategies and Trade of Medicinal Plants in Uttaranchal: Present and Future Prospects'. *Indian Forester* 131(3): 438–48.

Sujatha, V. 2007. 'Pluralism in Indian Medicine: Medical Lore as a Genre of Medical Knowledge'. *Contributions to Indian Sociology* 41(2): 169–202.

Sujatha, V., and Leena Abraham (eds). 2012. *Medical Pluralism in Contemporary India*. Hyderabad: Orient BlackSwan.

Trawick, Margaret. 1992. 'Death and Nurturance in Indian Systems of Healing'. In *Paths to Asian Medical Knowledge*, eds Charles Leslie and Allan Young, 129–59. Berkeley: University of California Press.

Turner, Bryan. 2004. *The New Medical Sociology: Social Forms of Health and Illness*. New York: W. W. Norton and Company.

Utkarsh, Ghate. 1999. 'People's Biodiversity Register'. COMPAS newsletter, October, 16–17.

Young, James. 1981. 'Non-use of Physicians: Methodological Approaches, Policy Implications, and the Utility of Decision Models'. *Social Science and Medicine* 15B: 499–507.

Zhan, Mei. 2009. *Other-Worldly: Making Chinese Medicine through Transnational Frames*. Durham, NC: Duke University Press.

eight

Documentation of Traditional Health Knowledge

To What End?

Arima Mishra and Devaki Nambiar

Documentation and codification of traditional knowledge has emerged as an important initiative for several countries including India, Korea, China and those in Africa that boast of a rich heritage of such knowledge, specifically in the context of a global intellectual property regime and the Rio de Janeiro declaration on conservation of biodiversity, sustainable use and equal distribution of benefits (Correa 2001; Johnson 2002; McNulty 2012; Poorna, et al. 2014; Wekundah 2012). Thus, globally, documentation has emerged as an important armour to preserve and protect traditional knowledge including traditional medical knowledge. Following the World Intellectual Property Organization's (WIPO)[1] guidelines on preservation (documentation and promotion of knowledge) and protection (against misuse), several countries have set up mechanisms to protect and preserve traditional knowledge in their respective country contexts. The TKDL in India is one such initiative that emerged as a follow-up of revocation of patents in turmeric and *neem* (Gupta 2005; Poorna, et al. 2014). Documentation in a form that is accessible to an international audience is a key feature of the TKDL, which records information in five foreign languages for ease of patent examination in international settings. The intention of this is to prevent misappropriation and misuse of traditional knowledge.

While the TKDL may have emerged as a response to the immediate threat of bio-piracy, there have been other efforts and recent initiatives by the State to document specifically the non-codified forms of knowledge called local health traditions/folk medicine as reflected in the State policy texts. As stated in the Introduction to this volume, the Indian Systems of Medicine and Homeopathy (Government of India 2002) acknowledges the knowledge available with the individuals, communities and tribes, which needs to be fully tapped, documented and validated. The policy expresses concern over the erosion—a natural yet human-prone geographic process—of knowledge in the face of the unfinished agenda of documentation. While this agenda gets reinforced in the NRHM document (Government of India 2005), the Draft National Health Policy (Government of India 2015) has sought to take it further, to articulate the need for documentation and validation for multiple objectives. These objectives range from empowering marginalised groups to realising the potential of India as a world leader in drug discovery to institutionalising medical pluralism as a value in guiding India's health policies. In all these cases, local health traditions are nested within the larger stated logic of 'mainstreaming AYUSH', as evidenced in the following excerpts from the Draft National Health Policy (ibid.).[2]

> The contribution of several organizations across the country is also visible in documenting, validating and promoting home and community based traditional practices and practitioners, especially *providing recognition* to the special knowledge held by various caste groups and adivasis, thereby *empowering the marginalized groups* (emphasis added). (ibid.: 10)
>
> India's strengths in AYUSH can also be leveraged for becoming a world leader in drug discovery as also in integrative medicine and this needs not only research as pure and applied science but also creating institutional structures for *documentation, validation and accreditation of community health practices and practitioners* (emphasis added). (ibid.: 11)
>
> ... *Pluralism*: Patients who so choose and when appropriate, would have access to AYUSH care providers based on validated local health traditions. These systems would also have Government support and supervision to develop and enrich their contribution to meeting the national health goals and objectives. *Research, development of models of integrative practice, efforts at documentation, validation of traditional practices and engagement with such practitioners would form important elements of enabling medical pluralism* (emphasis added). (ibid.: 12)

As seen here, these pronouncements point to at least three rationales—the recognition of subaltern knowledge, which in turn can be seen to empower the otherwise marginalised communities possessing it; the creation of institutional structures for community practices and practitioners; and thereby, the enablement of medical pluralism. As can be seen here, multiple communities—the marginalised, the general, the local and the global—are implicated in the project of pluralising medicine. These actors, rationales and objectives are appealing as it is perhaps rare for any health policy to provide devoted space to non-codified health knowledge, practices and their practitioners. Yet one needs to exercise caution, as each of these objectives, that is, empowerment of marginalised communities, role in drug discovery and pluralism as value, evokes different kinds of demands on the processes and outcomes of documentation. For example, while India's role in drug discovery would necessarily subject the documentation process and products to standardised, biomedically codified parameters of evidence (clinical trials, phytochemical tests, etc.), the pluralism objective connotes the contrary—acknowledgement and accommodation of plural forms of evidence in the spirit of dialogue and enquiry.

These ambitiously stated rationales, however, are absent in the final version of the National Health Policy (Government of India 2017). Somewhat ambivalent and ambiguously, this policy advocates for research and validation of tribal medicines within the larger objective of strengthening primary health services. Halfway through the policy, we see another statement under Item 9: Mainstreaming the Potential of AYUSH:

> ... the development of sustainable livelihood systems through involving local communities and establishing forward and backward market linkages in processing of medicinal plants will also be supported by this policy. The policy seeks to strengthen steps for farming of herbal plants. Developing mechanisms for certification of 'prior knowledge' of traditional community health care providers and engaging them in the conservation and generation of the raw materials required, as well as creating opportunities for enhancing their skills are part of this policy. (ibid.: 15)

Prior knowledge among local practitioners/healers has to be 'validated', 'researched', and 'certified' and 'conserved'. The intent of this policy begins with research and validation of plants. For practitioners, there is certification, engagement in conservation of raw materials and opportunities for skill enhancement. Practitioners must on the one hand preserve raw materials, but need also have their skills enhanced. Yet, this stated intent is a step up from such knowledge and practice considered illegal/quackery (by the State)—it affords tribal medicine and other traditions a kind of primordial value that has to be recast in contemporary reality. This chapter closely follows this context of the policy intent and the myriad efforts by the State as well as NGOs and research organisations involved in the documentation of local health traditions as part of a larger strategy of revitalisation by examining objectives, processes (methodologies) and outputs of documentation. Foregrounding the views of the traditional healers, it discusses the who, what and why of documentation.

This chapter draws on data collected as part of the larger study on policy lessons of and for the revitalisation of local health traditions: an ethnographic study (2014–16).[3] The methodology involves (a) discourse analysis of policy texts, (b) in-depth interviews with NGO (involved in revitalisation of local health traditions) representatives, academic experts and traditional healers (N = 120), case studies built around 10 healers (practising through the generations) with repeated follow-ups, and (c) observations of practices of healing, meetings of folks healers' associations/sangams and tribal conclaves (N = 15). We focus specifically on data collected in the two states of Karnataka and Tamil Nadu in the southern part of India.

Who Documents?: 'Documentation Cannot be Everybody's Business'

Our modest effort at mapping existing documentation efforts indicates the involvement of a range of stakeholders. These include governmental AYUSH institutions (research and teaching), national and state biodiversity boards, university departments (pharmacy, botany, forestry, life sciences), NGOs, regional centres of ICMR, state knowledge commissions, as well as smaller collectives and individual research studies drawing on researchers from diverse disciplines. Some efforts are part of a long trajectory of work, while most others are *ad hoc* or one-off exercises. The former are crystallised through forging alliances among different partners anchored by a bigger NGO and/or government department/ institution (AYUSH, Department of Forest). For example, FLRHT has steered the documentation of local health traditions through several local partner organisations, including community-based organisations (CBO), NGOs, local communities and with the support of state forest departments, in the southern states of India in the late 1990s (Hafeel, et al. 2004a, 2004b; Unnikrishnan and Hariramurthi 2012).[4] Other such alliances in the state of Kerala are discussed by Madhavan and Lal in Chapter 6 of this volume. The Ministry of AYUSH has recently been supporting documentation efforts by local NGOs, as well as more unique research collectives like the Jeeva Project, which seeks to understand the perspective of traditional midwives.[5]

In response to an upfront question on who should/could document local health traditions, the traditional healers (*paramparika/nati vaidyas*) interviewed in our research study categorically stated that they themselves should do it and/or be closely involved in the process as important stakeholders than as mere informants. There are two important rationales for this. First, the healers drew attention to the composite body of such knowledge, explicable and knowable only through practice. The apprenticeship mode of training for intergenerational/interpersonal transfer that rests on extensive observations, use of senses and gradual induction into the practice of local health knowledge bears significance in this context.[6] Healers spoke of how such knowledge is linked to the local ecology, cosmos, culture and biodiversity. One of the healers explained in an interview:

> Documentation cannot be done by anyone. Those who practise the knowledge need to be involved in documentation. How can someone who does not know the context and has never practised the knowledge even understand what it is all about and document? (A fourth-generation healer, Karnataka)

> Documentation is very important for the next generation. When we leave, our knowledge will go with us. The plants about which are written in the books are available to everyone, but the vaidya picks plants by smell, by taste and by touch. Hence, documentation needs to be done by healers. There are healers' associations that can be roped in for this purpose. (A third-generation healer, Tamil Nadu)

The second rationale submitted by healers for their involvement in the documentation process was that such knowledge, as much as the process of acquisition, training and practice, is considered sacred. Sacredness is linked to the value orientation within which local health tradition is practised. Such knowledge and its practice are characterised by a *service* orientation. Thus, as healers emphatically explained, not everyone can legitimately inherit, convey or even possess such knowledge. Only those who have the calling, as well as passion, sincerity, dedication and perseverance, can learn to practise local health traditions. Not everyone even within the same family can be a candidate for training in local health traditions. Such reasoning is not peculiar to the Indian context but prevails in other Asian countries, including China (Hsu 1999). Such attributes are extended to those who document it as well. Documentation without a real appreciation of such knowledge and/or commercial and profit motive sits uncomfortably with local health traditions, which are driven by notions of service or 'seva'. Thus, for the healers, documentation is no mere material exercise of cataloguing information. A healer thus summed up the concern:

> Documentation of local health knowledge cannot be everybody's business. Someone who is sincere, dedicated and who has a respect and passion for such knowledge can and should document. It should not go into the hands of those with selfish motives. (A fifth-generation healer, Karnataka)

Healers whose families had been practising for generations talked about *gharana-parampara* (a specific family lineage), which has been handed down through the generations using mostly family manuscripts (referred to as *mane pustaka* in Karnataka). Thus, documentation of local health knowledge was being done by family members themselves for internal use or when imparting knowledge to a disciple outside the family. Recently, we came across individual healers who have published books in regional languages for larger circulation in the local communities. The print media has always been an important site for the articulation and revival of indigenous medicine (Girija 2017). The current discourse and demand for documentation does not take such efforts into consideration. Though greatly valuing the role of various institutions, university departments and individual researchers in documentation, some healers expressed concern over an externally induced model of documentation, which relies on a survey technique of asking a series of questions on names of plants and remedies and a process and product that decontextualises the meanings and practices associated with that knowledge.[7]

What and How of Knowledge Documentation: 'Not Everything Can be Documented'

This section discusses the methodological processes involved in documentation, eliciting different kinds of engagement with healers/

knowledge holders ranging from mere one-off informants to closely participating in the processes of dialogue and exchange of knowledge to being the sole architects of documentation.

Considering the diversity of efforts and actors involved in documentation, methodological processes expectedly differed. One set of documentation efforts was in the nature of ethno-botanical/ethno-biological or ethno-medicinal surveys, not only in India but also in other contexts (Nair 1995; Rajasab 2011; Saranappa and Vidyasagar 2014; Sen, et al. 2008; Teklehaymanot and Giday 2007),[8] carried out by individual researchers or academic institutions. Such surveys focused on the name of medicinal plants, its parts, collection and the nature of ailment they were used for by the community. This also entailed recording of cultural practices and beliefs that guided the use of plant medicines or others. Usually, such information was elicited through rapport building with one or a community of healers through intermediaries (healer associations, government forestry departments or local government officials). The information was recorded through semi-structured interviews. These were published as books and journals for audiences in the field of botany, ethno-pharmacy, the life sciences or physical anthropology. The intent of these surveys was typically to publicise the local health knowledge as it is practised, pointing towards its potential for further phyto-chemical or phyto-pharmacology research to address public health concerns. Such studies did not involve further validation of such knowledge. The intent is to give a voice and ear to the knowledge shared by the local communities.

A second type of documentation largely followed the guidelines and methodology of government research councils in India. Such methodology relied on collection of knowledge on medicinal plants, their properties and treatment, with dual validation by both the sciences of botany and ayurveda. It was usually undertaken by a team consisting of representatives of AYUSH institutions, the forest department, botanists, and ayurveda practitioners. Names of hundreds and thousands of healers are identified and recorded in the states that we worked in. Such surveys identify eligible healers whose knowledge is to be documented through various informants, including the forest guards, community health workers and through snowball sampling. Survey questionnaire included information on the knowledge of plant, its parts, local name, scientific name and textual name, name of the healer, and mode of preparation and the specific ailment treated. Some of these were strictly in the form of medicinal plants survey alone. Healers mattered to the extent of identifying the names and use of medicinal plants and, thus, were projected as valuable informants.[9] Notwithstanding this, such methodologies were sometimes marked by suspicion (about the motive of those who document and oblivious to the objectives of documentation) and lack of trust. As a senior ayurvedic personnel involved in documentation shared with us:

> It is hard to collect all the relevant information. Healers might be using 4–5 ingredients but while sharing, they will leave out one of these. Sometimes they are able to tell only the local name and don't show the plant. It is difficult then to identify the scientific name. Without this, it is difficult to document. This will be incomplete documentation. Healers are also hesitant as they feel their knowledge might get misused. (Senior personnel involved in documentation in Karnataka)

Further, another government personnel candidly acknowledged:

> Actually such surveys are not an efficient means of collecting data. One needs to do a more anthropological (ethnographic) kind of research of spending time, observing, gaining the trust of the community and sharing with them the objectives, processes and products of documentation. Then only documentation can be trustworthy and useful.

Apart from incompleteness of information shared, such a mode of documentation screened and recast knowledge through validation. Thus, only that information on medicinal plants which had a reference in ayurvedic pharmacopeia passed the test of eligibility for recording. In the absence of such validation, documentation was considered meaningless. As explained by a senior government personnel, 'Basic validation is done here from ayurvedic pharmacopeia. If information is not validated, we do not pass on this information to the AYUSH department.' Another official added:

> The total number of diseases recorded for which medicinal plants were used was 55. They (traditional healers) had their own language for describing diseases. We had to correlate to the disease that was mentioned in our shastras (classical texts). There were uncommon uses of common medicinal plants, one for jaundice. Some traditional healers gave information worthy of a clinical trial.

As these testimonies demonstrate, the knowledge that was both worthy and visible to them was that which dialogued with existing codified systems of medicine or met the eligibility requirements of clinical, biomedical evidence, that is, clinical trials. In this way, documentation was, by design, supplanting local health traditions in a format and language that suited the socialisers of codified systems of medicine (AYUSH or biomedicine). As Torri and Laplante (2009) write, such validation is intended to convert the language of local health traditions to established systems of medicine for greater acceptance of the former, but in the process it may run the risk of creating false dichotomies of subjective-objective and scientific-experiential evidence, unless the methodologies accommodate different modes of evidence and the healers are as much important as stakeholders as the AYUSH/biomedicine team. Such validation often leads to a new and reinvented knowledge, which may speak to a different set of audience (local traders, pharmaceutical companies and the new elite, who can capitalise on herbal medicine products). Given this litany of requirements and users, validation has never been an easy or simple task, particularly in the rub between AYUSH and biomedicine—where there was clearly a tension not just between these two, but what that tension meant for the practice of local health traditions. One of the senior personnel from a government biomedical research centre reflected thus:

> We have some data with us, we are getting new data. But we don't know what to do further. Because one way people are saying scientific validation/ scientific assessment should be done. What is scientific assessment? That is again a question. Because again going to molecule phytochemicals, how they act, pharmacodynamics, pharmacokinetics is a kind of drug development. But for traditional practice where they are mixing so many plants together and looking at synergic activity, it is not possible. So what, we cannot go to clinical trials even though it is time tested and people are using it. For scientific evaluation, that is not the base.
>
> We don't know where to draw [a] line between [the] science part and [the] usage part. What science is to modern science is not science to ayurveda. If you say to isolate a compound and see the chemical activity. It is not a way of ayurveda which is based on synergetic actions. So pharmaco-kinetic will not work for single disease, single molecule for single conditions. If we cannot do that, then where is science? Because everybody says scientific evaluation is necessary ... Practice is entirely different from plant or compound. Again we need to think about practice or product. If we have to look into product, then pipeline is completely different. For practice, [the] approach is entirely different. What exactly we are looking at we don't know ... Revitalisation approach with product development and community empowerment have different approaches.

Healers we spoke to, while fully empathising with the efforts of the government, did share this concern about delimiting the scope of local health traditions in the form of registers of plants and remedies. They categorically state that local health traditions needed to be documented as community-based health knowledge, and not merely by botanic properties or nosologies of disease. The points of tension here were between documenting local health traditions in a format (capturing the immediate and tangible forms of knowledge) that rendered it bounded and limiting, while many healers would draw attention to the expansive nature of local health traditions, where worshipping the god of the forest (*vana debta*) is as important as the preparation and dispensation of herbs as well as other ritual prayers, chanting of hymns, diet (including the role of specific seasons) and other aspects of lifestyle. In this view, the forest as the source of healing properties (medicinal herbs) was sacred, as collection of plants was integral to conservation and replenishment in the practice of local health traditions. It only followed that there were elaborate rules about modes, timing, techniques of collection of herbs and their preparation, which the healers shared with us in the general terms they felt were integral to understanding, acquiring and recording knowledge (Nambiar and Mishra 2017). Harmony was an epistemological principle in local health traditions (as in AYUSH), of the individual body with the symbolic as well as body politic. The healers, hence, contest the narrow and confining vision of documentation, admittedly the first and easiest attempt that limits focus on the tangible, that is, medicinal plants (name, usage and ailments), and possibly excludes those whose practice may not exclusively rely on medicinal plants alone (for example, bone-setters or dais).

Why Document?: 'Documentation Must be Linked to Practice'

The key issue at stake has always been: Why document? The methodologies speak directly to the objective and rationale of the documentation process. The healers we spoke to were sceptical about the documentation exercises that transport the knowledge either to a library or the filing cabinet of a government department. They felt that the who, what and how of documentation needed to be aligned with the objectives linked to the continuing practice of such knowledge. As one of the healers in Karnataka put it:

> Documentation cannot be a mode of revitalisation of LHT if this is not linked to its practice. Everyone values such knowledge and documents it, no one is bothered about us, the knowledge holders. Our knowledge is valued but not us. We are not recognised as legitimate practitioners and are continuously harassed by either AYUSH officials or the police. Somewhere the objective of the documentation is either not clear or misplaced.

This was, in fact, echoed by a senior proponent of revitalisation of local health traditions (trained in AYUSH). He said:

> There will be real documentation when the documented knowledge is transferred/taught to the next generations. Like the use of tulasi plant shouldn't only be documented but it should be taught to the next generation in a practical manner.

Such a concern is shared and seriously taken up by the Amazonian tribal community, the Matsé people of Peru and Brazil, who have prepared their own 500-page encyclopaedia of their medicinal knowledge. Here, the elderly *Shamans* (five of them) were the sole architects of this exercise. The objective for documentation for the Matsé community was clear and simple—to improve and ensure health and health care through the use of local resources and remedies (Hance 2015). Thus, the community's objective of self-reliance was explicit. The need for documentation was not so much bio-piracy, but the erosion of this knowledge, as typified by the fact that one of the elderly Shamans died without systematic transfer of his knowledge. This was the turning point for this isolated and confined community, the Matsés, to seriously think of documentation. What methodology did they adopt? What circumstances, local and contextual, shaped this turn of events? The fact that documentation was done so that this knowledge is continued in practice is loud and clear and, hence, this was done in the mentorship and apprenticeship model, where each Shaman was attached to an apprentice (a younger educated member of the community), who learned while documenting. Thus, the methodology is a practice-based documentation, which documents all aspects of the knowledge-practice. Repeated conversations and discussions of the drafts happen among the entire Shamans' team as well as the Acaté (the conservation organisation) that facilitates this. The content follows categorisation of disease, learning of symptoms of the specific disease, its causes, which plants to use and how, and the mode of preparation of medicines and other therapeutic options. Since it is written by the Matsé themselves, the language embodies the worldview of the community, drawing on the interconnectedness of life and healing. Hence, medicinal knowledge is not independent of rainforest conservation, which defines life for many of these communities. Is such an encyclopaedia limiting because of the potential of drug discovery to address global public health problems? Christopher Herdon (2015, cited in Hance 2015), the Acaté representative, in an interview succinctly put it as, 'Comparatively, we live in a world of health care abundance. If there is to be a dialogue, in my view it should begin with how we can support them in the present rather than how they can help us in the future' (Hance 2015). Healers in our study repeatedly shared the spirit of such a documentation exercise and drew our attention to the mode of learning and ways of knowing through gradual initiation into the world of practice. It is true that such a mode of documentation might work better with communities that are in some sense bounded. Yet, this documentation effort reinforces the importance of having clarity in objectives of documentation, involving the healers themselves in this exercise, as well as linking documentation of knowledge to its practice.

Documentation of Local Health Knowledge as a Space for Pluralism?

If documentation is an expression of the recognition of the value of local health tradition, what kind of documentation efforts instil the spirit of pluralism? Is documentation by itself anomalous to the spirit of pluralism? While several well-meaning efforts establish the need for layered validation of local/community health knowledge, there are others which conceive of documentation in the spirit of a dialogue and provide a space for pluralism (in spirit and practice) of different systems and practices of knowledge. These efforts, as we discuss below, are a response to the limitation of the externally induced, top-down models of approaching local health knowledge. We discuss some of these initiatives and how these advance our understanding of medical pluralism.

Documentation is a Social Process: RALHT

While for many efforts, the process has been to identify, establish rapport and elicit information on the practice, several other initiatives have taken active steps to make documentation 'participatory', taking into consideration the worldviews, contexts and taxonomy of local health traditions.[10] FRLHT, since the 1990s, has been involved in experimenting with a participatory process of documentation, seeking to adopt a bottom-up approach to the process (Hafeel, et al. 2004a). The model, called Rapid Assessment of Local Health Tradition (RALHT), sought to address some of the concerns of the 'externally driven', top-down documentation process. RALHT, to begin with, privileged community local health priorities, commonly used remedies and their notions of efficacy as the starting point. In terms of knowledge, it documented the 'expert' knowledge of the healers and the more diffuse or miscellaneous knowledge residing within households. Along with details of medicinal plants, its properties and uses, RALHT took into account information on their economic and social contexts.

After elaborate documentation of local priority conditions, symptoms, diagnosis and mode of treatment, the second stage entailed validation by a team consisting of AYUSH/modern systems of medicine and healers. Information that is passed by the former gets validated and scope for further research is identified, and those that cannot get validated are set aside, calling for more research. It is at this stage that local health traditions encounter the language of standardisation and codification. Limitations notwithstanding, as Torri and Laplante (2009) have documented in Tamil Nadu, such a mode of documentation has allowed innovations in building ethno-medicine capacity managed by local community-level networks.

FRLHT's documentation exercise had multiple objectives. These include the protection of traditional knowledge as much as its active promotion in the community itself (specifically the younger generation) and sustenance through exploring livelihood opportunities, thus making local health traditions commercially viable too. Validation had a dual-purpose: to identify (a) sound health practices for promotion in the community, and (b) a product in future for potential larger use. On the former, validated practices were promoted in the community through herbal kitchen gardens and community health registers, with details on how to use local resources (herbs and others) to address common ailments. In such a model, the community healers were not merely informants. Rather, their worldviews represented a given community's notions of efficacy as a yardstick for consideration, though the validation process was not necessarily an overly technical exercise. One of the senior personnel involved in developing the RALHT methodology shared that validation has more than a technical aspect to it:

> The validation which we did through AYUSH had technical side to it but the main function is to build confidence in the healers. The validation spoke as much to the AYUSH/State as to the healers and community themselves. This confidence would allow healers to practise their healing without any fear (of being illegal or inferior). So it is like a public marriage. When a marriage takes place in front of so many people, the collective presence legitimises the couple's status. It is the same logic for why one needs to validate. Validation would also help to scale up the practice and the use of knowledge.

Thus, documentation in this regard is a social process serving social legitimacy than merely being tested for efficacy through given standards in biomedicine or AYUSH alone.

Documentation a Mode of 'Active Listening': Jeeva

The Jeeva (translated as 'life') project (2010) was led by a team of feminist researchers seeking to advance a participatory ethos in a manner that is non-hierarchical, consciously privileging the voices of the *dais* through an 'active listening' approach (the report is aptly titled, 'Entering the Dai's World'). Jeeva is not strictly a documentation project; it is a research initiative that seeks to strengthen the dai system of knowledge and practice, enabling their linkage to formal health care services.[11] Its approach of empathy and active listening was significant for the pluralism space as the team had people trained in biomedicine (gynaecology and paediatrics) as much as social science and the humanities. 'We agreed upon the need to elicit the dais' experiences, perspectives and assessments and to accept their words as given. As little empathetic research on *dais* exist, it was important to refrain from trying to prove something or to test whether it works' (Jeeva 2010: 10). The documentation process (with elaborate open-ended questions relating to learning and becoming a dai, practice of the skills, handling of complications, continuum of care and specific challenges) took care to capture the non-tangible aspects of their knowledge and practice that dais explain through demonstrations. Such demonstrations as non-verbal communications were seen as important, both to avoid risks of premature translation into the existing language of medicine and to understand a hands-on art that involves senses of sight, touch and feel. This is very different from an exercise of documentation that separates knowledge from the worldviews and contexts in which it is practised and assumes a singular way of knowing and learning. The ritual aspects that play an important role in midwifery were given as much importance as the technique of placenta stimulation, thus bringing the physical therapeutics and metaphysical aspects together. Thus, photography, as much as oral text, was an important mode to capture the knowledge and practice of the dais. The documentation in this case was a dialogical process, where the research team and the dais presented the knowledge (to a larger public) in a language that was legible to others but not at the cost of excluding any aspect of the dais' knowledge. What this methodology advances to our understanding of documentation is that while many aspects of the dais' knowledge and practice had references to existing literature, including ayurveda, and could, thus, be 'validated' (ibid.: 35–43), included in the record was also knowledge that was at the time beyond the codification or fathoming of current medical sciences and public health. The detailed documentation of placenta stimulation to revive neonates was one such contribution to knowledge on maternal health. Through a dialogical process, the Jeeva team could document the best practices that have continued relevance, while cautioning against some of the limitations of the dais' practice (ibid.: 75).

Documentation Process as a Cooperative Enquiry: Shodhini

Furthering a participatory and empowering methodology, the Shodhini experiment in Tamil Nadu propounds a research lens on seeking to understand and document women healers' knowledge on health that rests on 'cooperative enquiry whose goal, as it seeks, truth must be the empowerment of women' (Khanna 2004: 4). Shodhini was facilitated by a group consisting of several grassroots organisations and women's health activists under the banner of Action Research on Alternative Medicine and Women's Health. Shodhini sought to understand women healers, their herbal and non-herbal practices in relation to common women's health problems, and 'to help women take charge of their bodies through a process of self-help so that they understand the body, its rhythms as well as its power' (ibid.: 2). The research and documentation process here had an explicit objective of allowing women to have greater control over their own bodies, health and healing. Thus, here documentation did not aim to mainstream or conform to established systems of medicine, rather to see this as an alternative to the dominant systems, namely allopathy. Through a range of workshops eliciting women's stories, observations, select physical examination and illustrations, women's common health problems were identified. Information sheets on the use of plants were collected, based on the healers' information, and referenced through existing data by members of the Shodhini team. The field testing of the herbs (for which there is reference in ayurvedic literature) was done by the community members (self-help groups) with the Shodhini team. The specific use of herbs and experiences in treating specific ailments and the limits to such experiences were not merely documented but diagnosed. For example, the treatment of vaginal infections could not prove to be effective (as per the women's experiences) despite the use of herbs because of the specific circumstances of women's everyday lives (lack of nutritious diet, continued stress, lack of cooperation from their husbands who never used condoms). Thus, herbal practices could not have been looked at in isolation.

Since Shodhini largely framed itself as feminist action research, the cooperative inquiry developed an innovative mode of enquiry. It witnessed the coming together of the folk, classical and modern systems of medicine not in a hierarchy, but acknowledging that all forms of knowledge, including biomedicine, is socially constructed and it operates in a subjective-objective reality (Gupta, et al. 1997). The spirit of reflection in engaging with different knowledge systems in such a process of documentation itself was empowering for women when health became the subject of discussion and concern. Validation, thus, entailed three stages: ascertainment of wide use, reference in standard ayurvedic classical texts and triangulation based on women's experiences with the use of these plants-based medicines. The continuous dialogues among these three modes of knowledge helped as much to look for local sustainable solutions to women's health problems as to identify toxicity and, thus, the harmful effects of some of the herbs. Shodhini admits that it is not the scale (as the work could be done on limited plants and practices for specific known ailments), but the idea itself that has important ramifications, nurturing many barefoot gynaecologists who render women's health visible and heal through locally available remedies in their respective communities.

Lessons from Documentation Efforts

This chapter has discussed myriad documentation efforts, which have important lessons to offer in light of the State's recent intent to revitalise local health traditions through documentation, codification, validation and promotion. Several documentation efforts supposedly suggest a turn towards the community (tribal) and their knowledge, thus revisiting the space that may have earlier been eschewed given its ritualistic superstitious nature, and the conception of it as being outside the boundary of the science of medicine. And yet, there is no one coherent narrative about why and how to document tribal medical knowledge; one wonders if the turn is to the community that holds and practices the knowledge *or* the ingredients or components of that knowledge (possibly independent of the context of practice and the community) to serve the needs of science (drug discovery). Lurking here is also the danger of fragmenting what are composite bodies of knowledge through efforts to capture it in terms of plants and remedies—a kind of disciplining that sequesters practice, while also articulating and amplifying a disjunction between knowledge and knowledge holders, and critically decoupling knowledge from practice. This (over)simplification abets the delay in documenting or recognising other aspects of the knowledge or the social context in which such knowledge is produced and practised (timing, space of collection of plants, prescriptions and proscriptions regarding diet, other aspects of lifestyle, chanting of hymns that are believed to add effectiveness to the therapeutic process). Ultimately, this serves to invisibilise these other forms and practices. Styles of knowing are deeply connected to styles of learning and the fact that social contexts of the practice of a specific body of knowledge matter (Hsu 1999). It is not surprising that healers themselves are deeply ill at ease with this. In many cases, healers are indifferent to this as perhaps they know the limits of documentation and harbour lower expectations than these intermediaries, the State or even us researchers.

In the context of pluralism, does documentation suggest acknowledgment of plural forms of knowledge (including tacit knowledge), modes of training and practice (the paramparaik mode of dissemination of knowledge) and ways of understanding of epistemology (rooted in local ecology), or are we instead homogenising by subscribing to established modes of understanding of science, evidence and medicine (either biomedicine or AYUSH)? Are we then missing out on revitalising the study of pluralism itself? At the core of it, the objectives of documentation need to have much more clarity. If community self-reliance, recognition and valuing of different forms of health knowledge are key to documentation and revitalisation, methodologies must be sensitive and empathetic to such forms of knowledge and knowledge holders. The language of validation and promotion need careful translations that should not exclude and slice the local health knowledge. Such translations require conversations across disciplinary and methodological boundaries, a fact that is increasingly being acknowledged (Garcia 2010; Srinidhi 2018). The experiences of Jeeva, Shodhini (both these are limited to women healers) and FRLHT offer select lessons to advance the understanding of engaging with plural forms of knowledge through more reflexive methodological processes.

Notes

1. Available at http://www.wipo.int/pressroom/en/briefs/tk_ip.html (accessed 1 June 2015).

2. The Draft National Health Policy was placed in the public domain for comments, suggestions and feedback before this was finalised and approved by the cabinet in 2017.

3. Details of the study are provided in the Introduction to the volume.

4. See Hariramamurthi (2000).

5. Available at www.ayush.gov.in/lhtschemes (accessed 11 April 2016).

6. For more details on the acquisition and transfer of knowledge, see Menon and Spudich (2015) and Hsu (1999).

7. Select healers in Tamil Nadu also discussed how revealing the names of plants risked diminishing the power of healing of these plants.

8. Journals like *Studies on Ethno-medicine, Journal of Ethnobiology and Ethnomedicine* and *Journal of Ethnopharmacology* have several such articles published.

9. The regional Indian Medical Research Centre at Belgaum in Karnataka has come up with a database of ethno-medicinal plants of the Western Ghats that documents 500 medicinal plants, addressing more than 200 ailments.

10. India is not alone in this. The Ara Irijita Project among the Anangu indigenous community in western and central Australia is a community-based multimedia digital archive, available at http://www.irititja.com/ (accessed 16 May 2016). It produces a living archive that seeks to address the needs and concerns of the present generation. Documentation involves the recording of the oral knowledge in multiple formats—photographs, artefacts, films, videos, sound recordings, etc. The project format (software) is developed in consultation with the community to reflect the local cultural specificities and categories of thought (gender-specific information, sacred and secular, etc.).

11. For details of this research initiative, see http://www.jeevaresearch.org (accessed 29 March 2014).

References

Bhange, P. V., and Y. S. Bhatambre. 2016. 'A Conceptual Overview of TKDL'. *International Journal of Ayurveda and Alternative Medicine* 4(2): 75–79.

Chakravarty, R. 2010. 'Preserving Traditional Knowledge: Initiatives in India'. *IFLA Journal* 36(4): 294.

Correa, C. M. 2001. 'Traditional Knowledge and Intellectual Property: Issues and Options Surrounding the Protection of Traditional Knowledge'. Discussion paper, QUNO, Geneva.

Fokunang, C. N., V. Ndikum, O. Y. Tabi, R. B. Jiofack, B. Ngameni, N. M. Guedje, E. A. Tembe-Fokunang, P. Tomkins, S. Barkwan, F. Kechia, E. Asongalem, J. Ngoupayou, N. J. Torimiro, K. H. Gonsu, V. Sielinou, B. T. Ngadjui, F. Angwafor III, A. Nkongmeneck, O. M. Abena, J. Ngogang, T. Asonganyi, V. Colizzi, J. Lohoue and Kamsu-Kom. 2011. 'Traditional Medicine: Past, Present and Future Research and Development Prospects and Integration in the National Health System of Cameroon'. *African Journal of Traditional, Complementary and Alternative Medicine* 8(3): 284–95.

Garcia, R. 2010. 'The Relevance of Traditional Knowledge Systems for Ethnopharmacological Research'. *Theoretical and Methodological Contributions* 6(32): 1–12.

Ghatapanadi, S. R., N. Johnson and A. H. Rajasab. 2011. 'Documentation of Medicinal Plants in Glubarga Region, Karnataka'. *Indian journal of Traditional Knowledge* 10(2): 349–53.

Girija, K. P. 2017. 'Interface with Media and Institutions: The Reordering of Indigenous Medical Practitioners in Twentieth-century Kerala'. *History and Sociology of South Asia* 11(1): 1–8.

Government of India. 2002. 'Indian Systems of Medicine and Homeopathy'. Ministry of Health and Family Welfare, New Delhi.

———. 2005. 'The National Rural Health Mission 2005–2012'. Ministry of Health and Family Welfare, New Delhi.

———. 2015. Draft National Health Policy, Ministry of Health and Family Welfare, Delhi. Available at https://www.mygov.in/frontendgeneral/pdf/draft-national-health-policy.pdf (accessed 3 November 2015).

———. 2017. National Health Policy. Ministry of Health and Family Welfare, New Delhi. Available at https://mohfw.gov.in/sites/default/files/9147562941489753121.pdf (accessed 30 November 2017).

Gupta, Anu, Bharati Roy Choudhury and Indira Balachandran. 1997. 'Touch Me, Touch-me-not: Women, Plants and Healing'. Shodhini: Insights and Issues. Available at http://www.womenstudies.in/elib/health_care/hc_shodhini_insights.pdf (accessed 16 April 2016).

Gupta, V. K. 2005. 'Traditional Knowledge Digital Library'. Asia-Pacific Cultural Centre for UNESCO. Available at https://www.accu.or.jp/ich/en/pdf/c2005subreg_Ind1.pdf (accessed 16 April 2016).

Hafeel, A., T. S. Suma and P. M. Unnikrishnan. 2004a. 'A Participatory Approach in Assessing Health Traditions'. In *Challenging the Indian Medical Heritage*, eds D. Shankar and P. M. Unnikrishnan, 114–27. New Delhi: Centre for Environment Education.

———. 2004b. 'Documenting and Revitalizing Local Health Traditions'. In *Challenging the Indian Medical Heritage*, eds D. Shankar and P. M. Unnikrishnan, 95–113. New Delhi: Centre for Environment Education.

Hance, J. 2015. 'Amazon Tribe Creates 500-page Traditional Medicine Encyclopedia'. *Mongabay*. Available at http://news.mongabay.com/2015/06/amazon-tribe-creates-500-page-traditional-medicine-encyclopedia/ (accessed 1 November 2016).

Hariramamurthi, G. 2000. 'The Genesis of the Medicinal Plant Conservations Network (MPCN)'. Available at http://www.bgci.org/education/article/428/ (accessed 10 April 2015).

Herndon, C. N., M. Uiterloo, P. M. J. Melvin, G. Emanuel-Smith and Jeetendra Jitan. 2009. 'Disease Concepts and Treatment by Tribal Healers of an Amazonian Forest Culture'. *Journal of Ethnobiology and Ethnomedicine* 5(27): 1–22.

Hsu, Elizabeth. 1999. *The Transformation of Chinese Medicine*. Cambridge: Cambridge University Press.

Jeeva. 2010. 'Entering the Dai's World'. Report of the Jeeva pilot project. Available at http://www.jeevaresearch.org/pilot-project.php (accessed 18 March 2016).

Johnson, O. 2002. 'Venezuelan Project Establishes Indigenous Plant Database'. *British Medical Journal* 325(7357): 183.

Khanna, Renu. 2004. 'Women's Health through Self-help and Traditional Remedies: The Shodhini Experience'. Lokayan. Available at planningcommission.nic.in/reports/sereport/ser/seeds/seed_helth.pd (accessed 12 January 2015).

McNulty, N. 2012. 'How to Build an Indigenous Digital Library through Community Participation: The Case of the Ulwazi Programme'. Proceedings of the Standing Conference of Eastern, Central and Southern African Library and Information Associations (SCECSAL), conference in Nairobi, 400–11.

Menon, Indudharan and Annamma Spudich. 2015. 'The Ashtavaidya Physicians of Kerala: A Tradition in Transition'. *Journal of Ayurveda and Integrative Medicine* 1(4): 245–50.

Muqbil, I. 2011. 'India Leads Battle against Bio-piracy of Traditional Knowledge'. *Travel Impact Newswire*, 25 March. Available at https://www.travel-impact-newswire.com/2011/03/india-leads-battle-against-bio-piracy-of-traditional-knowledge/ (accessed 20 April 2015).

Nair, Vishwanathan N. (ed.). 1995. *Anthropology of Tribal Health and Medicine in a Forest Environment*. Thiruvanthapuram: KIRTADS.

Nambiar, D., and A. Mishra. 2017. 'In Defense of Traditional Healers: Not What They Are Quacked Up To Be'. *eSSay*, esocialscience.com 30(January): 1–5.

Ngarivhume, T., Van't Klooster Charlotte I. E. A., J. T. de Jong and Jan H. Van der Westhuizen. 2015. 'Medicinal Plants Used by Traditional Healers for the Treatment of Malariainthe Chipinge District in Zimbabwe'. *Journal of Ethnopharmacology* 159: 224–37.

Omawumi, M. O., and Oludare A. Shorunke. 2013. 'Exploiting the Values of Indigenous Knowledge in Attaining Sustainable Development in Nigeria: The Place of the Library'. *Library Philosophy and Practice* (e-journal), paper 908. Available at http://digitalcommons.unl.edu/libphilprac/908 (accessed 20 April 2015).

Panghal, Manju, Vedpriya Arya, Sanjay Yadav, Sunil Kumar and Jaya Prakash Yadav. 2010. 'Indigenous Knowledge of Medicinal Plants used by Saperas Community of Khetawas, Jhajjar District, Haryana, India'. *Journal of Ethnobiology and Ethnomedicine* 6(4): 1–11.

Poorna, L. R. M. Mymoon, and A. Hariharan. 2014. 'Preservation and Protection of Traditional Knowledge: Diverse Documentation Initiatives Across the Globe'. *Current Science* 107(8): 1240–46.

Rajasab, A. H. 2011. 'Documentation of Folk Knowledge on Medicinal Plants in Gulbarga Ddistrict in Karnataka'. *Indian Journal of Traditional Knowledge* 10(2): 349–53.

Saranappa, R., and G. M. Vidyasagar. 2014. 'Documentation of Traditional Knowledge on Medicinal Plants Used in Treating Candidiasis in Hyderabad Karnataka Region, India.' *World Journal of Pharmacy and Pharmaceutical Sciences* 3(7): 739–51.

Sen, Prabal, Mihin Dollo, Manabendra Dutta Choudhury and Dhrupad Choudhury. 2008. 'Documentation of Traditional Herbal Knowledge of Khamtips of Arunachal Pradesh'. *Indian Journal of Traditional Knowledge* 7(3): 438–42.

Srinidhi, V. 2018. 'Engagements between Biomedicine and Ayurveda: Policy, Practice and Philosophy'. Unpublished doctoral thesis, FMP, IIMB, Banaglore.

Theophilus, Yeboah. 2000. 'Improving the Provision of Traditional Health Knowledge for Rural Communities in Ghana'. *Health Libraries Review* 17: 203–08.

Teklehaymanot, T., and M. Giday. 2007. 'Ethnobotanical Study of Medicinal Plants used by People in Zegie Peninsula, Northwestern Ethiopia'. *Journal of Ethnobiology and Ethnomedicine* 3(12): 1–11.

Torri, M. C., and T. M. Herrman. 2011. *Bridges between Tradition and Innovation in Ethnomedicine: Fostering Local Development through Community Enterprises in India*. London: Springer.

Torri, Maria-Costanza, and Julie Laplante. 2009. 'Enhancing Innovation between Scientific and Indigenous Knowledge: Pioneer NGOs in India'. *Journal of Ethnobiology and Ethnomedicine* 5(29): 1–12.

Udgaonkar, S. 2002. 'The Recording of Traditional Knowledge: Will it Prevent "Bio-piracy"?'. *Current Science* 82(4): 413–19.

Unnikrishnan, P., and G. Hariramurthi. 2012. 'Local Health Practitioners in India: Resilience, Revitalization and Reintegration'. In *Medical Pluralism in Contemporary India*, eds V. Sujatha and L. Abraham, 279–304. New Delhi: Orient BlackSwan.

Wekundah, J. M. 2012. 'Why Protect Technical Knowledge?'. Special paper series no. 44, African Technology Policy Studies Network Biotech Trust, Nairobi, Kenya.

Yearsley, C. 2015. 'Amazonian Tribe Compiles 500-page Traditional Medicine Encyclopedia'. *Herbal Gram (The journal of American Botanical Council)* 108: 54–59.

———. 2015. 'The Biopiracy Issue: To Document or Not to Document?'. American Botanical Council. Available at http://cms.herbalgram.org/herbalgram/issue108/hg108-feat-amazonencyclo.html?ts=1497182034&signature=a4e4dd3b8ed63e87257dfb7a56f842af (accessed 16 April 2016).

III

Gender in Healing

nine

Nested Marginalities

Women in Healing in South India

Arima Mishra, Maya Annie Elias,
Devaki Nambiar and Rajeev B. R.

During the research dialogue on revitalisation of local health traditions that we had organised in January 2016 (details of which are mentioned in Chapter 1), a feminist researcher rightly asked: 'Where are the women healers? Why are they not part of this dialogue?' This question resonates with Flueckiger's (1997) work on female healers in the city of Hyderabad. She had similarly asked: 'Why are there so few female healers in public domain?' Our dialogue had only one young woman healer who had accompanied her father, a reputed healer in Kerala. This question on the absence (or limited presence) of female healers led to much introspection, as much on the part of the research team as other participants. It forced us to ask: Is the field of folk medicine/healing gender-neutral? Are women in the field of healing restricted to being *dais*? Could existing categories of nature/culture, public/private dichotomies render gender visible in the field of healing? This chapter was born out of these critical queries.

We argue that the statist frame of approaching local health traditions' marginality, though critical, has rendered many other pertinent issues within local health traditions non-problematic. Within this (or in addition to) broader frame of marginality, we argue that women's role(s) in traditional healing are marked by further layers of marginalities, rendering them invisible or selectively visible. Local health tradition/folk medicine has always been approached in a gender-blind way, as if such forms of knowledge and practice are gender-neutral. Yet, local health tradition is supposed to be integral to local culture, ecology and, hence, cannot be devoid of the social norms that characterise relationships of gender, caste, kinship and class. Our data, as we discuss later, suggest that a gender lens allows us to decode layered complexities in the social space of healing which need not conform to either given binaries or stereotypes. Our healers have spoken in much more ambivalent ways.

Women's roles in healing have always generated curiosity and controversies in traditional/alternative healing spaces around the world (Nenno 1997; Whaley 2011). Women healers were always part of indigenous/traditional healing, if in smaller numbers, and mentions of women healers cover a broad range, from magicians to witches, herbalists, spiritual healers and dais, engaging in various forms of healing practices (Ehrenreich and English 1973; Semenya and Potgieter 2014). While in many cultures, women were considered the custodians of traditional knowledge and their connection with the divine sources was acknowledged, in due course, this seemed to diminish with the rise of patriarchal systems and colonisation (Achterberg 1990; Munshi 2001) in varied contexts and configurations of caste, class and ethnicity. One set of literature has extensively dealt with women as witches (Levack 1992; Nathan, et al. 1998; Stewart and Strathern 2004; Willis 1995), while another highlights their role as spiritual healers where they transgress gender boundaries to heal others (Carrin 2009), and yet another set of rich literature exists on traditional midwifery/the dai role of women (Chawla 2006; Jeffery, et al. 1985; Lang and Elkin 1997; Pinto 2008; Sadgopal 2009, 2013; Soman 2011; and Troski 1997, to cite a few).

In the Indian context, studies on women healers, apart from the work on dais, are very few (Flueckiger 1997). The women healers we spoke to in our study are engaged in a variety of healing tasks including bone-setting, dai, tantric healing and herbal/folk ayurveda. Drawing from their diverse life histories and experiences, we discuss what it means to be a woman healer or a woman in a healing role (without necessarily being identified as a healer). We show how the sacred circumscriptions of traditional healing establish a hierarchy of healing tasks, wherein women are involved in supportive activities (like preparation of medicines) while the front-stage consultations are done by men, specifically in family practice. Gendered roles are reinforced through outlining the spaces of healing, with women healers treating only 'women' patients or not entering the forest to collect herbs during menstruation. Yet in some other contexts, some women healers express how healing is beyond gender; rather, what matters is divine power, the chosen ones who not merely practise but sustain it effectively. Thus, we had women healers who sat next to their husbands to treat 'women' patients while another healer in an unconventional role of a bone-setter got felicitated by a retired High Court judge in a healers' association meeting (that has 300 healers from different parts of Kerala).

Who is a Woman Healer?: Locating Healers

We did not specifically set out to study gender in healing. We were interested in listening to healers' perspectives and experiences pertaining to revitalisation of local health traditions. We initially approached the organisations that were our primary contacts and informants, having longstanding engagement with documentation and revitalisation of local health traditions, to lead us to the healers they have worked with. We were introduced to members of healers' associations, to those whom the organisations had identified for the purpose of documentation and, hence, in some sense, they were part of the official registers (though not necessarily resulting in official State recognition). We then used a snowball sampling method, asking each of these healers, 'Are there other traditional healers (known locally as *paramparikavaidyas*, *nattu* or *nati vaidyas*, *siddha vaidyas*, *gram vaidyas* or tribal healers, as they are locally known in our field sites) with whom we could interact?' Despite occasional frictions among the healers' community, we were referred to many other healers. We also followed success stories of healers and reached out to them to understand their experiences of visibalising their stories. Interestingly, about half-way through our study, we had spoken to close to 35 healers and noted that they were all men, even as we had asked and checked about referrals to women healers. This relative invisibility struck us.

We observed that any specific query on women healers was responded to as automatically being a question on healers of 'women's problems'—dais. Dais who deal with 'women's problems only' have an insular trajectory and fate due to the State's insistence on institutional deliveries and, hence, the usual response is: "They were there earlier but now dais hardly help in childbirth due to the government's focus on hospital births through cash incentives', says a senior official in an organisation involved in documentation.

Others saw a limited role for women healers and/or as having an important healing role in the domestic space as an extension of kin relations, but not necessarily as healer-practitioner.

> Women are also here. I treat all kinds of problems. Certain women also treat but they deal with women's problems; women's problems women will know and treat. (A fourth generation male healer from Karnataka)
>
> Yes there are ladies, but they don't do full-fledged practice. There is one woman who treats only kidney stone, there is another one who treats jaundice. (A senior male healer from Karnataka)
>
> My mother used to make *rasam* (a spicy, thin soup popular in south India) with neem fruits at least once in a week. There were many such *paatti vaidhyam* (traditional medicine given by grandmothers) in those days and now the situation is that there is no grandmother at home and hence there is no traditional medicine practised by them. (President of a healer's association in a welcome address to a large congregation of healers in Tamil Nadu)

While grandma's knowledge is valuable as part of home remedies, she may not be visible as a healer if one were to ask to identify one. Within the field of local health traditions, attention is drawn to specialised or guided knowledge and generalised/household knowledge (Unnikrishnan and Hariramurthi 2012; Sujatha 2007). While the former indicates specialised modes of knowledge transmission and rules of practice at a community level, which the paramparikavaidyas are involved in, the latter is more diffused. While the sacred and bounded character of the former is highlighted, the latter is more routine, and the possession and transmission of knowledge there is wide and open. We also found that elderly women having knowledge on food, nutrition and medical plants used for common ailments, etc., and women who practise ottamooli[1] treatments are not considered as having any specialised knowledge and, thus, do not become part of the healers' community. In the same vein, myriad documentation efforts rarely have documented knowledge and practice of women healers. For example, we noticed that the biodiversity register of one taluk in a north Karnataka district has all *vaids/hakims* (traditional practitioners of medicine) as male members.[2] This listing is done through what the village identifies and certifies as practitioners having traditional knowledge in the field of health and medicine. Organisations carrying out documentation identify healers through either the forest department, healers' associations or local organisations.

Women healers, thus, get systematically excluded through this gendered process of identification of 'practitioners' or 'healers'. The exceptions are very few women healers who are recognised by KIRTADS[3] as part of its mandate of promoting the welfare of tribal communities.

Nordstrom (1995) echoes a similar problem in identifying women healers. In an aptly titled essay, 'It's All in a Name: Local Level Female Healers in Sri Lanka', she discusses how, despite the valuable role of local healers (predominantly women) in primary health care, they are not known through any specific or generic name (either as exorcists, shamans, ayurvedic practitioners or any other), and hence they are unrecognised in the survey conducted on the mapping of practitioners or health care utilisation. She adds that 'the location of local level healing in the domestic contexts both perpetuates its invisibility and explains why its practitioners are predominantly women' (ibid.: 56). Both by conscious efforts (approaching through the woman healer who participated in our dialogue, visiting tribal villages to specifically ask for women having knowledge on healing) and by accident (through casual conversations with women members of the male healers' team), we uncovered the social space of healing by women. We listened to the experiences of 12 healers with varied profiles—old and young, tribal and non-tribal, a few living very close to the forests and others practising in semi-urban and urban neighbourhoods, practising with their husbands to reversing the gender role, where the husband supported the woman healer. Few pursued healing as a full-time commitment, while others also engaged in agriculture as an income-generating activity (see Table 9.1). It is interesting to learn that they are known by their gender identity than by profession. Barring a few, who practise folk ayurveda and would be called *vaidyar*, others were known as *amma* (referred to as 'mothers'). Thus, what brings them together is their gender rather than their professional roles.

Table 9.1: Profile of Women Healers in our Study

No.	*Age*	*Ethnicity*	*State*	*Nature of Treatment*
1	75	Soliga tribe	Karnataka	Maternal health services—deliveries, infertility treatment.
2	65+	Gowda	Karnataka	Jaundice.
3	80+	Brahmin	Karnataka	Maternal and child health services.

(Contd)

Table 9.1 (Contd)

No.	*Age*	*Ethnicity*	*State*	*Nature of Treatment*
4	70	Kattunayaka tribe	Tamil Nadu	Generalised service, including stomach and skin-related problems, fever, etc.
5	65	Not known	Tamil Nadu	Mainly oral health and fever, headache, cough.
6	60	Bettakurumba tribe	Tamil Nadu	Treats fever, diarrhoea and offers maternal health services.
7	80	Kurichia tribe	Kerala	Bone-setting.
8	35	Kani tribe	Kerala	Asthma, ulcers, arthritis, cancer, etc. Also offers massages and steam baths.
9	32	Kani tribe	Kerala	Massages and steam baths, asthma, poison-treatment.
10	58	Malasar tribe	Tamil Nadu	Siragadithal (a special treatment method) for dysentery in children, headache, fever and cough. Also gives medicine for scorpion bites, other poisonous bites and skin allergies.
11	80+	Badaga	Tamil Nadu	Dai, used to conduct deliveries, currently not practising due to old age.
12	42	Not known	Tamil Nadu	Skin diseases, menstrual problems for women, general weakness, ulcer, piles, asthma.

Source: Authors' fieldwork.

Healers Speak: The Divinity of Practice and Knowledge Transmission

While the divine nature of traditional medical practice runs through the accounts of healers irrespective of gender, its articulation does differ. Women healers tended to underplay their own agency unless it was in the context of the sacrifices and negotiations they had made to sustain their practice. Most of them attributed their ability to heal to a 'gift of god' and considered their practice to be a 'divine 'calling', thus beyond gender, age or any other criterion. They believed that more than their own ability, it was the power of god and the blessings of their ancestors that were key to the healing process.

> I healed the person and corrected the physical ailment. It is not my power. It is god's power. I will do it, I will touch, but the wisdom to do and orders are given by god. (Healer 4, Tamil Nadu)

For healers, especially those from tribal backgrounds, pleasing the gods was very crucial in healing, and prayers and *mantras* (incantation) were as important as the medicines. A few healers clarified this:

> I think that the turning point in my life is that I learnt *siragadithal*[4] which is considered a holy practice in our community. Our community people will respect the healers who practise siragadithal as it is considered a gift from god. (Healer 10, Tamil Nadu)

All healers, irrespective of gender, in our study talked about the specific qualities required in a learner to acquire knowledge and be allowed to practise. This is in line with traditional medicine practice elsewhere too (Hsu 1999; Flueckiger 1997). Thus, even within the family, not everyone is evidently eligible to learn and practise. Qualities like sincerity, perseverance, passion and devotion to the art are important, but our women healers added the divine element here too, saying this had to be god's calling. Here, interestingly, god need not be the supernatural/otherworldly figure, but personified through the master/guru, be it one's father, mother or grandfather. A non-tribal elderly healer who is proficient in oral health problems clarified:

> We were three sisters and all of us observed our father doing his practise. This is a family tradition. But my sister could not pick it up. My younger sister's hands used to shiver when she tried her hand at assisting my father in healing. My father taught me everything and before he died, asked me to go ahead and practise. (Healer 5, Tamil Nadu)

In this context, becoming a healer has a divine calling and, more importantly, possesses specific qualities. The aforesaid healer added, 'I would know who has the right set of qualities—kind of *kai raci* (healing hand), I would be able to judge by observing the way they talk, behave and possess *gunas* (qualities), and these should be good. I had these qualities, so my father taught me.' While the need for such qualities was clearly articulated and determined the healing trajectory, in other contexts this happened more organically and naturally, specifically with our dai healer. One healer, well-known for her healing hand, claimed to have conducted more than 2,000 deliveries in her community. She recalled:

> At a young age of 10, I would accompany my mother when she went to conduct deliveries. Gradually I assisted her before I did it on my own. This is my only education. This is an art (*kala*) which has been handed down through generations. (Healer 1, Karnataka)

While several studies show that transmission of knowledge usually happens along male lines (Hsu 1999; Chand and Shukla 2003), the life histories of our healers and their trajectories of becoming a healer in one sense defy this, as in several cases they learnt healing from either or both parents and grandparents. One tribal healer had gone to other villages to learn the practice from others.

> It is being practised for generations in our family. I learnt it from my father when we were in Ceylon. If you take my family, my grandma used to treat for stomach related problems in small children. She used to put the drops of the extract of a plant into the ears. People will bring their children to my grandmother after undergoing various treatments. This is followed as a tradition in my family. Next my mother did that and now my wife is using that. This is passed on from generation to generation. (A male healer from Tamil Nadu)

Yet, when asked if they themselves would pass on this knowledge to their sons/daughters, they were more inclined towards daughters, as they felt the sons were not interested. Thus, daughters/granddaughters (subject to qualities of kai raci)[5] became candidates because the sons/grandsons were not sufficiently interested in the form of knowledge and practice. Women's responsibility in maintaining indigenous knowledge was, thus, due to lack of interest on the part of the younger men and/or economic advancement and urbanisation (Pidatala and Khan 2003). Exceptions were in those cases where the continuation of this knowledge and practice had better economic incentives. For example, among the Kani tribal community, whose knowledge came into the limelight through the documentation and production of Jeevani (an ayurvedic drug), practising *vaidyam* is a natural trajectory for everyone in the family. In one such family, we met the father, son, two daughters and their husbands practising vaidyam. The father, who was in his 80s, is a well-established healer inviting several patients in and around the village and is the master/guru for his family.

Adding to this diverse set of familial trajectories, we have the story of another woman who could not become a 'healer' for easy identification, despite performing a healing role and teaching her own son (we discovered her erstwhile healing role by accident while we did repeated spells of fieldwork with her son, who is a reputed healer). This healer is in her late 80s and was curious about our continuous observing of practice and long hours of conversation with her son, who is known for his healing ability, depth of knowledge, as well as public articulation.[6] She then proudly narrated how her son had surpassed the knowledge she had imparted to him by learning further from his uncle, having the chance to walk through the forest while learning to identify, collect and prepare herbs.

> I was interested in going out, identifying plants, learning more, but the need to take care of the family and young children did not make this possible. People came to me with queries on caring for their children and delivering. I began to do deliveries and attend to mothers and young infants. I have done many deliveries for our relatives. I have not written anything in the *mane pustaka* (home book which has records of diagnosis and remedies) as I do not know how to write. (Healer 3, Karnataka)

She was involved in healing, but was not a practitioner. Hers was more like an extended kinship role. Thus, even when women healers talked about the divine character of healing, their precise role was gendered.

Social Space of Healing

Most of the healers practised in the domestic space, except two, who had a designated space near their homes. We noted that the women who practised independently were supported by either family members or assistants, who helped them in collecting the medicinal herbs and/or accompanied them if they had to go out for consultations. While male traditional healers moved around and organised their treatment camps, female healers offered their treatment only to people who approached them, and visited patients who were not able to move around because of their health condition. Female healers did not have any promotional activities, and it was usually by word of mouth that they got new patients. To quote the healers:

> I treat a girl and she becomes all right, then this girl will tell others that she recovered well. She will give my number to those who are suffering and ask them to call me. They will call me and come here. (Healer 4, Tamil Nadu)

> You cannot take it outside. The medicine will go dry. It will lose its power. We shouldn't go out and give the medicine. A patient should come searching for a doctor, right? (Healer 5, Tamil Nadu)

> Those who came here and got treated have spread the word. Not by any advertisements. They come here and get cured from our treatments and speak about us. That is how many patients come. (Healer 8, a young woman healer in Kerala)

Traditional healing was often guided by the cultural values and social norms in particular communities. Women healers who practised alongside their husbands or other male members said that they attended to female patients themselves. To quote one of the healers:

> Yes, treatment for man is done by men and for woman it was women. (Healer 8, who practises with her husband in Kerala)

Westerman (2004) reported a similar trend in her study among aboriginal communities of Australia, where she found that clients felt 'shame' in engaging in intimate discussions with healers of the opposite gender, but interestingly, we found that age and years of practice neutralise such strictly gender-based expression. For example, an 80-year-old tribal healer in Kerala who treats mainly sprains and fractures attends to patients irrespective of gender and offers treatments, including massages, to men. She is well-known as the 'amma' for her healing hands in this part of Kerala. A 65-year-old healer in Tamil Nadu further clarified:

> Someone will think, how to touch men while treating, we shouldn't think like that. Even you also shouldn't think, I also shouldn't think. Whoever comes to my house, I will give medicines.

This is echoed by other elderly women healers too, whose clientele and mode of practice had a gender-neutral tone. This reinforces earlier anthropological findings that 'the onset of menopause releases women from the symbolic associations and social obligations of fertile women. Postmenopausal women enter the public domain, exercise authority and acquire prestige in the same way as men do' (McClain 1995: 7). It is no wonder that our younger women healers (two of them) described the age-specific rules about entering sacred spaces (temples and specific rituals) for healing purposes. This was not an issue for older women.

Beyond or within gender norms? Story of Radha Kuttikrishnan (fondly known as Radhamma), a bone-setter in Kerala

Radhama is a tribal healer aged around 80 years. She belongs to the Kurichia tribal group from Wayanad, Kerala. She is temporarily settled in Ambalavayal in Sultan Bathery, Wayanad district (for treatment purpose). She lives in a small house, along with two of her female assistants. She has four children, and three of them practise independently in their hometown, which is about 45 km from her current residence.

She is very well-known in the area for the treatments for backache, fractures and other related ailments. She regularly attends to patients coming from different parts of Kerala. The day the interviewer went to meet her in the morning, 5–6 patients were already waiting for her. She allowed the interviewer to observe her while she attended the patients. She was very pleasant and all patients fondly called her 'amma', which means 'mother'. She was patiently listening to patients' complaints and then examined them carefully. She applied a herbal paste for most of their patients and supplemented it with some herbal medicine, or oil.

Radhama got married at the age of 16 years, and after her delivery she developed an illness and became paralysed. She remembers that she could not sit or stand and had to be carried by her husband even for her daily activities. Her husband belonged to a family of traditional healers and decided to take up the challenge of treating her. It took a long time for her to get cured and in the meantime, she learned the healing practices—how they massage, etc. She says she has not undergone any training, but learned it only by observing her husband while he was treating her.

During those days, her husband used to travel and would come home only once in two or three days. When he was not around and if a patient came, she started attending to them. She remembers that she was not so confident initially, and her logic was that if anything went wrong her husband would be back in two days and could set things right. Initially, her father-in-law showed her the medicines and herbs, and explained which medicine was used for what condition. But what her husband used to treat her was a medicine combination of herbs that he learned from his father, added with a few others he used as an experiment, and to treat her he used a peculiar method of massage, which she now practises.

Over the years, she has become a renowned healer in the area and many people come to her. She has taught about the herbs and the massage to her sons as well as daughters-in-law. Each of them practises independently in their hometown.

(Contd)

Along with her practice at home, she participates in traditional healing camps, organised with other traditional healers, conducts a monthly camp in Thiruvananthapuram, the capital city of Kerala, on fixed dates. She was the only female healer who was recognised in the traditional healers' meet in 2016—a meeting organised by traditional healers' associations and sangams in Kerala, held at Palakkad.

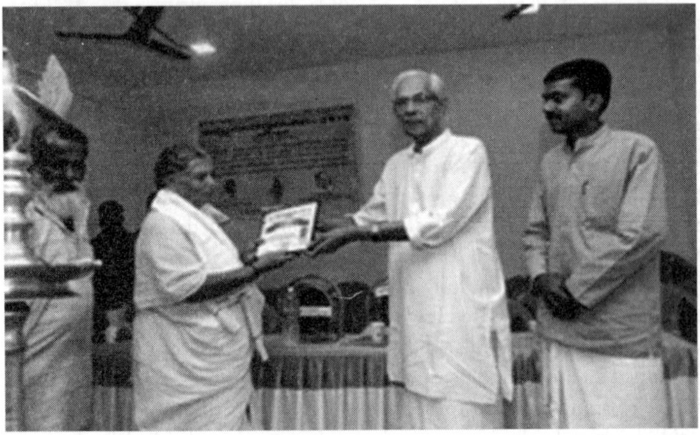

Image 9.1: Radhamma being felicitated at the Palakkad meeting, 2016

Source: Shine Vaidyar, Thadesya Paramparya Chikitsha Vibhagam, Kerala.

Negotiating or Reinforcing Gender Norms?

In an upfront question on why there are so few women healers, one of the older healers shared:

> Yes, it is only me. There is no one else who does this in our community. No one likes to come forward and do this. I do this from early days; it is only me who sustained this. There were a few, but did not sustain, they just go, attend some meetings and that's it.
>
> Q: Is it because it is difficult?
>
> No, it is not difficult, it is because they [women] are not interested or some of them could not sustain.
>
> Q: You haven't seen other ladies, when you go to the camps, also?
>
> No.

> Some ladies are there who work in some centres. There are not many who do it on their own.

This healer's narrative suggests that independent practice requires pushing gender and healing boundaries; courage (to come forward to do the work) and perseverance (she says 'interest' in this sense during the conversation) are key to this. This again echoes the women in Flueckiger's (1997) study who do not think that the healing abilities of Amma (the Muslim woman healer in her study) are exceptional—anyone who can read the Quran should be able to do it and yet no one has emerged as a healer like Radhamma. While the need to push routine boundaries to successfully heal might be true of all healers, these attributes take on a different meaning for women who need to stretch the boundaries of gender symbols and roles, including domestic responsibilities, role of the support network at home along with avenues for continuously honing one's skills, like in the case of Amma. She was encouraged by her husband to treat patients, including his own (in his absence), a supportive father-in-law who taught her about medicinal herbs and an organisation (KIRTADS) that has recognised her as a healer, and she is invited to attend camps on a monthly basis in the capital town of the state.

This is different from the experiences of younger women, whose boundaries are naturalised (linked to their bodily events). For example, during menstruation they are usually not allowed to go inside forests or to offer treatments. In a few places, only men are allowed to go. The same restrictions are applicable to female patients; often treatments are paused during their menstruation. Healers felt that following such customs is important for a positive treatment outcome.

We learned that one of the key reasons for women not to be very active and take on 'independent practice' was that their domestic roles and responsibilities took priority, and an added disadvantage was poor, or the lack of, an effective familial support network. This was reinforced when we spoke to male healers.

> They would have learnt but got married and never practised. (A male healer from Tamil Nadu)

One of our respondents explained that the healers themselves go out and fetch medicinal plants, which is an important component of authentic practice, and this is often not possible for women.

> Established women healers are only a few, maybe a handful in Kerala. There are some risks involved, and hardships, it is difficult to fetch medicines and mix them. So a family would be hesitant to push them to vaidyam; they are only asked to assist. (A male healer from Kerala)

Similar observations have been reported by Semenya and Potgieter (2014), where they found that due to social responsibilities, women entered the healing profession late in their lives compared to male healers. Thus, women's supportive role in healing is encouraged and practised as an extension of the kin role rather than outside it. For most of the male healers who are full-fledged practitioners, their wives 'assist' in healing in terms of medicine preparation; male healers also acknowledge their wives' knowledge about medicinal plants and other modalities of treatment. Few of them practise alongside their husbands or fathers, especially when the treatment involves massage or other kinds of treatment involving touch (for example, as prevalent in the Kani tribe from Thiruvananthapuram, Kerala). Women's healing role (supportive or as an independent healer) is dependent on family circumstances and support as seen in the following anecdotes.

> My wife assists me. She knows everything. (A male healer from Karnataka)

> I am a fifth-generation healer. I have been learning it from my mother since 2001. It has been more than 10–12 years. My father was a very famous vaidyar (the entire conversation had several references to the popularity of his father as a vaidyar). He used to treat 400–500 patients daily. Some people came and stayed here for six months to study his practice. But he died when I was very young. Then my mother took over the practice. She was practising along with father when he was alive. She used to treat female patients and father was treating male patients. (A young male healer from Karnataka)

> My husband and I are *parambarai siddha vaithyars* (lineage-based traditional healers). My father and grandfather were practising. We are a vaithyar family for about three to four generations. My husband also comes from a vaithyar family. Their family is practising for an even longer period. Now we both together treat the patients. We prepare the medicines needed for treatment on our own. (Healer 12, Tamil Nadu)

Familial ruptures have led some women to emerge as independent practitioners, or discontinue completely. We met an older woman healer in Karnataka, who specialised in the treatment of jaundice (the community members led us to this healer; her popularity was well-known) and discontinued treatment due to circumstance—she lost her husband, was disowned by her sons and had to support a divorced daughter. She had a lot of resentment and anger at this spate of unfortunate events and expressed it to us first by refusing to talk, denying that she was ever treating jaundice and later reasoning her discontinuation as a result of an overall distrust of people and their changing lifestyles, which are not suitable for indigenous medicine treatment. She felt that women would be easy scapegoats for patients' discontentment if medicines fail.

The women healers we met were not very active in the healers' associations and seemed focused on their own practice, rather than collective engagements. During the course of our fieldwork, we got the opportunity to attend many such healers' sangams and noticed that women's participation in such sangams was minimal. Even when they participated, they were just passive spectators of such events than being actively involved. During one such meeting organised in Kerala, in which more than 300 traditional healers participated, only a handful of women healers were present. While asked about the healers' associations and its activities, one venerable female healer responded:

> I go there only to attend some meetings. They conduct meetings there, once a month to discuss some topics related to our practice. (Laughing) I don't know how to say that. They discussed many issues. I go once in a while. They say we need to take it forward in a good way, like that ...

However, their healing roles through a public/private (domestic) binary cannot be stretched too far. As the elderly women healers noted, healing roles emerged organically through everyday observing, doing and learning of such knowledge in and around the family (from parents, grandparents or any other). Such a role is not consciously nurtured to practise at a 'public' space as to promote self-reliance within the immediate family and extended kin network. Due to the erstwhile bounded nature of some of these indigenous communities, the extended kin network would stretch to the entire village. The belief that such knowledge has a service orientation and, thus, should be accessible to those who seek it also meant that no deliberate promotional exercise would be needed (at least, such promotion leads to commercialisation, which is an antithesis of traditional knowledge worldviews).

Women healers, in addition to challenges of specific gender norms, shared the larger challenges of the folk medicine healers. These included increasingly difficult access to medicinal herbs (decline of green cover due to increasing urbanisation that has reduced the growth of wild plants, which have medicinal properties) and changing patient lifestyles (food habits, consumerism culture) that were deemed to be unsuited to the ethos of traditional medicine. This had important ramifications for their practice—many chose to underplay their expertise or discontinue it completely. Earlier studies on traditional healing systems have reported modern lifestyles, including food habits, affecting treatment outcomes (Ramshankar and Sharma 2015). One healer expressed concern, saying:

> Nowadays, the plants are not easily available. One of the causes is the growth of Lantana, which has destroyed the local plants. You need expertise in taking it, or it would be destroyed. When you pick a root/tuber, you need to dig a few inches away from the stem, pluck the root and then cover it with mud. This will rejuvenate the root. Now, people just dig up the roots and then leave it exposed. This kills the plants. (Healer 1, Karnataka)

What Do Women Healers' Experiences Tell Us?

Through diverse trajectories and experiences, our women healers conveyed a set of common messages. The first was that we do need a gender lens to understand the nature of the role women play in healing. Due to the gender-blind/gender-biased way of identification of women healers, they often remain obscure from the public gaze, thus getting limited visibility in the reams of documentation efforts by several organisations. Such a gendered lens also projects women healers as restricted to their role as dais—treating it as an insular and separate issue within the revitalisation debate, including documentation, certification and validation. This leads to a hierarchy of knowledge and knowledge holders, relegating women's role to a limited and limiting one.

Second, we learned that given binaries may help but do not adequately capture the nuances of the everyday realities of the women's lives in their myriad roles in the household and community—as daughter, mother and healer/amma. Though in some sense gender norms seem reinforced through their supporting role in healing, subscribing to rules of biology, in select cases, norms were redrawn when gender roles were relaxed within the family sphere. The gender lens also needs to be situated within the worldviews of indigenous medicine, in which ways of learning and doing (at least among some of the forest-dwelling communities we spoke to) revisit public/private binaries that are so common in women's health literature. In this context, primary health care ideology (thus, self-reliance) might be more empowering than practising in a 'public' space for attempting to achieve gender equality in local healing. It is no wonder that when probed, many women healers cited pragmatic reasons for why they did not attend either our dialogue or even other collective forums. At the core of this, then, is the dire need to have a conscious gender lens that helps uncover and decode the layered complexities and marginalities—to begin with, making healers visible either as 'healer-practitioners' or in a healing role is important. The fact that they perform a diverse set of roles, negotiate gender and healing boundaries and extend their kai racis would be important to making a meaningful contribution to any debate and discussion on the revitalisation of knowledge, and knowledge and recognition of the knowledge holders.

Notes

1. Ottamooli is a Malayalam word, which means 'single ingredient'. The ottamooli practice is very common for certain diseases such as jaundice, and usually this knowledge is kept guarded by the vaidyas.
2. Exceptions are in the state of Manipur, which has the *maiba-maibi* mode of healing involving the joint expertise of both husband and wife in healing.
3. For more details, check http://www.kirtads.kerala.gov.in/ (accessed 19 February 2017). See also *The Hindu* (2012).
4. It is a healing practice by blowing air to one's body with the help of some leaves or a cloth.
5. Kai raci, kai guna and *kai punyam* are words in south Indian languages, which mean 'gifted hands'.
6. We read about him in the newspaper, and his powerful statement was: 'we are not quacks, recognize our knowledge' (Chatterjee 2014).

References

Achterberg, J. 1990. *Woman as Healer*. Boston: Shambhala.

Ayyanar, M., and S. Ignacimuthu. 2005. 'Traditional Knowledge of Kani Tribals in Kouthalai of Tirunelveli Hills, Tamil Nadu, India'. *Journal of Ethnopharmacology* 102(2): 246–55.

———. 2008. 'Traditional Healing Potential of Paliyars in Southern India'. *Ethnobotanical Leaflets* 1(37): 311–17. Available at http://opensiuc.lib.siu.edu/ebl/vol2008/iss1/37 (accessed 27 January 2015).

Bakker, J. 1992. 'The Rise of Female Healers in the Middle Atlas, Morocco'. *Social Science and Medicine* 35(6): 819–29.

Carrin, Marine. 2009. 'Women's Agency: Recasting Distress in Two Therapeutic Cults of India (Bengal and Karnataka)'. In *Restoring Mental Health in India: Pluralistic Therapies and Concepts*, ed. Brigtte Sébastia, 125–54. New Delhi: Oxford University Press.

Chand, V. S., and S. R. Shukla. 2003. 'Biodiversity Contests: Indigenously Informed and Transformed Environmental Education'. *Applied Environmental Education and Communication: An International Journal* 2(4): 229–36.

Chatterjee, Pritha. 2014. 'Folk Healers Say We are No Quacks, Recognise our Knowledge'. *Indian Express*, 10 November. Available at https://indianexpress.com/article/cities/delhi/folk-healers-say-we-are-no-quacks-recognise-our-knowledge/ (accessed 4 October 2016).

Chawla, J. (ed.). 2006. *Birth and Birth Givers: The Power behind the Shame*. New Delhi: Har-Anand Publications.

Ehrenreich, B., and D. English. 1973. *Witches, Midwives and Nurses: A History of Women Healers*. New York: The Feminist Press.

Family Health and Development Research Service. 2004. 'Evaluation of the Impact of Kitchen Herbal Garden Program'. Madhurai.

Flueckiger, J. B. 1997. 'There are Only Two Castes, Men and Women: Negotiating Gender as a Female Healer in South Asian Islam'. *Oral Tradition* 12(1): 76–102.

Gadon. E. W. 2004. 'Annapurna Ma, Priestess and Healer: Women's Agency in Folk Culture of Rural Orissa'. *Journal of Social Science* 8(2): 87–92.

Hsu, Elizabeth. 1999. *The Transformation of Chinese Medicine*. Cambridge: Cambridge University Press.

Imperato, Pascal James. 1981. 'The Role of Women in Traditional Healing among the Bambara of Mali'. *Transactions of the Royal Society of Tropical Medicine and Hygiene* 75(6): 766–70.

Jeffery, P., R. Jeffery and Lyon, Andrew. 1985. 'Contaminating States and Women's Status: Midwifery, Childbearing, and the State in Rural North India'. Issue 22 of the Monograph Series, Indian Social Institute, Delhi.

'KIRTADS Aid for Select Ethnic Healers'. 2012. *The Hindu*, 1 June. Available at http://www.thehindu.com/todays-paper/tp-national/tp-kerala/kirtads-aid-for-select-ethnic-healers/article3478988.ece (accessed 23 June 2016).

Lang, J., and E. D. Elkin. 1997. 'A Study of the Beliefs and Birthing Practices of Traditional Midwives in Rural Guatemala'. *Journal of Midwifery and Health* 42(1): 25–31.

Levack, B. P. 1992. 'Introduction'. In *Witchcraft, Women and Society*, ed. B. P. Levack, *vii–xii*. New York: Garland Publishing.

McClain, C. S. 1995. *Women as Healers: Cross-cultural Perspectives*. New Jersey: Rutgers University Press.

Moeng E. T., and M. J. Potgieter. 2011. 'The Trade of Medicinal Plants by Muthi Shops and Street Vendors in the Limpopo Province, South Africa'. *Journal of Medicinal Plants Research* 5(4): 558–64.

Munshi, I. 2001. *Women and Forest: The Study of the Walis of Western India—Gender, Technology and Development*. New Delhi: Sage Publications.

Nagaraj, N. M. 2009. 'Traditional Healing Gets a Big Boost'. *The Times of India*, Bangalore, 30 November.

Nathan, D., G. Kelkar and X. Xiaogang. 1998. 'Women as Witches and Keepers of Demons: Cross-cultural Analysis of Struggles to Change Gender Relations'. *Economic and Political Weekly* 33(44): 58–69.

Nenno, N. 1997. 'Between Magic and Medicine: Medieval Images of the Woman Healer'. In *Women Healers and Physicians: Climbing a Long Hill*, ed. L. Furst, 43–63. Lexington: University Press of Kentucky.

Nordstrom Carolyn. 1995. 'It's All in a Name: Local Level Female Healers in Sri Lanka'. In *Women as Healers: Cross-cultural Perspectives*, ed. C. S. McClain, 42–57. New Jersey: Rutgers University Press.

Pelicci, G. 2008. 'Growth and Transformation among Women Healers'. *ReVision* 30(1): 46–52.

Pidatala, Krishna, and Aisha Rahman Khan. 2003. 'Women and Indigenous Knowledge: A South-South Perspective'. IK notes no. 63, World Bank. Available at http://web.worldbank.org/archive/website00297C/WEB/IMAGES/IKNT63.PDF (accessed 3 March 2016).

Pinto, S. 2008. *Where There is no Mid-wife: Birth and Loss in Rural North India*. New York: Berghahn Books.

Piper, J. 1997. 'Is There a Place for Traditional Midwives in the Provision of Community Health Services?' *Annual Tropical Medicine Parasitology* 91(3): 237–45.

Popper-Giveon, A. 2009. 'Adapted Traditions: The Case of Traditional Palestinian Women Healers in Israel'. *Qualitative Social Research* 10(2), Article 11. Available at http://www.qualitative-research.net/index.php/fqs/article/view/1205 (accessed 2 April 2015).

Ramashankar, Deb S., and B. K. Sharma. 2015. 'Traditional Healing Practices in North East India'. *Indian Journal of History of Science* 50(2): 324–32.

Ranabir, P., K. M. Pradip, G. Sarker, N. Rustagi and A. Ghosh. 2015. 'Traditional Healers and Evidence-based Medicine'. *American Journal of Public Health Research* 3(5A): 194–98.

Sadgopal, M. 2009. 'Can Maternity Services Open up to the Indigenous Traditions of Midwifery?' *Economic and Political Weekly* 44(16): 52–59.

———. 2013. 'Towards Recognition of Traditional Midwives (Dais): The Jeeva Study'. Newsletter of the International Institute of Asian Studies 65, 26.

Semenya, S. S., and M. J. Potgieter. 2014. 'Bapedi Traditional Healers in the Limpopo Province, South Africa: Their Socio-cultural Profile and Traditional Healing Practice'. *Journal of Ethnobiology and Ethnomedicine* 10(4): 1–12.

Shukla, S., and A. J. Sinclair. 2009. 'Becoming a Traditional Medicinal Plant Healer: Divergent Views of Practicing and Young Healers on Traditional Medicinal Plant Knowledge Skills in India'. *Ethnobotany Research and Applications* 7: 39–51.

Soman, K. 2011. 'Women, Medicine and Politics of Gender: Institution of Traditional Midwives in Twentieth Century Bengal'. Institute of Developmental Studies, Kolkata.

Stewart, P. J., and A. Strathern. 2004. *Witchcraft, Sorcery, Rumors and Gossip*. Cambridge, UK: Cambridge University Press.

Sujatha, V. 2007. 'Pluralism in Indian Medicine: Medical Lore as a Genre of Medical Knowledge'. *Contributions to Indian Sociology* 41(2): 169–202.

Troski, T. R. 1997. 'The Importance of Traditional Midwives in the Delivery of Healthcare in the Republic of South Africa'. *BMC Journal of Health Services* 20(1): 15–20.

Unnikrishnan, P., and G. Hariramurthi. 2012. 'Local Health Practitioners in India: Resilience, Revitalization and Reintegration'. In *Medical Pluralism in Contemporary India*, eds V. Sujatha and L. Abraham, 279–304. New Delhi: Orient BlackSwan.

Westerman, T. G. 2004. 'Engagement of Indigenous Clients in Mental Health Services: What Role Does Cultural Difference Play?'. *Australian e-Journal for the Advancement of Mental Health* 3(3): 88–94.

Whaley, L. 2011. 'The Wise-woman as Healer: Popular Medicine, Witchcraft and Magic'. In *Women and the Practice of Medical Care in Early Modern Europe, 1400–1800*, 174–95. UK: Palgrave Macmillan.

WHO. 2003. 'Women and Indigenous Knowledge: A South-South Perspective'. TK Notes, 30454.

Willis, D. 1995. *Malevolent Nurture: Witch-hunting and Maternal Power in Early Modern England*. Ithaca, NY: Cornell University Press.

ten

Ritual Pollution and Women's Blood

Listening to Dais

Janet Chawla

It is provocative to note that both the 'outcaste' and women at the time of menstruation and postpartum share the category of 'untouchable' or polluted. In 1992, I interviewed an older, wealthy Delhi woman originally from Amritsar, Punjab, who shared the experience of her mother being 'touched by the sweeper', meaning she was menstruating.

> I am one of eight children. In those days people had big families and women had lots of work. Only on the days she was menstruating could the woman rest. When she had her periods they'd say she was 'touched by the sweeper'—that's how they'd explain it to us as young children. The woman would be secluded, sitting separately on a cot, doing nothing—neither kitchen work, nor children's work. How I hated not being able to be touched by my mother, not to sit on her lap or be held by her! I was very naughty. I'd touch her cot and say 'Now I am also *chhu jana*' (untouchable; impure).
>
> On the third day she'd have a bath. She wouldn't touch anything, but would call me or one of my sisters to prepare the bath. I'd burn incense in the bathroom and arrange the wooden platforms and the partition, separating her from me. Then I'd take out her clothes and change her sheets. Things that couldn't be washed like the blanket and mattress were put in the sun. Tubs of hot and cold water were put in the bathroom and a glass of milk. I'd pour the water into her mug across the partition. I had to be sure not to touch her or even allow my mug to touch her mug. She'd wash, rinse with milk and then I'd pour a bucket of water over her. Her mug had to be washed with ash and put in the sun to dry. Then I'd heave a sigh of relief that now I could again touch Bibiji and get things done by her. I didn't like all this at all. I thought, 'When I grow up I will never do this (she speaks intensely). I'll never believe in this *chhu chhat*.'

In modern discourse, the concepts of 'untouchability' and 'pollution' have been *only* associated with structures and spaces of hierarchy and oppression. This writing in this chapter takes another track—that is, to highlight the skill, practice and knowledge of the body held by low and outcaste women (the dais) who attend births as well as heal along the maternal health care continuum. I do not deny the oppressive aspects of the social categories reflected in the term Dalit, meaning 'broken' or oppressed, nor the humiliation and exclusion of women from the spiritual at the height of their bodily power. Rather, I am attempting to place another interpretation and valuation of this bodily social space, and those who negotiate it are both outcaste and women—the *dais*. Anthropological literature contests the reductionist lens of approaching taboos/seclusion related to female blood (menstruation and post-partum bleeding) through the category of pollution or symbolic contamination, that is dangerous and, hence, oppressive (Buckley and Gottlieb 1988; Furth and Shu-yueh 1992; Lamp 1988; and Sobo 1992, to cite a few). There is increasing recognition that the social functions of cultural taboos related to female bodily substances vary in different contexts. Ritual taboos have no universal explanation. In many societies, menstruation or taboos connected with childbirth rituals are a means of accessing gender-exclusive ritual power (Lamp 1988), and in some others, it might be more ambivalent, having shades of both suppression and liberation (Buckley 1988). These cross-cultural studies indeed suggest that an understanding of the social, political and symbolic significance of the knowledge and practices related to childbirth, and related rituals and taboos must liberate itself from given binaries—traditional/modern, religious/scientific, expert/lay knowledge, etc. In this context, this chapter enters into the worldviews of the dais and family caregivers (other women) in seeking to understand what bodily events and rituals associated with childbirth convey, both literally and metaphorically.

Dais (or *bais* or *sulagithis*—addressed through various names in different regions in India) are mostly women from the lower castes.[1] Dais are outcastes in so many senses of the word—poor, illiterate, female, mostly of the lowest castes and not recognised by the State. They were excluded in 2005 from the then government's flagship programme, the National Rural Health Mission (NRHM),[2] that has sought to focus so much on maternal health. Unfortunately, due to changing policy priorities and other related factors, dais have not been an important mandate of several NGOs' women's health programmes either. Ironically, it seems that the only groups that appreciates dais are the communities whom they serve! (Jeeva 2016).

Although there are caste, cultural and geographical specificities, Jeeva researchers observed that dais are culturally rooted in their communities and are, thus, accepted and appreciated by the families whom they serve (ibid.). An important part of this rootedness is the commonly felt importance of ritual during the birthing process. One important ritual is that both dais and families reported the observation of (ritual) pollution and separation of the mother from normal household life—especially during the postpartum phase.

Meanings and significance of 'pollution' have been interpreted differently. Louis Dumont (1966), in his classic Orientalist work *Homo Hierachicus*, identified only the hierarchical aspects and structure of caste. His hierarchical model of caste (Brahmins were the 'pure', thus highest, and Dalit or untouchable were 'impure', thus the lowest—outcaste) has dominated historical, sociological and anthropological studies of India for a century. This dominance has made any reclamation or reworking of the values, knowledge and skills of those who negotiate this 'polluted' social space challenging. As I have discussed elsewhere (Chawla 2013), anthropologist Frédérique Apffel-Marglin (1977) disagrees with Dumont's theorising and points out that the categories of auspiciousness and inauspiciousness have, under the hierarchical paradigm, been wrongly put together with those of purity and impurity. She differentiates these categories and points out that the terms *auspiciousness* and *inauspiciousness* speak of different values and a different sort of power. Purity and pollution as Dumont interpreted them are inherently hierarchical. But auspiciousness and inauspiciousness refer to a non-hierarchical form of power (Chawla 2013). Han and Das (2015) add that while childbirth is polluting, requiring the services of lower-caste dais, it is considered auspicious, while death as a polluting event (which also involves the services of the lower castes) is inauspicious.

My experience of 25 years of fieldwork among the dais supports Apffel-Marglin's assertion. Childbirth is considered an auspicious event, even though a 'polluted' one, not really a paradox. As Apffel-Marglin (1977) argues, when it is a matter of regenerating life (childbirth), those at the lower end are foregrounded and needed by all, including the Brahmins, who are at those moments out of the picture and helpless.

During our recent research in Jharkhand, the dais stated that they are invited to social events of families (whom they have helped in the birth of the child) and gifted different items, including sarees (Chawla 2013). They have been instrumental in the auspiciousness of the child's birth and must be honoured during the wedding, so the auspicious gift of fertility is passed on to the next generation. Dais, in Apffel-Marglin's words, enact the work of auspiciousness—that is, 'the regeneration of life and wellbeing'. They are not 'pure' but the work that they do is 'auspicious'—irrespective of the caste groups they serve.

Yasumasa Sekine (2002: 16), a Japanese scholar, also rejects the 'homo hierarchicus' theory of Dumont. Sekine, drawing upon fieldwork in a south Indian village, asserts that in the 'pure-impure' ideology, polluted phenomena are only seen as objects of 'repression and rejection', and argues that the very marginal nature of pollution makes it a creative space, potentially radically changing one's own sense of given order through encounters with others.

He views pollution as a concept indicative of a chaotic situation that destroys the conventional order. Sites of pollution require a renewal of order. This 'chaotic situation', the fluidity inherent in ritual pollution where normalcy is suspended, is the site for the power and practice of low-caste dais—those who can negotiate the chaos of body and spirit presence, the phase of *narak* (menstruation and postpartum bleeding, and the related ritual pollution). As I have discussed elsewhere (Chawla 2007: 154–55), narak is not merely a hell or demonic place, but as the dais and women understand, it is the site or energy of the unseen inner world—of the earth and of the body, particularly the fertile and bleeding female body. It has a connotation of dirt but also of the fertility of earth and women. Narak is used in congruence with terms like opening (labour), open (birth) and closing (postpartum) of the body during birth. This phase also connotes the nature of female bodily energy to be out of usual social control, where women may be more vulnerable, emotional and needing care, thus suspending mundane demands on women's bodies and lives. The practice of dais is a subaltern therapeutic[3]—marginal in a statist and patriarchal sense, but they exercise cultural and therapeutic power in facilitating births and regenerating lives.

The women's and dais' voices discussed later have emerged from two research endeavours—one from Motherhood and Traditional Resources, Information, Knowledge and Action (MATRIKA) in the late 1990s and the other from Jeeva Research Project 2008–12. MATRIKA was a three-year research project on traditional Indian midwifery in collaboration with four NGOs in north India. We came together to generate and analyse data gathered from workshops, role-plays, interviews, folklore and songs.[4] The Jeeva study, on the other hand, was a multi-centric research project carried out in four regional sites, including Jharkhand, Himachal Pradesh, Karnataka and Maharashtra, covering a total study population of 41,621, comprising about 10,000 in each of the four locations. The Jeeva initiative began in 2007 to strengthen the evidence base in support of systemic inclusion of dais and their skilled traditions in formal health care services. The four study locations were selected for their remoteness, diversity, lack of development and the presence of a suitable and willing local partner organisation.[5] Both these studies attempted to capture the culture of birthing at home from the perspectives of dais, mothers and families, rather than biomedical practitioners. This research perspective inverted the usual paradigm that begins with top-down presuppositions.

Women's Voices: The Cultural Code of Pollution

The custom of 'pollution' or '*chhu chhat*' functions both to do patriarchal violence to women and to create inviolable spaces for femaleness and the female body to play out and 'speak'. Reams of writing is devoted to the oppressive characteristics of pollution but our modernist orientation prevents us from discerning the wisdom, skill and gentler gender norms embedded in this idea of the 'polluted'.

Both Muslim and Hindu women living in a poor neighbourhood in Delhi described their experiences of the ritual impurity ascribed to women during childbirth:

> In our religion, without taking bath nobody is purified. My grandmother used to give bath to both mother and child after six days, give them clean new clothes to wear, and call the priest to read holy texts. The sacred water is brought from the nearby mosque and sprinkled on them. Then the woman starts doing the household work. After feeding all the relatives, the child's name is kept, Riyazuddin. (Sahana from Jehangirpuri, MATRIKA)

> Women don't cook food in the kitchen during this period, but they do the rest of housework. Both the menstruating woman and the one who has recently given birth are considered untouchable. They can do household work, but can't enter the kitchen. If she washes a vessel, others touch it only

> after it is dried in the sun. The woman who recently delivered is considered polluted for a month and a quarter. I don't know why this is, but the elders consider it so. (Kanta from Seemapuri, Delhi, MATRIKA)

Ritual impurity customs obviously have serious implications for the caste status of the dai. Not only are the signs of women's procreative power defined as defiling, but also the midwife herself remains in that state of 'pollution', whereas for the menstruating woman or new mother, the state is temporary. The often caste-based work of dais, and the stigma of handling 'untouchable' bodily substances (placenta, blood, cord, amniotic fluid), renders the dai herself as 'permanently' polluted. A belief in the impure and polluting nature of the birth process was widespread and deeply held in each of the Jeeva study areas. Ritually observed, this belief affected community understandings of the dai's abilities, as it was she who could negotiate this process or period of pollution. However, this view often considered the dai herself as polluted. The impure period lasted from the birth itself, or cord-cutting in particular, until the rite celebrating the end of the ritual impurity, allowing the woman back into everyday life (Jeeva 2016).

Female blood, both menstruation and postpartum bleeding, are marks of female power and the capacity to manifest new human life. These biological phenomena are by and large outside of normal social control, or have been before the dominance of biomedicine. We can understand priestly injunctions (Leviticus and Dharma Shastra) as attempts to control the uncontrollable, or at least banish them from 'spiritual' life. Rachel C. Newell (2007) writes that the rite of the purification and thanksgiving of women after childbirth found its way into the Christian prayer books by the eleventh century. This rite is the only ritual in the Western Christian church to address women specifically, and at a time of considerable significance—women who have recently given birth. She points out that the placenta, which has separated from and been expelled by the uterus (which sustained the intrauterine life of the baby), is now dead and will decay. In childbirth, life and death coalesce, she suggests. I personally have viewed priestly attitudes towards female bleeding mainly in terms of misogyny, womb envy and constructing laws and customs to control women—but not in terms of men's fear of their own embodied mortality—a fear of death. Women have periods and sometimes babies—we know about blood and body—perhaps we know, in a way men do not, that we are going to die. It is inviting to view the reverence with which dais handle and bury the placenta in terms of their own comfort with the whole lifecycle and the fact that whatever is born will die. Prevalent across all four Jeeva study areas is the ritual burial of the placenta. This custom showed respect for the role the placenta played in the baby's growth and development. Care is always taken to protect the buried placenta from being dug up and eaten by animals or taken by a malicious person for the practice of black magic.

> We put the placenta in a vessel with betel leaf, betel nut, three types of grains and one-two rupees. A pit is dug and we put it in there and cover it. One should not throw it. (Mallaamma, Karnataka, Jeeva)

Interestingly, Newell (2007) claims that in Christian 'churching', the maternal body is again rendered symbolically clean or pure, as it is within the Indian postpartum rites. However, she points out that in England, within a secularised National Health Service maternity system, post-natal women undergo the ritual practice of the 'six-week postnatal examination'. The maternal body is again 'clean' or given a 'clean bill of health'. She claims that the practice of churching with its concepts of dirt, uncleanness and pollution, as once practised, is not obsolete. It has emerged disguised within a secular health service. In the Indian context, *chhati* ritual (observed on the sixth day after the child is born) observances also end the period of 'pollution', but less under the influence of religious authorities and more under the watchful eye of female relatives and particularly the dai. This is an all-women ritual, usually observed at night. Both birth and chhati rites are domestic activities and the cultural code of 'pollution' ensures that women are in charge. Priests are not officiates at chhati ritual performances. Birth is a female process and the dai is often the ritual practitioner. In Himachal Pradesh, the Jeeva team learned that the post-birth rite to remove pollution involved a ritual fire and the dai may be the one to light it.

Since the chhati rites involve 'cleaning', women are central. A new mother describes the process:

> On the third day after the birth, the dai and the women in the house together do the cleaning and plastering of the house. Dai bathes the baby and the mother and does massage with hot oil. She also washes the dirty clothes and the bedding. Then the dai takes a bath herself and sprinkles sacred water in the entire house. She lights the ritual *havan* or fire. The mother along with the baby crosses over it. After that the house becomes

purified. We then feed rice to all our relatives and give money, clothes to the dai.

It seems paradoxical that the dai, although polluted, lights the ritual fire and orchestrates the rite that ushers the new mother into cleanliness.

Voices from the Ground: Postpartum Experiences

Although the worship of the Goddess Shashti (considered the benefactor and protector of children and worshipped on the sixth day of the lunar month of the Hindu calendar) crept into the Manva Griva Sutra (the Hindu text concerning domestic ceremonies), women and men earlier had also marked the sixth day of the bright fortnight of the lunar month. Sociologist Veena Das (1988) discusses how menstruation is symbolic of the regularity of nature. The rhythms of the body and that of the cosmos are in harmony. The ritual code of female blood, thus, has cosmological links and not merely an ordinary bodily substance. Furthering this, Sitapati, a dai, speaks about another rite related to postpartum practice and its underlying philosophy:

> We cannot take water from the well after childbirth until we perform the well-worship ritual. If for some reason I cannot do it in the first month, then I'd worship it in the third month, not in the second or the sixth months. We don't do any auspicious work in the even months ... I think that during childbirth, God's *shakti* (power) is there. If this shakti was not there, then this child, a whole human being, how could I help bring the child to the world? But if I don't do anything, just sit or sleep, and think that child would be born—this too is not correct. God is the one to give. To do the rest is in our hands. Without one's own strength, nothing is done. One can't sit, relying on God alone. (Sitapati, Delhi, MATRIKA)

Apart from this bodily event being endowed with power (with god's shakti), it also has social significance. The 'polluted' period during the postpartum phase traditionally functioned not only as marking an 'unclean' time, but also offered the new mother rest, relieving her of social, ritual, domestic and family responsibilities. The isolation of the mother and newborn protected them from infections or evil spirits. It also established the dai, or whoever cut the cord, as the person who had the skills and responsibility to negotiate the time and space.

Hemkala describes her experience of postpartum in terms of customary 'untouchability':

> The baby was born in the evening. After a while I drank milk, then ate *halva* (sweet). We buried my daughter's placenta inside the house. When she was 11 days old, we called a priest, had the ritual fire and kept the child's name. The first milk was given when she was five days old. We gave food to the villagers through inviting five young girls (virgins).
>
> After 11 days we purify the new mother with Ganga water. My sister cooked all the food. For 21 days I remained in bed. When my sister went away, my husband did all the work, my own and the children's, for a month quarter. Amongst us, we practise untouchability for 11 days. People of the house stay away from the new mother for a month and a quarter. After that the woman takes a bath in Ganga water and goes to the temple. I, too, visited a temple and then came home and cooked food. (Hemkala, Delhi, MATRIKA)

On the sixth day, the narak period (period of pollution) ends, as the dai does her work of cleaning and of lessening the pollution. In Bihar, the *narak upwaas* or 'fasting' during postpartum ideally is congruent with the mother's diminished ability to digest heavy food. Her energy has been directed towards birthing and lessens the digestive fire. However, in situations of poverty and food scarcity, this fasting cannot be valorised. We can understand 'untouchability' or pollution only in terms of ideas of physiological processes that are foreign to us. The 'dirty blood' or lochia fluid that slowly exits the body during postpartum is thus explained by a dai: 'It is called dirty blood because it has collected over nine months in the body. It is dark, smelly and clotted' (Chawla 2007: 154). The reference to `dirty' is not meant to highlight its polluting aspect. Instead, this is an expression of concern for the woman's health as such dirty blood must come out to restore her body to cleanliness and health, both physically and socially. The mother experiences postpartum contractions of the womb as it reduces in size. Often painful, especially after repeated childbearing, these contractions are sometimes called *gola* (or ball) and are understood as the womb 'searching' for the baby. As one dai from Punjab explained:

> *Gola* is the baby's home. When the house becomes empty, only dirty blood is left. When this comes out, there is pain. Hot drinks (with herbs like ajwain, dry ginger, pepper and jaggery) are given. This drink cleans the belly. After the baby is born, the *gola* roams around. This *gola* has taken care of the baby, now it must leave. If the pain is intense then warm fomentation

> is done so that the *gola* melts away. This is dirty blood and needs cleaning up. (Cited in Chawla 2007: 154)
>
> On the 13th day after birth, the new mother is allowed to enter the kitchen. Some do it on 7th or on 11th day. Everybody celebrates. There is singing and dancing. On this day the new mother and the baby bathe and wear new clean clothes. She comes out to get everyone's blessing. Friends and relatives are invited and eat food together. The dai is given clothes, food and grain. (Cited in ibid.)

Another dai from Rajasthan describes their ritual celebrations and the worship of a birth goddess, Bemata, known to be the deity associated with protecting children and facilitating childbirth:

> On the day of the birth ritual chhati, the sixth day, the women wear everything that was taken off at the time of the birth. She puts on *bindi*, bangles, henna and nose ring. We make ritual drawings of Swasthik, worship Bemata and light a lamp. We make a foot impression of the mother on the floor and then the woman enters the main house. Till the fifth day the Bemata roams around in the house. After the birth celebrations Bemata leaves, she goes to another house. The dai also goes to serve others. (Paana, Rajasthan, MATRIKA, quoted in Chawla 2007)

From Jharkhand, Subhadra describes a post-birth rite at the pond that is analogous to the well-worship ritual:

> We work a lot on the sixth day, bring earth, and plaster the house where the placenta is buried, take the new mother's clothes to the pond and bring back the washed clothes, wash the cot and then give the baby a bath. After finishing the tasks at home, we take the woman to the pond, where she bathes with soap and oil. From home we take vermilion, *kaajal* (kohl), turmeric, rice. When she has finished her bath, then she does *ghaat* (edge of the pond or water) puja and gives those things and milk from her breasts on the stone at the pond and bows to that stone and then washes it. This is all offered to god. What our elder women started, we follow that. (Subhadra, Jharkhand, quoted in Jeeva 2016)

Accompanying some postpartum rites is the birth goddess writing the baby's fate on the third day after birth. The goddess has different names in different places. In some areas of north India, she is called Bemata, other places Vidhmata. Old gazetteers recorded that Brahmins would place a notebook and pen for a boy, or cooking implements for a girl. For fisherfolk, it would be a fishing net. Following is a rather humorous report of this process from Karnataka:

> On the third day, below the cradle, one pot of water is kept and around the cradle puffed rice is spilled, one coconut is broken at the door. On the third day Vidhimunde comes and writes the fate of the child and when she comes, children should not make noise and trouble Vidhimunde so that she can write the fate of the child without disturbance. If children are disturbing, how can she write the fate? She will write something wrong, so they do like that.

In the Bellary district in Karnataka, the Hole Puja (worship) is equivalent to chhati in the north. In our Jeeva data, it was repeatedly said that besides giving thanks, this puja is done to pray that the new mother's bleeding would stop.

Gupasing is the Bondo postpartum ritual equivalent to chhati. I learned about this from Bondo women and relate it here:

> Till gupasing the mother is not supposed to do any work at home. Her plate, the pot in which they give hot water for her to take bath and the gourd for drinking are kept separately. Others are not supposed to use those. The old ladies will tell her not to carry heavy loads for three weeks, or she will get a prolapsed uterus.
>
> Those who helped in delivery won't give food to guests till gupasing. Neighbours won't take fire from that new mother's house because then they can't give food to their guests.
>
> The shaman will do puja and sprinkle turmeric water on mother and baby. They give the turmeric water and food to those who helped her. Then everyone does all the normal work.

I asked a Bondo tribeswoman about the significance of women who helped at a birth 'washing' before resuming normal activities. She said that participating with a woman in labour and birthing changed a person. She put it quite succinctly, saying that she would be different from her normal self. 'My spirit would be different from your spirit.' I think this is a most eloquent way of putting women's seclusion or 'confinement' and the notion of uncleanness. Birthing energies can affect those attending profoundly. If one allows those energies to enter ones' consciousness, then ones' psyche-self becomes different from that of the person walking down the street or cooking dinner. Bathing is one way of literally and figuratively washing away or changing those energies.

Washing and 'purification' rituals are also required after attending a cremation. The beginning and end of a human life are messy bodily affairs, not amenable to social or even religious control. Both birth and death are literally handled by low or outcaste people. Dom men are the ritual specialists of death. Dais, *bais*, *suins*, almost always female, are the expert handlers of birth. Our Jeeva data from Himachal Pradesh confirm an association I have always made—that the fertility of women and the fertility of the earth are analogised. A woman who has recently given birth explains that the 'untouchability' after the birth also extends to the fields. That is, the fields are also ritually untouchable.

> In our village when the *prasoota* (birth) is done no one goes into the fields to work as we consider it *jooth* (untouchable) for 3 days in the entire village. On the 3rd day we clean the house, plaster the house and also wash the clothes. Only after that can people go into the fields to work.

A new mother's father-in-law, also from a Himachali village, stated:

> If a birth happens in anyone's house then we call it out in the same way the night guard calls out at night. A family member gives the call that *jooth* (pollution) has fallen and then no one goes to the fields to work as the fields are god's land. Even if someone dies, we don't work in the fields. It is so in our hills.

Another ritual enactment which was common among agricultural communities points towards the conflation of the fertility of women and the earth—that is, of placing the baby in a winnowing basket, just as grains are after harvest. From Karnataka, this account came:

> Hole includes a prayer so that her bleeding will stop. As soon as they come from the hospital within third day they make *holepuje* after giving bath to the mother and to the baby. After the bath they put the baby in the *mora* (winnowing basket). On the third day they keep coconut, betel leaves, betel nuts, sickle, dry dates and one measure of jawar and make puja. After the puja, they give all these things to sulagithi (traditional midwife). They give money also. They prepare sweet dishes for the puja. They must give all the things in the winnowing basket to the sulagithi (dai). Empty basket should not ever be given to dai, so we will put all these things and give to dai.

Conclusion

From dais themselves, we have learned of their long, gradual and experiential learning process. As the chapter shows, an approach of 'active listening' to dais (and community knowledge) enables us to understand the underlying philosophical, ontological, symbolic and social bases of knowledge and practice related to birthing. A reductionist lens of pollution as inherently dangerous/oppressive obscures such an understanding. The elaborate postpartum rites corroborate that birthing is as much a physical as a social process. Their knowledge and practice, specifically during postpartum, bear added significance, as this phase is completely neglected in the global biomedical discourse on safe motherhood. This is despite the evidence that postpartum hemorrhage is an important cause of maternal deaths. Dais share an understanding of bodily functioning with families, although this is being eroded with the incursion of allopathic medicine. In fact, several of the dais' practices are consistent with current globally recommended best practices in childbirth.[6] Relooking at ritual pollution through the dai's worldviews was an entry point to bring home the point that we need a critical and reflexive gaze to make sense of community/local health knowledge. Liberating ourselves from the rudimentary science/ritual, traditional/modern dichotomies (a concern reinforced in several chapters in this volume) would help us uncover the values of knowledge systems, both in terms of their scope and limitations. Thus, understanding how dais and community birthing traditions are learned, retained and adapted may make it possible for the State to make use of dais effectively. This, however, rests in reframing the lens to approach the community model of childbirth.

Notes

1. Among the Garo community in Assam, dais, of course, mean anyone, including men, as childbirth and care are necessarily collective affairs (Sharma 2016).

2. Launched in 2005, the NRHM was the United Progressive Alliance (UPA) government's flagship programme that sought to undertake architectural corrections of the public health system to improve access to quality, and affordable and equitable health care. One of several that constituted such corrections was community ownership of health, thus instituting several mechanisms to promote the same. One of NRHM's key goals was to achieve millennium development goals (MDG) 4 and 5 and, thus, had put in place elaborate measures to improve maternal and child health services.

3. See the use of this term in Hardiman and Mukharji (2012).

4. For more details, see http://matrika-india.org (accessed 28 April 2019).

5. For details of the Jeeva project's objectives, methodological process and findings, see http://www.jeevaresearch.org/dias.php (accessed 28 April 2019).

6. Abiding presence and continuous care; emotional support and encouragement; massage and touch; movement during labour; food and drink as mother desires; no routine episiotomy; choice of birth position and delayed cord cutting.

References

Apffel-Marglin, Frédérique. 1977. 'Power, Purity and Pollution: Aspects of the Caste System Reconsidered'. *Contributions to Indian Sociology* 11(2): 245–70.

_____. 2008. *Rhythms of Life: Enacting the World with the Goddesses of Orissa*. New Delhi: Oxford University Press.

Buckley, T. 1988. 'Menstruation: The Power of Yurok Women'. In *Blood Magic: The Anthropology of Menstruation*, eds T. Buckley and A. Gottlieb, 187–209. London: University of California Press.

Buckley, T., and A. Gottlieb (eds). 1988. 'Introduction'. In *Blood Magic: The Anthropology of Menstruation*, 1–50. London: University of California Press.

Chawla, Janet, and Renuka Ramanujam. 2000. 'Hearing Dais' Voices: Learning about Traditional Birth knowledge and Practice'. Plan India, MATRIKA.

Chawla, Janet, and Sarah Pinto. 2001. 'The Female Body: As the Battleground of Meaning'. In *Mental Health from a Gender Perspective*, ed. Bhargavi V. Davar, 155-80. New Delhi: Sage Publication.

Chawla, Janet (ed.). 2006. *Birth and Birth Givers: The Power behind the Shame*. New Delhi: Har-Anand Publications.

_____. 2007. 'Understanding "Narak": Reinterpreting Pollution'. In *Exploring the Dirty Side of Women's Health*, ed. Marvis Krikham, 165–76. London: Routledge.

_____. 2013. 'Outcaste Women and Caste Out Birthing Knowledge: Dai's Accounts in Central India'. In *Multiple Voices and Stories: Narratives of Health and Illness*, eds A. Mishra and S. Chopra Chatterjee, 75–93. New Delhi: Orient BlackSwan.

Cohen, Michael H. 2007. *Healing at the Borderland of Medicine and Religion*. Hyderabad: Orient Longman Private Ltd.

Das, Veena. 1988. 'Feminity and the Orientation to the Body'. In *Socialisation, Education and Women*, ed. Karuna Chanana, 193–207. New Delhi: Orient Longman.

Das, Veena, and Clara Han. 2015. *Living and Dying in Contemporary World: A Compendium*. London: University of California Press.

Dumont, Louis. 1966. *Homo Hierarchicus: The Caste System and its Implications*. Chicago: University of Chicago Press.

Furth, Charlotte, and Ch'en Shu-yueh. 1992. 'Chinese Medicine and the Anthropology of Menstruation in Contemporary Taiwan'. *Medical Anthropology Quarterly* 6(1): 27–48.

Han, Clara and Veena Das (eds). 2015. 'Introduction'. In *Living and Dying in the Contemporary World: A Compendium*, 1–37. California: University of California Press.

Hardiman, D., and P. Mukharji. 2012. *Medical Marginality in South Asia: Situating Subaltern Therapeutics*. London: Routledge.

Jeeva. 2016. 'Jeeva Project Study Report: Establishing the Scope and Pattern of Care by Dais During and After Childbirth in Four Cultural and Geographical Settings in India (2016)'. The Shepherds of the Jeeva Collective, Centre for Women's Development Studies, New Delhi.

Lamp, F. 1988. 'Heavenly Bodies: Menses, Moon and Ritual of License among the Temne of Sierra Leone'. In *Blood Magic: The Anthropology of Menstruation*, eds T. Buckley and A. Gottlieb, 210–31. London: University of California Press.

Newell, Rachel C. 2007. 'The Thanksgiving of Women after Childbirth: A Blessing in Disguise?'. In *Exploring the Dirty Side of Women's Health*, ed. Mavis Kirkham, 44–59. London: Routledge.

Sekine, Yasumasa. 2002. *Anthropology of Untouchability Impurity*. Osaka: National Museum of Ethnology.

Sharma, S. 2016. 'Maternal Health among Garo Community in Assam'. Masters field project report, Azim Premji University, report available on request

Sobo, Elisa. 1992. 'Unclean Deeds: Menstrual Taboos and Binding "Ties" in Rural Jamaica'. In *Anthropological Approaches to the Study of Ethnomedicine*, ed. Mark Nichter, 101–26. Switzerland: Gordon and Breach Science Publishers.

eleven

Dais

Transforming the Traditions

Renu Khanna*

Despite policy pressures for institutional deliveries, large numbers of home births still happen in India. In states like Meghalaya, Chhattisgarh, Uttar Pradesh, Uttarakhand, Bihar and Himachal Pradesh, home births continue to be high.[1] Many community health organisations in remote parts of India find that despite the current conditional cash transfers schemes by the Indian government for institutional births, many women continue to prefer home deliveries conducted by a traditional midwife or *dai*. A survey conducted by Jan Swasthya Sahyog (JSS) in 2006 in Chhattisgarh showed that 77 of the 159 women surveyed had delivered at home (Jan Swasthya Sahyog 2015).[2] The preference for home delivery is due to a variety of factors,

*This chapter is a result of insights gathered over three decades of community-based engagement with women's health in the tribal districts of Gujarat and intense conversations with collaborators and fellow-travellers. Discussions with friends in several different fora are used to support the arguments given in this chapter. They are acknowledged wherever possible. Any inadvertent omissions may be excused.

Acknowledgements: Thanks to all the dais and traditional healers, many of whom I have known since 1985, who taught me that I needed to unlearn many things, and from whom I learned how to listen—Nirmalben in SARTHI, Neeta, Arundhati, Pradeepa, Rita and Sheela in ANANDI, Sunanda and Pallavi in SAHAJ; friends in Shodhini, Women and Health (WAH) and CommonHealth; and Kamakshi Thareja, an advertising executive who helped brainstorm on the title.

including poverty, accessibility of care (poor condition of roads, lack of transportation), limited decision-making by women, community trust and negative perceptions of government health facilities (Sarker, et al. 2016). A study conducted by SAHAJ and ANANDI in 2015 in the Dahod district of Gujarat showed very interesting factors (Saha, et al. 2015). Table 11.1 shows that there are several factors that lead to such preference. These include low level of health literacy and poor birth preparedness, gender issues and lack of decision-making power, beliefs and cultural factors (that hospitals are meant only for complicated deliveries or first pregnancies), fear of hospitals due to previous bad experience, either their own or someone else's, and finally, poor contact with the health system representatives.

TABLE 11.1: Reasons for Home Deliveries

Serial No.	*Reasons for Home Delivery*	*Woman/Family*
1	Prolonged labour/ woman is not aware of pains or does not recognise the symptoms of labour.	1. The woman had started crowning very quickly, so there was no time to call a doctor home or even go to a hospital, even though there was complete mental preparation for it. **(I-1)** 2. The woman said that she did not realise when labour pains set in. And also that the time between the labour pain setting in and the delivery happening was extremely short. **(I-12)** 3. The woman already had longstanding issues with her reproductive system, so there was a lot of general pain and did not realise the gravity of the labour pain when it kicked in. **(I-8)** 4. The delivery happened very suddenly. There was no time to even consider going to a hospital. **(I-16)** 5. The 108 (ambulance service) had already been called. And the delivery occurred the moment it arrived. Though labour pains had started at midnight, the phone call to 108 was only made at 3 pm, and then it took an entire hour to arrive from the Gamani primary health care centre. **(I-21)**

(Contd)

Table 11.1 (Contd)

Serial No.	*Reasons for Home Delivery*	*Woman/Family*
2	Husband is away—lack of decision-making, no one to take care of the children if she goes to the health facility.	1. There was no one to call 108, no one to take her to the hospital and no one to even lend her money, to do it herself. So the dai was called through a child, and they did the delivery at home. **(I-2)** 2. There was no one at home (as in, no male member of the family was present) to call 108, or to really do anything about the situation, so the dai was called, and the delivery was conducted in the house. Also, she did not want to bother everyone at home and disturb the routine by going away. **(I-5)** 3. Did not want to bother everyone at home and disturb the routine by going away as there was no one to take care of the children. **(I-19)**
3	Perception that when there are complications, only then hospital deliveries should be done.	1. It happened without any complication so what was the need to do it in a hospital? **(I-3)** 2. The general belief that she should stay home until complications arise. **(I-4)** 3. The general belief in the household seemed to have been that only if complications arose would there be a need to go to hospital. All eight deliveries in the family had happened at home. **(I-6)** 4. The general consensus among the respondents was that there are two primary circumstances that usually result in making a trip to the hospital: (a) If it is the first child, and (b) if the labour lasts for really long. The fourth delivery happened with ease, so there was no reason to go. **(I-13)** 5. If it could be done at home, there was no need for a hospital. **(I-14)** 6. Common tradition/belief that hospitals are needed only in the case of complications. **(I-23, 24 and 27)**
4	In transit—108	The delivery happened when 108 was still on its way, so there was an intention to go to the hospital, despite reservations that the woman had. **(I-9)**
5	Fear of hospitals	1. The women did not like the idea of hospitals because of their smell, so she wanted to avoid going there at all costs. **(I-10)** 2. Was scared of going to a hospital. Had heard terrible rumours in the village about how they treat people in the hospitals and how they give stitches. Did not want all of that. She is scared of hospitals, had heard all sorts of terrible things. **(I-15, 17 and 18)**

(Contd)

Table 11.1 (Contd)

Serial No.	*Reasons for Home Delivery*	*Woman/Family*
6	No contact with Anganwadi worker/ ASHA/ ANM.	The woman said that she did not really know otherwise. She had had no interface with the whole Anganwadi system, or any of the workers, and had not even considered that going to a hospital was a possibility. **(I-11)**
7	Multiple reasons	1. (a) Was hesitant to call 108 because was unsure of how to speak to them, and what to say. Wanted the ASHA worker to make the call, but she wasn't immediately available. **(I-7)** (b) Had had the two hospital deliveries in Vadodara because there are no dais in the city. In the village, there is always the dai to take care, so only if complications arose would there be a cause to go to a hospital. (c) In the two deliveries that they had done at a hospital in Vadodara, they had a bad experience with government doctors (wouldn't specify in what way even upon probing). Rumour plays a big part in this—she gave an example of the woman in a nearby house who delivered in a hospital and lost a lot of blood due to neglect, and died. This has led to a deep lack of faith in the village folk about government institutions. 2. Reasons were four-fold: **(I-22)** (a) Had generally thought it would be best if a safe delivery happened at home. (b) Earlier, on the day of the delivery, there was a marriage in the house (the daughter), and so by the time labour pains kicked in at night, everyone was tired, and the woman wasn't sure how to bring it up in the middle of all the general chaos. (c) The woman was not entirely sure that the pains she was feeling were labour pains, since it was her first delivery. (d) The woman had heard all sorts of rumours in the village about the behaviour of the hospital staff during deliveries, and this affected her decision to not go to a hospital. 3. Reasons were multi-fold: **(I-20)** (a) Were scared of the hospital establishment and its non-approachability for 'people like us' (this point was repeatedly made by the mother-in-law). (b) When the pain kicked in, the woman did not tell her mother-in-law and sister-in-law, who were present, immediately. (c) The husband was not at home, so there was no one available to call 108, so the natural recourse was to just call the dai and do a home delivery.

Source: Saha, et al. (2015).

Home births typically have been conducted by traditional birth attendants (TBA) or dais. The WHO's definition of a TBA is 'a person who assists the mother during childbirth and who initially acquired her skills by delivering babies herself or through apprenticeship to other traditional birth attendants by working with other TBAs' (WHO 1992: 4). The actual tasks of the dais vary across different contexts. In some places they are the persons who support the woman through labour, deliver the baby, cut the cord and provide care for the baby and mother after delivery. In other contexts, the 'cord cutters' and 'baby catchers' are different persons performing these functions (Pinto 2006). In many contexts, the dais are from the lower castes, performing polluting functions like cleaning and disposal of the placenta. In some places and communities, there are also men who perform the role of dais and assist in childbirth.

While there is widespread recognition at the community level that dais have a significant role when it comes to cultural competence, empathy and psychosocial support at birth, with important benefits for the mother and the newborn child, they have been systematically sidelined and derecognised. TBA training programmes that were widespread in the 1970s and 1980s, and which resulted in 'trained dais' or 'trained birth attendants', have been discontinued. Based on our work with dais for three decades and other available research and advocacy on a community model of maternal and child health care, we make an argument for policy support, including recognition of dais.

What Does the Evidence Tell Us?

Research on the effectiveness of trained dais presents a mixed picture. Sibley, et al. (2007) state that the research has largely remained inconclusive. They argue that while TBA training has a lot of potential in reducing peri-neonatal mortality when combined with improved health services, unfortunately the number of studies meeting the inclusion criteria is insufficient to establish training effectiveness. Bergstrom and Goodburn (2001) highlight that the evaluation of the TBA training programmes that assessed outcomes, such as decrease in maternal mortality and morbidity, was fraught with problems. They point out that there are methodological issues in the measurement of mortality and morbidity. It is difficult to prove reductions in mortality in the absence of vital registration systems. Similarly, there are methodological difficulties in measuring morbidities, especially in community-based studies. One meta-analysis shows that perinatal and neonatal deaths were significantly reduced with interventions incorporating training and support of traditional birth attendants (Wilson, et al. 2011). Another study cited in the *Cochrane Database of Systematic Reviews* (Hodnett, et al. 2013) shows that when continuous labour support was provided by *doulas* (who do a part of the work done by the traditional dai, such as providing emotional and physical support to the woman in labour at the time of childbirth and in the postpartum period), women experienced a 31 per cent decrease in the use of oxytocin, 28 per cent decrease in the risk of C-section, 12 per cent increase in the likelihood of a spontaneous vaginal birth, 9 per cent decrease in the use of any medications for pain relief, 14 per cent decrease in the risk of newborns being admitted to a special care nursery and 34 per cent decrease in the risk of being dissatisfied with the birth experience. These research findings are supported by other researchers and community-level activists who argue that in resource-poor settings where health systems are not equipped to provide 'skilled attendance', it is important to engage the traditional birth attendants, as they are an important part of society and enjoy respect and trust of the families they serve (Jan Swasthya Sahyog 2015).[3]

Other researchers go further to say that the value of dais lies not only within resource-poor settings, but also within a worldview that challenges the medicalisation of childbirth and institutional deliveries. Citing examples of Sweden, the Netherlands and Malaysia, Sadgopal (2013) points out that women are choosing to birth within the familiar surroundings and comfort of their homes, and a cadre of trained professional midwives assists them to do so, thus ensuring 'safe births' as opposed to the 'institutional births' which are being emphasised by global and national policies. This begs the question: Can traditional dais at all contribute to 'safe births'? The global policies assert that traditional dais cannot be upgraded to fit the criteria of trained professional midwives or skilled birth attendants (SBA),[4] mainly because of their lack of literacy and formal education. Yet there is an opinion that trained traditional dais can perform 90–95 per cent of the functions of SBAs.[5] Thus, irrespective of the effectiveness-based studies and the resource-poor context arguments, traditional dais continue to be preferred, and this in itself is a form of social legitimacy requiring research and policy attention to approach dais' knowledge and skills in a value-neutral way.

Policy Context

Globally, since the 1970s, when 'primary health care' and 'health for all by the year 2000' was the policy focus, TBAs were actively promoted. A larger number of countries adopted TBA training programmes to reach out to pregnant and birthing women. The decline in maternal and infant mortality slowed down in the 1980s. Hence, there was a rising global pressure to shift to institutional births through skilled birth assistance to address maternal mortality. This shift systematically excluded TBAs. This was reinforced in 1997 at the 'Safe Motherhood: The Next Ten Years' technical consultation in Colombo, Sri Lanka. It was suggested that TBA training neither decreased maternal mortality or morbidity, nor had any effect on referrals. The policy focus, thus, shifted to an emphasis on 'skilled attendance at birth' and improved obstetric services in health facilities as key interventions to reduce neonatal and maternal mortality. The Averting Maternal Death and Disability programme went further to argue for a primary focus on the development of emergency obstetric care at district hospitals. In the discussions on who could be defined as SBAs, as stated earlier, dais were found to not fit the bill.

In India in the Reproductive and Child Health Programme (1997), traditional dais still had a place. TBA training programmes were organised in most states. There was a provision of dai kits for 'clean' home deliveries. However, it was in Reproductive and Child Health Programme II (and the NRHM) in 2005 that the emphasis shifted significantly and explicitly to SBAs and on incentivising institutional deliveries through the Janani Suraksha Yojana schemes.[6] Home deliveries were actively discouraged, even though institutions were ill-equipped to handle institutional deliveries. Although SBA training was launched in earnest, many evaluations showed that the results were not as expected (Bali n.d.; Chaturvedi, et al. 2014).[7] Chaturvedi's study in Madhya Pradesh in India showed that trained SBAs had a poor emergency obstetric care competence score. Similarly, Bali's evaluation showed that the SBA training quality was poor—the trainers themselves were not updated and did not follow the curriculum and schedule. Interestingly, in addition to the achievement of Millennium Development Goals (MDGs) 4 and 5, the NRHM has the goal of revitalising primary health care. In this spirit, it spoke of the mainstreaming of AYUSH and revitalisation of local health traditions, carrying forward the twin agendas stated in the Tenth and Eleventh Five-Year Plans. The revitalisation of local health traditions included indigenous midwifery. However, the NRHM did not spell out what the revitalisation of local health traditions would entail. Among the different local health traditions (including herbal healing, bone-setting, folk ayurveda, etc.), the dai tradition sat uncomfortably, with the State's insistence on institutional deliveries and its active promotion through mobilisation by ASHAs and conditional cash incentives, among others. TBAs or dais were regarded as 'unskilled' within this mandatory institutional delivery model and had no place in NRHM. In 2017, home births were still treated as a matter of shame and sign of backwardness, and frontline health care providers are answerable for the same (Sadgopal 2012).

Since the initiation of the NRHM in India and the implementation of the ASHA programme, some dais have been sought to be absorbed as ASHAs. However, many do not fit the bill because of the educational criteria laid out for the ASHA's position. In many states, there is now a cadre called Mamta or Yashoda[8] at the facility level to support the woman and her family during institutional delivery and the postpartum phase, providing support in immunisation, breastfeeding, family planning counselling and psycho-social support. She is a birth companion, a role traditionally performed by dais or elderly women in the community. Many of these roles continue to be performed by dais who do assist in deliveries in these facilities as there is a shortage of nurses.[9] Thus, even in an unfavourable policy climate, dais perform, or potentially can play, a role in the maternal health care continuum. The dais' stories discussed here draw our attention to such a role.

Dais' Stories

The stories of dais that we present here are from two time periods, the late 1980s, when the health services and infrastructure were weak in the Panchmahals district of Gujarat, and more recently in 2015, when there was considerable improvement in accessibility, roads and communication. The first set of stories is excerpted from a process documentation of a women's health programme implemented by Social Action for Rural and Tribal Inhabitants of India (SARTHI), in a tribal district in Gujarat in western India. The second set is from progress reports of the field staff of ANANDI working in the same area.

Dais' Stories: Panchmahals (Khanna 1992)

Navalben: Goalie Mahadev

She lives with her husband, daughter, and two sons and their families. She is not educated, because girls were not allowed to study earlier. Her husband works as a carpenter. He also works as a traditional healer if called upon. Their economic condition is good enough to allow them to keep other people's land and ornaments on mortgage. She is Damor[10] by caste.

Navalben says that both good dais and dais with the evil eye are called for the delivery. This is to avoid the curse of the dai with the evil eye. She described an instance when a dai had gone for a delivery and returned home, where the woman died because a dai with an evil eye had cursed her.

During delivery, Navalben describes, the woman is made to sit on the edge of the cot. She is also made to sit on her haunches on the ground. The dai gives courage and support to the woman. She asks her to bear the pain. Then when the sac bursts, she puts force on the stomach and the child is delivered. After childbirth, the placenta is forced through and then buried. The cord is cut with a pair of scissors and tied with a clean thread.

If any problem occurs during delivery, the woman is taken to the hospital. She checks the position of the child first. In case the child's position is not normal, she advises going to the hospital.

Sumitraben: Village Doli

Sumitraben has seven children—four daughters and three sons. The family owns about 2–3 acres of land. Her husband's main occupation is farming. He also helps her in her work as a dai when it is a difficult delivery and 'extra force is required'. She also works on land. Their economic condition seems to be bad. From her remarks about their living conditions and food, it seems that they have always lived in poverty.

Her elder sister is also a dai. Sumitraben has always accompanied her sister, to assist her with deliveries. She learnt from her sister about handling deliveries. Initially, she would simply go along with her, helping her perform small tasks. As she picked up the skills required, she grew more confident and now she goes alone. She started delivering children on her own around 1985–86.

Once the labour pain begins, she is called. She goes with two or three other women. The practice here is that all the women in the village who are available go to the pregnant woman's house. Sumitraben checks the position of the child first—feels the woman's stomach and the child's body. She calculates if nine months are over and, thus, knows if a premature delivery is about to take place. If the positioning of the child is not normal, she manipulates it with her hands and tries to rectify it. In the case of delayed labour pain, she helps the woman by holding her hand and walking her around the place. This is said to speed up the delivery. She then puts her palms flat on the contracting womb with each palm facing downwards and pushes the child downwards. Soon the baby comes through and she holds it. After the placenta comes out, she cuts the umbilical cord and bathes the mother and child.

After attending to a delivery, she cannot enter her own kitchen and cook for a period of 10 days. There is no nurse in the village, and neither is there any nurse to help with the deliveries. She has access to a doctor and she can call him for difficult deliveries. Only in the case of very prolonged labour is the woman taken to the hospital.

Dariyaben: Village Doli

After the birth of her first son, Dariyaben started accompanying her husband's paternal aunt (*kaki-sasu*), who is a dai, to assist her in deliveries. In those early days, she says, she went along to help her out or just keep her company. She started working alone very soon, and this was for economic reasons. And, she says, once a woman has attended a delivery alone, she is obliged to go and assist anyone who comes to her seeking help.

Dariyaben says that she is called only after the labour pain begins. She says that other women are required during the delivery and she needs at least two or three women to help her. Once she is with the pregnant woman, she checks the position of the child. If the pain is slight, she walks around with the woman. To speed up delivery, she makes the woman sit on her haunches, with her palms on the ground, to push the baby downwards. With this, the pain accelerates, after which she makes the woman lie on her back. She presses the stomach wall as the contractions occur. And the baby is soon out of the womb. After the child is born, she cuts the umbilical cord. She then places the cord with the placenta in a hole dug up where the cattle are tied.

Dariyaben says that there are some beliefs that may indicate the sex of the baby. If the woman has become weak during pregnancy (lost weight, feels tired, etc.), it will be a girl. On the contrary, increase in the weight of the mother is a sign of a boy-child.

If the delivery is difficult and needs more force, men are called to help. She says she has called men in several cases. She says that the other women will not touch the mother and child after delivery—they are considered polluted.

She is willing and has gone to the houses of people outside her caste as well.

Sukhiben: Village Godhar

Sukhiben lives with seven members of her family—her two sons, their wives and three daughters. They are Barias by caste. She is not educated. Sukhiben says that she is the main decision-maker in the family, because she feels she cannot rely on her husband, especially during emergencies or at times when quick decisions and actions need to be taken.

Her grandmother was a dai. Sukhiben used to go with her to help with deliveries. She gradually learnt how to handle deliveries and soon started going on her own. She has also undergone government dai training in a nearby village. She had to take an examination for this training in Kadana. She has received a certificate, which is fixed on top of a door in the house. She works for the government.

She describes her own deliveries. The deliveries took place inside a house in a corner of an inner room. She says that it is not advisable to keep the mother and child in the open or near the cowshed—it affects their health. Describing labour pain as she experienced them, she says she felt as though her body was being torn into two. She also started bleeding at the beginning of the labour pain.

Her father then called her grandmother, who was a dai. Her paternal aunt and mother were present at all deliveries. In most cases, her mother cut the cord. She also bathed the child, wrapped it in clothes and then blocked her vagina to prevent entry of air in her body. She says this also prevents pain during the post-natal period, and supports the waist and hips. During and after the first delivery, she says that she felt scared and also very strange. She did not know what to do with or feel about the child. After that, she gradually relaxed and was happy.

Kaliben: Village Navmovada

... Generally a dai who is respected is called, but one with the evil eye has to be called too.

... Ghee and *gur* (jaggery) are given to the woman to speed up the delivery. The stomach is kneaded/massaged if the delivery seems difficult. The woman is made to sit and walk alternately. Delivery takes place lying down. After childbirth, the cord is cut after the placenta comes out. If a thread is available, it is used to tie the cord, or else a strip of cloth is used.

... In case of the death of the child/mother during delivery, it is assumed to be the machinations of fate. The dai is not blamed for anything ....

Kum Kumben Gomabhai: Village Limdi

... She likes her work as a dai. Once she learnt the work she had to go for deliveries whenever called upon—people call her work religious, and she likes it.

She has never been to the hospital for a delivery case. The nurse does not come too frequently, and she has never met her. Her family is supportive of the dai's work, so is the community.

These stories show that in this tribal district in 1988, there was hardly any presence of government nurses. Even at that time, without the fear created by the emphasis on institutional deliveries and the push of the Janani Suraksha Yojana, and contrary to the prevailing belief amongst health system representatives, the dais seem to be aware of their own limitations, and when to call upon a doctor or take the woman to the hospital. There is a whole birthing system with components like space, nutritional beliefs, practices and rituals, including massages and manipulation, birthing positions, dealing with the placenta and so on. As highlighted by Van Hollen (2003) and Jordan (1988), all this makes birthing more than a physiological process—birthing is a process that includes social, cultural and spiritual elements. The dai is the central actor in this process. While other women are around to provide support to the woman in labour, it is the dai who provides continuous care to the baby through childbirth and postpartum. She 'catches' the baby, cuts the umbilical cord several minutes after the birth, and handles the placenta and buries it. Many of these women regard their work as divine and spiritual—'*dharam nu kaam*'—and will go to whoever is in need, no matter what the caste. While some of the practices of the dais appear to be doubtful (putting abdominal pressure, for example), there are others that are helpful, like supporting the woman to walk around, encouraging her to squat to bear down, cutting the cord after the placenta is out and so on.

Dais' Stories: Dahod District (2015–16)

Here are some recent stories of dais of the Dahod district. Many of these women were originally traditional dais. Subsequently, as a result of the TBA training they underwent, they came to be recognised as trained dais. They are also leaders and active members of the local women's collective, Devgadh Mahila Sangathan, nurtured by a women's organisation, ANANDI. As the case stories show, these women have emerged as powerful change agents and influencers within their communities. Families rely on them and so does the health system.

Kesliben

Kesliben, a traditional dai and member of the Devgadh Mahila Sangathan, visited Geetaben Ranjitbhai Nayak in Kasatiya village, Baria Taluka on 29 May 2015. She found that Geetaben was three months pregnant and had fluid discharge. She explained the risks to the family members and advised them to admit her to the hospital, but they did not take any action. On 30 May, she went again to emphasise the risk to the mother's life. After much persuasion, they took her to Dr M's private hospital at 5 pm. They were asked to pay Rs 1,500 for sonography, but they did not have that much money with them. Kesliben, who was with them, convinced the doctor to attend to the patient. She also asked the family members to pay Rs 200 to the doctor. Dr M examined Geetaben, gave some medicines and asked them to go home. Geetaben went to her mother's place in Ankli village. Because of the medicines, her fluid discharge stopped, but the next morning at 6 am, Geetaben noticed blood discharge. Geetaben informed Kesliben about it. Kesliben asked her to call 108 (number for the ambulance) and get admitted in Baria Civil Hospital. Kesliben reached there by 10.30 am.

The doctor advised them to go to a private hospital. Once again, they took her to Dr M's private hospital. He charged Rs 1,500, but they had only Rs 800 with them. Kesliben gave Rs 400 from her own pocket, and then everyone went back home in a *chhakda* (a roofless three-wheeled motorcycle rickshaw used in rural areas).

From the field organiser's report: Kesliben says in the film *Hoyani* (CommonHealth, SAHAJ and ANANDI 2016):

> I give women complete information on nutrition and I also ensure that she eats properly. I encourage her to eat everything—curd, milk, groundnuts ... things that older people in the community discourage her from eating because they think these would cause difficulty in childbirth ... They may make faces and complain, but I ensure that she eats frequently .... (ibid.)

Kesliben describes a difficult case that she handled:

> Jayantaben's ... 10–12 people of her family came along. We took her to Baria, to many hospitals. Wherever we took her, they refused to admit her because she was in a very bad condition—she was stinking and dripping ... Finally, the family took her back home. I managed to convince them that she needed hospital care. Took her to Godhra where they cleaned her up and treated her. Finally, on Monday they said please take her to Baroda (150 km away). There, they did her sonography. And in the evening a caesarean was done. The baby had to be kept in an incubator. We were there for 10 days. It was difficult. I left home in just the clothes that I was wearing ... there was no arrangement for food or for bathing ... I kept my courage and handled the situation ... How many of such cases I have *supported* .... (ibid.)

The female health worker from the government health system tells us:

> Kesliben visits all pregnant women, helps them in many ways ... accompanies them to open their post office accounts, get all their identity documents in order—the BPL card, the Aadhar card, caste proof—she gives me all the documents so that they can receive all the entitlements like the Janani Suraksha Yojana, the Kasturba Poshan Sahai Yojana. Her contribution is enormous ... Two years ago there was an epidemic of Chandipuram virus. She went with our staff house to house. Even in ordinary diarrhoea and vomiting she gives ORS, lemon juice. (ibid.)

Leelaben: Moti Mangoi (in the film Hoyani)

Leelaben, a dai, describes a case that she handled:

> Her pain started at night, and her brother called me. I said we have to take her to the hospital. I am trained, but will not do delivery at home. But before we could get her to the hospital, she delivered at home. This was her first baby and the baby did not cry. The family, her mother were scared

> and started crying. I told them—don't cry. Give me a clean cloth. I have received training, I know what to do. With the clean cloth, I cleaned the baby's mouth, nose, and eyes, and gave breathing support, the baby started breathing. Now this boy is this tall!
> ... After delivery, we visit the mother to check whether she has any fever, is she bleeding too much, does she have pain?
> ... When women are sitting and waiting, I explain to them that the child's vaccinations and polio drops are very important to prevent the child from getting diseases. Now they understand ....

Both the stories show that dais help women in multiple ways. Their role has expanded from the traditional dai who 'caught the baby' to a multifarious health worker who is women-centred. These dais provide nutritional advice, help with reproductive health issues like menstrual problems or need for hysterectomy, some are DOTS (Directly observed treatment, short course) providers, and much more. They negotiate on behalf of the women to help them get the necessary documents, like below poverty line (BPL) cards or Aadhar cards, which are so necessary for poor people to access the entitlements that the government has provided for them. They negotiate with private providers who tend to deny treatment to the poor families who arrive at their doorstep in states of desperation. The families trust them—for many, they are the first source of support and advice. There are several stories from our field areas where young and new medical officers have relied on traditional dais to handle complicated deliveries within the 24 × 7 primary health centres. Similar to our experience, which shows that traditional dais are recognised as community leaders, Baxter, et al. (2010) suggest that traditional birth attendants as authoritative community leaders could play an important part in appropriate health communication messages, and, thus, community women would benefit from relevant training and improved links with the formal health systems. Piper (1997) cautions that such a role needs to ensure the existence of the necessary health resources, local consultations and training to be a two-way process of learning.

Discussion

The powerful stories of dais, all the reasons for continuing preferences for home births, as well as concerns about the increasing medicalisation of childbirth (and recent evidence on obstetric violence), all point to the need to create a transformed role for the traditional dai—a role that values them as repositories of many 'good' cultural and spiritual birthing practices, and their role as community leaders. In justifying such a role, Barnes (2015) argued that the dai is the one person who is the common denominator and ensures continuity of maternal health care for a pregnant woman. Left to the health system, her care would be fragmented between the auxiliary nurse midwife (ANM) [iron folic acid (IFA) and tetanus toxoid (TT) provisions], ASHA for logistics for institutional delivery, family members (especially women) for providing care and support, doctors for complications and maybe TBAs for postpartum care. Much of the time, she states, there is no collaboration between these many providers and there are conflicting health messages and care advice.

There is an additional argument for preserving and transforming the traditional dais' role. The current human resource reality in India is that the maternal health cadres are seriously compromised (Maheshwari and Mavalankar 2016). There are not enough SBAs with the requisite competencies; the ANMs have been systematically deskilled (ibid.) through the reduction of their basic training period and changes in their basic curriculum, overburdening of recording and reporting responsibilities and so on. The MBBS doctors do not feel confident to handle even normal deliveries (as evident from our field engagement). In this scenario, it makes practical sense to preserve and nurture the valued local maternal health resource that is the traditional dai.

How would the transformed role of the traditional dai be different from that of ASHAs? It could be argued that Kesliben and Leelaben are performing what could be termed as the ASHA's role. However, ASHAs are not organic community leaders like many of the dais—ASHAs are 'selected' based on certain criteria. The roles defined for the ASHAs are health care facilitators, service providers and social activists, with maternal and child health as one of their many responsibilities (National Health Systems Resource Centre 2013). They have been vested with multifarious tasks—creating awareness about determinants of health, counselling community members on a wide range of health issues (including sexually transmitted diseases and gender-based violence, all requiring a high level of understanding and expertise, for which they would require repeated capacity building), providing community-level curative care for common health problems like diarrhoea or childhood illnesses and so on. The natural advantage that dais have in the domain of culturally sensitive maternal health should be utilised, which is more than mobilising women for hospital births, as is done by ASHAs. By doing so, there will be greater complementarity between their roles, rather than the competition that exists at present (our field experience indicates that there is a constant tussle over the incentives for institutional delivery, with both the ASHA and the dai claiming that each took the poor, hapless woman to the health facility!).

A second issue that deserves attention is the training of the maternal health cadres. From the two sets of dais' stories, it appears that the training of the traditional dais has undergone many changes over the decades. The formal TBA training, sponsored by the health system, seemed to have focused on the 'bad' practices of the dais—delivering with unclean hands, cutting the cord with a kitchen knife or scythe, bathing the baby immediately after birth, applying fundal pressure, etc. This kind of 'official' training largely taught them antenatal care and the '5 Cleans' (clean hands, clean surfaces, clean blades, clean cord ties and clean cord stumps), to transfer to first referral unit, immediate newborn care including immediate breastfeeding, immunisation and family planning. The newer training imparted by community health organisations [like JSS and Society for Education Welfare and Action (SEWA) Rural] focuses more on technical content that contributes to decreasing maternal and neonatal mortality, like identifying danger signs and providing first-aid before ensuring access to emergency obstetric care. The ongoing training that organisations like ANANDI have provided to the dais appears to be more about claiming entitlements and rights or providing woman-centred holistic health education, including nutrition. Most of the recent training, therefore, typically seems to come from a biomedical perspective and does little to examine the positives in the dais' traditional knowledge and reinforce this. Thus, while the dais' traditional role is expanding and they are acquiring new knowledge and skills to negotiate with the increasingly complex health systems' contexts, the effect on their 'good' traditional practices is not known.

Sadgopal (2013) shares her concern about the lost opportunity for the health system that could incorporate the strengths of the dai in a positive and natural way. She argues that harmonising the best of the dais' knowledge, outlook and skills with facility-based obstetric care would humanise childbirth (Sadgopal 2009). Based on her work as part of the Jeeva collective devoted to strengthening the indigenous midwifery knowledge and practice, she strongly advocates the role of dais towards a community model of childbirth and child care, whereby dais are not seen in opposition to the health system but as part of a more decentralised mode of health care organisation. Dais in this role complement the work of frontline health workers through their hands-on skills (Sadgopal 2012). Others[11] suggest that a separate professional midwifery cadre should be created. Midwifery training, as well as ANM, SBA and MBBS training curricula, should incorporate the 'good' of the dais' cultural practices to enhance the biomedical content, and make these curricula and, therefore, obstetric care more woman-centred.

This implies that more research is required to understand and assess dais' practices. Or perhaps more visibilisation of the existing research (Jeeva 2010; Matrika 2004) is required. We also need to reflect on the question: How do we judge what is 'good' in the dais' practice? Some kind of interpretation of dais' practices and their 'validation' would be useful and, in fact, is necessary. Lessons learnt from Shodhini (1997)[12] may help here. Shodhini used the following criteria to assess the traditional remedies and plants that local women healers were using for their gynaecological problems:

- Is there repeated use of a particular practice/plant across time and space for the same condition? (For example, making a woman drink ghee and gur during labour is prevalent across different states. Or, stimulating the placenta to revive a newborn is a practice prevalent across continents.) This implies that there is a universality to this piece of traditional knowledge.
- Is there any mention in ayurveda about this particular practice?
- Is there an explanation for a particular practice in modern medicine? Botany? Neurosciences? For example, dais wait to cut the cord. This practice is upheld by obstetrics. Or, the perineal oil massage given by the dais, according to obstetrics, stretches the perineum, reduces the need for episiotomy and thereby reduces blood loss and risk of infection.
- Is a particular traditional practice woman-centred? Does it promote her well-being? Or does it violate her human rights? An example from Shodhini is the labelling of certain women as *dakins* (witches) and then beating them to drive out the 'evil spirit'—this can certainly not be termed as a 'good' practice!

Any practice that addresses these is termed as a 'good' practice and should be promoted. Underlying these questions is an important mode of enquiry—cooperative and reflective—that is non-judgemental. The reference to ayurvedic texts or modern obstetric practice is not meant to demean this composite body of knowledge, but provides a lens that allows conversations between the different bodies of knowledge (thus not reducing women's lay knowledge to exotic/different/traditional). Just as we would like to question the *kinds* of evidence that would judge a dais' programme, we would like to question *how* the evidence is generated. Research methodologies to enquire into traditional childbirth practices and to interpret and validate them would need to be reflexive, participatory and require imaginative triangulation, as outlined in this chapter. Research should be supported to critically examine as well as interpret the dais' practices. The yardsticks used to measure dais' effectiveness should be appropriate and holistic, and not be limited to the reduction of maternal and neonatal mortality. Research methodologies should be reflexive and participatory.

There is another larger issue that needs to be discussed. In relation to the earlier discussion on the reasons for stopping TBA training, we need to ask: How fair is it to judge the success of TBA training programmes based on such macro-indicators like maternal mortality and morbidity? Especially when we know that maternal mortality is affected by health system factors as much as, if not more than, the social determinants. How fair is it, then, to try and attribute decreases in maternal mortality and morbidity to only TBA training? Can TBAs be held responsible for addressing and influencing *all* the factors that lead to maternal mortality and morbidity? So, then, what should our indicators be of judging whether investments in TBA programmes are worthy? This needs a wider discussion. We would begin by saying that if birthing becomes more respectful, humane, empathic and safe, it is certainly worthwhile to invest in programmes that integrate the TBA within maternal health cadres, and the TBAs' cultural practices within obstetric care.

We thus argue that the role of the dais and their contribution towards maternal wellbeing should be affirmed in maternal health policies and programmes. The emphasis should not be on 'institutional delivery' but on 'safe delivery' and the role of the dai to promote safe deliveries in different contexts should be explored and explicated. Where the health systems are weak and the dais are the only source of maternal health care, their contribution in birthing, pre- and post-natal care should be recognised and their technical skills should be upgraded and integrated within their existing practice, to provide rational maternal health care. Where skilled birth attendance is a reality within institutions, dais can be effective birth companions and health facilities should respect them and their cultural practices, facilitate their contribution and encourage their participation in the birthing process. The potential of dais as community leaders and mobilisers of community support for maternal health should be utilised. As mentioned above, dais and ASHAs can play complementary roles at the community level. We emphasise, the context should define the dais' role and appropriate training inputs.

Notes

1. Meghalaya (49% National Family Health Survey or NFHS 4), Chhattisgarh (40% Adolescent Friendly Health Services or AFHS 2011–12), Uttar Pradesh (57% Health Management Information System or HMIS 2015–16), Uttrakhand (36% NFHS 4), Himachal Pradesh, Bihar (35% NFHS 4).

2. See www.jssbilaspur.org/ (accessed 18 April 2015) for details of their work on maternal health and other related work.

3. Personal communication with Dr Satish Gogulwar (Aamhi Aamchaya Arogya Sathi).

4. An SBA is a midwife, physician, obstetrician, nurse or another health care professional who provides basic and emergency health care services to women and their newborns during pregnancy, childbirth and the postpartum period. Birth attendants are trained to be present at ('attend') childbirth, whether the delivery takes place in a health care institution or at home, to recognise and respond appropriately to medical complications and to implement interventions to help prevent them in the first place, including through prenatal care.

5. Personal communication with Dr Pankaj Shah, Sewa Rural, which has a longstanding engagement with working in community health.

6. Under the Janani Suraksha Yojana, women delivering in the public health facilities receive a cash incentive of Rs 1,400 in rural areas.

7. This is supported also by global studies and reviews. See, for instance, Harvey, et al. (2007).

8. This innovative concept of a birth companion, named after a legendary foster mother in Indian mythology, was introduced as part of the Norway–India Partnership Initiative in 2006. Initially, it was introduced in five high-focus states. For more details on this, see www.nipi.org.in (accessed 10 April 2017). For an evaluation of this initiative, see Varghese, et al. (2014).

9. Personal communication with Dr Subha Sri, a member of CommonHealth.

10. An ethnic community originally from a section of the Bhil tribe.

11. Deliberations with women's health activists at the National Consultation on Maternal Health, 5 January 2015, New Delhi, organised by CommonHealth.

12. Shodhini was a feminist collective, which undertook a field-based enquiry on the traditional remedies and plants used by local women healers for their gynaecological problems.

References

Bali, Surya. n.d. 'Evaluation of the Skilled Birth Attendant Training Program of Madhya Program Department of Community and Family Medicine, All India Institute of Medical Science Bhopal Saket Nagar, Bhopal (MP)'. Department of Community and Family Medicine, AIIMS, Bhopal.

Barnes, Lindsay. 2015.'The Role of the Traditional Birth Attendant'. Presentation at the National Consultation on Maternal Health, organised by CommonHealth, 5 January, New Delhi.

Baxter, Jennifer, K. F. Norr, C. P. Kaponda, A. Malata, R. Ngalande and L. C. Kumbani. 2010. 'Beyond Birth: The Role of Traditional Birth Attendants as Community Leaders'. Virginia Henderson International Nursing eRepository, Registry of Nursing Research Conference Abstracts, MNNRS Midwest Nursing Research Society.

Bergstrom, Staffan, and Elizabeth Goodburn. 2001. 'The Role of Traditional Birth Attendants in the Reduction of Maternal Mortality'. *Studies in Health Services Organisation and Policy* 17: 77–95.

Chaturvedi, Sarika, Sourabh Upadhyay and Ayesha De Costa. 2014.'Competence of Birth Attendants at Providing Emergency Obstetric Care under India's JSY Conditional Cash Transfer Program for Institutional Delivery: An Assessment using Case Vignettes in Madhya Pradesh Province'. *BMC Pregnancy and Childbirth* 14: 174.

CommonHealth, SAHAJ and ANANDI. 2016. *Hoyani: Traditional Birth Attendants Support People's Health* (film). Available at https://www.youtube.com/watch?v=rmLJBwCZjlE (accessed 10 April 2017).

Harvey, Steven A., Yudy Carla Wong Blandón, Affette McCaw-Binns, Ivette Sandino, Luis Urbina, César Rodríguez, Ivonne Gómez, Patricio Ayabaca and Sabou Djibrina (the Nicaraguan maternal and neonatal health quality improvement group). 2007.'Are Skilled Birth Attendants Really Skilled? A Measurement Method, Some Disturbing Results and a Potential Way Forward'. *Bulletin of the World Health Organization* 85(10), October: 733–820.

Hodnett, E. D., S. Gates, G. J. Hofmeyr and C. Sakala. 2013. 'Continuous Support for Women during Childbirth'. *Cochrane Database of Systematic Reviews* 7.

Jan Swasthya Sahyog. 2015. 'Dai Training'. Available at http://www.jssbilaspur.org (accessed 15 April 2015).

Jeeva. 2010. 'Entering the Dais World: Jeeva Pilot Project Report'. June.

Jordan, Bridgette. 1988. *Knowing by Doing: Lessons Traditional Midwives Taught Me*. Michigan: Michigan State University.

Khanna, Renu. 1992. 'Taking Charge: Women's Health as Empowerment'. SAHAJ, SARTHI.

Maheshwari, Sunil Kumar and Dileep Mavalankar. 2016. 'Human Resource Issues in Maternal and Neonatal Health in India'. Working paper no. 2016-03-51, Indian Institute of Management, Ahmedabad.

Matrika. 2004. *Hearing Dais' Voices*. New Delhi: Matrika/PLAN.

Mavalankar, D., and K. S. Vora. 2008. 'The Changing Role of Auxiliary Nurse Midwife (ANM) in India: Implications for Maternal and Child Health (MCH)'. Working paper no. 2008-03-01, March, Indian Institute of Management, Ahmedabad, India.

Mavalankar, D., K. Vora and M. Prakasamma. 2008. 'Achieving Millennium Development Goal 5: Is India Serious?'. *Bulletin of the World Health Organization* 86(4): 243.

National Health Systems Resource Centre. 2013. 'Guidelines for Community Processes'. NRHM, New Delhi.

Pinto, Sarah. 2006. 'More Than a Dai'. *Seminar* 558, February. Available at http://www.indiaseminar.com/2006/558/588%20sarah%20pinto.htm (accessed 1 May 2017).

Piper, J. 1997. 'Is There a Place for Traditional Midwives in the Provision of Community Health Services?'. *Ann Gp Med Parasitol* 91(3): 237–45.

Sadgopal, Mira. 2009. 'Can Maternity Services Open Up to the Indigenous Traditions of Midwifery?'. *Economic and Political Weekly* 44(16), 18 April: 52–59.

———. 2012. 'Why Dais Are Important: Community Model of Child Birth'. *The Alternative*. Available at http://www.thealternative.in/society/why-dais-important-community-model-childbirth/ (accessed 23 May 2017).

———. 2013. 'Towards Recognition of Traditional Midwives: The Jeeva Study'. The Focus IIAS Newsletter no. 65, Autumn.

Saha, Pallavi, Renu Khanna and Sunanda Ganju. 2015. 'Home Deliveries and the Role of Traditional Birth Attendants: Experiences from Rural Gujarat, India'. Unpublished report, SAHAJ and ANANDI.

Sarker, B. K., M. Rahman, T. Rahman, J. Hossain, L. Reichenbach and D. K. Mitra. 2016. 'Reasons for Preference of Home Delivery with

Traditional Birth Attendants (TBAs) in Rural Bangladesh: A Qualitative Exploration'. *PLoS One* 11(1): e0146161.

Shodhini. 1997. *Touch Me, Touch-me-not: Women, Plants and Healing*. New Delhi: Kali.

Sibley, L. M., T. A. Sipe, C. M. Brown, M. M. Diallo, K. McNatt and N. Habarta. 2007. 'Traditional Birth Attendant Training for Improving Health Behaviours and Pregnancy Outcomes'. *Cochrane Database of Systematic Reviews* 18(3).

Van Hollen, C. 2003. *Birth on the Threshold: Childbirth and Modernity in South India* (1st edition). Berkeley: University of California Press.

Vargheese, Beena, Reetabrata Roy, Somen Shah and Sidsel Roalkvam. 2014. 'Fostering Maternal and Newborn Care in India the Yashoda Way: Does This Improve Maternal and Newborn Practices during Institutional Delivery?'. *PLoS One* 9(1): e84145.

WHO. 1992. 'Traditional Birth Attendants: A Joint WHO/UNFPA/UNICEF Statement'. WHO, Geneva.

Wilson, Amie, Ioannis D. Gallos, Nieves Plana, David L. Lissauer, Khalid S. Khan, Javier Zamora, Christine MacArthur and Arri Coomarasamy. 2011. 'Effectiveness of Strategies Incorporating Training and Support of Traditional Birth Attendants on Perinatal and Maternal Mortality: Meta-analysis'. *British Medical Journal* 343: d7102.

twelve

May the Vital Force Be with You

An Indian Homeopathic Doctor's Approach to the Gendered Ills of Our Time

Cecilia Coale Van Hollen

'Homeopathy is effective for everything.' Dr Radha,[1] a homeopathic doctor whom I met in a small rural NGO clinic in Tamil Nadu, south India, was clearly confident about the benefits of her treatments. It was the summer of 2015 and I was conducting ethnographic research on the programmes for women's reproductive cancers. She was eager to explain how and why homeopathy was the most effective system of medicine to treat the ills of our time—including cancer—all of which she attributed to the increasing 'derangement' of people's 'vital force'. During our conversations,[2] she spoke passionately about the connections among homeopathy, cancer, social change and gender relations in India.

Dr Radha's dedication to homeopathic medical care as her life-cause was compelling. Like so many homeopathic doctors in India, she considered the practice to be a form of social service:

> With homeopathy, you are able to do service for the people with good quality and less cost. That is very important; it doesn't require so much cost to cure the patient. And it is permanent. It is a good thing we can do for people with homeopathy. That is the main thing.

According to her, no one in her family took any kind of medicine other than homeopathy. Although she said that homeopathy is widely used by the middle class[3] in cities and towns in Tamil Nadu, she wanted to extend its appeal to the lower-class rural populations, which she described as 'village people who do not have awareness'. She was working to this end through her jobs at an NGO, providing health care and educational services to rural Dalit women in Tamil Nadu and at a clinic attached to a nuclear power plant in the state.

Dr Radha felt that because of its low cost, homeopathy was a more sustainable and appropriate form of medicine for all people—especially for members of poorer communities—compared to allopathy[4] (biomedicine), or to other Indian systems of medicine such as siddha or ayurveda. More importantly, she claimed that stress is the primary trigger of all health problems that people are experiencing in the contemporary era and that stress is causing people's vital force to become deranged. For her, homeopathy is the only system of medicine based on strengthening the vital force, and which can, therefore, effectively combat diseases of the modern era caused by stress. Furthermore, she noted that most of her patients were women. She attributed this to the fact that although all people are experiencing increased stress in their lives, changing gender roles have led to disproportionate stress in the lives of women who, as a result, were experiencing more health problems than men. However, even though she locates the source of health problems in social change, she sees homeopathy and not further social changes as the only remedy.

In their 2004 article entitled, 'Towards an Ethnography of Indian Homeopathy', Robert Frank and Stephan Ecks point out that there is a surprising dearth of ethnographic studies on homeopathy in India despite its immense popularity, and they call for more such work. S. M. Bhardwaj made this exact same point as early as 1980, but to no avail. Frank and Ecks (2004) also say that there is consensus among homeopathic doctors in India that female patients far outnumber male patients, but they do not explore this issue further. In this chapter, I draw from my interview with Dr Radha to shed light on the views of a homeopathic doctor from the southern part of India on this form of medical practice, and on her analysis of the relationship between gender and health.

This edited volume seeks in part to extend the discussion of pluralism in health and medicine from the vantage point of a marginal space within an extraordinary heterogeneous medical landscape in South Asia by focusing on 'local health traditions', particularly those that that lie outside of the domain of formal 'systems of medicine' that are sanctioned by the State. Although homeopathy in India is a system of medicine that is recognised and supported by the State, it is also considered a local health system (despite its German roots), but it does not unequivocally carry the cultural capital of indigeneity that other systems of medicine such as ayurveda and siddha enjoy. Homeopathy is marginalised both in terms of the low level of State support and prestige granted to it, and in terms of the lack of attention given to it by medical anthropologists, making it an appropriate topic to explore within this volume.

This chapter considers how one practitioner of this marginalised system of medicine interprets and responds to the issue of gender inequality and its impact on health and health care. Although this doctor recognises the social causes and context of illness, it is interesting that her response lies solely with the individual and with homeopathic treatment. Although this is not a case of the misrecognition of the social context of illness typically found in analyses of medicalisation, nevertheless, the response can certainly be characterised as a process of medicalisation, in which the therapy includes both medicine and 'mind power'. This case provides a useful reminder that biomedicine does not have a monopoly on the phenomenon of medicalisation.

I want to be clear at the outset, that this chapter is not based on an in-depth ethnographic study of homeopathy. My larger study is on the social and cultural contours of cervical and breast cancer screening and treatment programmes in the southern part of India, and focuses on cancer patients. It was through that study that I came to meet Dr Radha, who had experience of treating women with cancer. For my broader project, I also interviewed allopathic doctors, a siddha doctor, a spirit medium and yoga therapists, all of whom were involved in treating cancer patients. I make no claims, therefore, that Dr Radha's views are representative of all homeopathic doctors in Tamil Nadu or in India. Rigorous ethnographic research is indeed needed, as Frank and Ecks (2004) state. At the same time, however, many (though not all) of Dr Radha's comments do resonate with the findings of scholars like Frank and Ecks who are engaged in deeper ethnographic studies of homeopathy in India.

Homeopathy in India: History and Anthropology

Homeopathy is used extensively throughout much of India. It originated in Germany with the founder, Samuel Hahnemann (1757–1843), and reached India in the 1830s where it first took root in Bengal before spreading *via* Bengali migrants to other parts of India, particularly to urban centres in Uttar Pradesh, Bihar, Kerala and Tamil Nadu (Bhardwaj 1980; Frank and Ecks 2004: 308). Over time there has been such a proliferation of homeopathic colleges and of registered homeopathic doctors that India has been dubbed the 'world capital of homeopathy' (Jütte 1996, cited in Frank and Ecks 2004: 308). Bhardwaj (1980) argued that the widespread popularity of homeopathy in India was due to two factors. First, he notes that 'Bengali physicians made serious efforts to harmonize the fundamental principles of homeopathy with that of Hinduism'. Second, he suggests that early on, homeopathy was perceived positively as 'modern' due to its European origins but that, unlike allopathy, it was not criticised for being a tool of British colonialism (Arnold 1993) because it was Bengali homeopathic physicians who were promulgating this form of medicine, which the British colonial administration scorned (Bhardwaj 1980: 214).

In his pathbreaking 1976 edited volume, *Asian Medical Systems*, Charles Leslie included homeopathy as one among several important systems of medicine that coexist within what he referred to as 'the pluralistic Indian medical system' (Leslie 1976b: 358). He considered homeopathic medicine in India to be 'a special form of popular culture medicine' (ibid.: 359) because of the fact that it is so widely practised in India and because, although originating in Europe, in India 'its practice assimilates elements from Ayurvedic and Yunani[5] traditions' (ibid.). By the time Leslie's book was published, the Government of India had already included homeopathy as one of India's distinct 'national' systems of medicine in 1973, warranting support through the public health system (Frank and Ecks 2004: 308).[6] Hausman (2002), however, suggests that historically homeopathy in India has occupied a much more complicated and shifting position in debates on how to situate it on the 'modern *versus* traditional medicine' and 'scientific *versus* spiritual' spectrums, and whether to consider it an 'Indian/indigenous' system of medicine or a Western system of medicine aligned more closely with allopathy/biomedicine. Hausman provides a fascinating historical account of the complex political processes through which homeopathy came to be recognised by many as an 'indigenous' system of medicine in the broader Indian context, while in southern India, it came to be understood as a 'non-Tamil Indian system' of medicine (along with ayurveda), but distinct from siddha medicine, which is deemed uniquely 'indigenous' in Tamil Nadu (ibid.: 320).

Today, homeopathy is one of the systems of medicine included in the Government of India's Ministry of AYUSH—an acronym for ayurveda, yoga, unani, siddha, homeopathy—which was founded in 2014 in order 'to provide focused attention for the development of Education and Research' in these medical systems.[7] This ministry grew out of what was initially called the Department of Indian Systems of Medicine and Homeopathy (ISM&H) when it was first established in 1995. It was later renamed the Department of AYUSH in 2003 before being elevated to the ministry status.[8] Note that in its first incarnation, homeopathy was included but, unlike the others, it was not considered an 'Indian system of medicine'. That distinction disappeared in the newer title. In addition to promoting health and wellbeing, the Ministry of AYUSH, established during Prime Minister Narendra Modi's Bharatiya Janata Party (BJP) administration, is one of this administration's initiatives to promote Indian nationalism. Homeopathy is, thus, sometimes associated with national identity, even if it is not viewed as indigenous.

Despite the prevalence of homeopathy, medical anthropologists studying medical pluralism and non-allopathic systems of medicine in India have, until recently, been relatively silent on homeopathy. Although Leslie included homeopathy in his list of important systems of medicine in India in his article published in his 1976 edited volume (Leslie 1976a), there is very little attention given to it throughout the book. The chapter by Edward Montgomery does include some discussion of homeopathic doctors, but it is within the context of a more quantitative analysis of the number of professionally trained homeopathic doctors within a broader system of medical care in Vellore, Tamil Nadu, and does not provide qualitative ethnographic insights into the meanings and practices associated with homeopathy (Montgomery 1976). In Leslie and Young's follow-up in the 1992 edited volume, *Paths to Asian Medical Knowledge*, there are only two passing references to homeopathy on pages 4 and 196. Moreover, in Joseph Alter's 2005 edited volume, *Asian Medicine and Globalization*, homeopathy does not appear at all in the index. By contrast, the medical anthropological literature on ayurveda, siddha and unani in South Asia is extensive (see, for example, chapters by Basham, Obeyesekere, Taylor, Gupta and Leslie in Leslie's 1976 edited volume; chapters by Obeyesekere, Leslie, Trawick and Zimmerman in Leslie and Young's 1992 edited volume; chapters by Alter, Habib and Raina, Kumar, and Van Hollen in Alter's 2005 edited volume; and many other works by anthropologists, including Halliburton 2009; Langford 2002; Nichter 1980; and Trawick 1992b).

The dearth of medical anthropological studies of homeopathy in India is particularly curious when we take into account the fact that according to S. M. Bhardwaj, although both allopathy and homeopathy made inroads into India during the colonial era, in rural areas of several states—including Tamil Nadu—by the 1960s there were more homeopathic than allopathic doctors (Bhardwaj 1980: 214). A WHO report indicated that in Tamil Nadu in 2005 there were 16,902 registered homeopathic practitioners, which was greater than the number of registered practitioners in siddha (16,192), ayurveda (3,542) or unani (980); there were 217,460 registered homeopathic doctors in all of India that year (WHO 2007: 12).[9] Bhardwaj argued convincingly in 1980 that despite its widespread use, homeopathy had been sorely neglected by scholars interested in medical pluralism in India. It has only been quite recently that medical anthropologists and other social scientists of medicine in India have begun to pursue ethnographic studies of the use of homeopathic medicine in India from the perspective of practitioners and patients (see, for example, Bhardwaj 2013; Ecks 2013; Frank and Ecks 2004). However, it still remains an understudied phenomenon.

The Body, Mind and Medicine in Homeopathy: One Doctor's Account

According to Dr Radha, homeopathy and psychology are two sides of the same coin. She, therefore, studied both fields. As she put it, 'The main thing is that homeopathy is based on the mind, the mind of the people. The reason I did the course in psychology was that homeopathy and psychology are very closely related.' First, she completed five-and-a-half years of medical training at a homeopathic medical college in Salem to receive a Bachelor of Homeopathic Medicine and Surgery (BHMS) degree. This training covered all of the same subjects as an MBBS training for allopathic doctors, except that the courses in medicine differed. It was her father who first urged her to pursue BHMS and she did so reluctantly. But once she began her studies, she became enthralled and convinced of the value of homeopathy. It was during her studies that she came to see the close links between homeopathy and psychology, leading her to then go on to complete a Masters degree in psychology from Madras University.

My research assistant Shweta Krishnan and I sat in the room where Dr Radha met patients at the NGO clinic as she described her theory and practice of homeopathy. She began by explaining that in homeopathy, the treatment for the same symptom will be highly individualised and vary from patient to patient, and that it is a holistic approach to treating the whole body and not simply one part of the body. As she put it:

> For example, you two people are sitting here. You have some natural characteristics and she has some natural characteristics. In homeopathy the medicine differs based on these characteristics. For you, if you have fever, the medicine may be different than for someone else with fever. Or if you have fever, the medicine for that may be the same as the medicine for ten people who do not have fever. Based on the type of behaviour they have, what they desire more, what they like to eat, what type of food they eat, where they get headaches, whether or not they get cold attacks frequently.... Like that we have to take a full history and based on the whole history, the medicine will be given. We don't give the same thing for all the patients with fever. So for leg pain, we are not saying that the leg is separate from the person; it includes the whole person. We will say that the whole person is diseased, not that just a part is diseased. So we take all of the data and based on that we give the medicine.

In this respect, homeopathy resonates with other non-biomedical systems in India, such as ayurveda, siddha, and unani. But some of the core philosophical and medical concepts in homeopathy that were developed by Hahnemann diverge from these other systems of medicine, such as the notions of the vital force, the view that highly diluted doses of medicine strengthen their effect and the law of similars. Dr Radha explained each of these concepts.

Vital Force and Mind Power

First, she emphasised the fact that underlying the homeopathic understanding of the body, health and treatment is the concept of the vital force. It is the condition of this vital force that determines how an individual will respond to the emotional and physical stressors that one encounters in life, and thereby determine one's ability to maintain health. For Dr Radha, this force has a spiritual dimension akin to the concept of the soul, as well as a psychological dimension akin to the concept of the subconscious. She explained:

> In homeopathy we say that a force is there in every person. We call this the 'vital force'. In Tamil we call it *āṉmā* (soul). It is that force inside you that we are not able to see. If a person is dead, every part of the person is there, but he is not alive. So some force has left and only this thing [she waves her hands along the sides of her body to refer to 'the body'] remains. In homeopathy we call that force the 'vital force'. So if the person's vital force is healthy, the person is healthy but if it is diseased, the person is diseased.

Dr Radha explained that the strength of the vital force is essential to maintain health because this force allows an individual to deflect aggravating stressors, whether they are emotional or physical, from weakening the body. But, if the vital force becomes 'deranged', the body will not be able to deflect such stressors; the body will then 'accept' diseases and become weakened as a result. As she put it:

> We say that the vital force can be deranged. That is what is causing the disease. So what this means is, for example, when I get angry, if my vital force is normal, I am able to control my anger. But if the vital force is deranged, I am not able to control my anger, then I will easily accept all the diseases. So that derangement is because that normal attribute has been disturbed and the person will be able to accept all of the diseases. That is the main concept. For example, in the environment there are a lot of microbes, everything is there. But if ten people are sitting in the same place, why are only two people able to accept the bacteria and get typhoid and things? The reason is that they have the capacity to accept things. That capacity is developed because of that derangement.

In some respects, this is similar to the preventative health ideas associated with the immune system in allopathy and with balanced *dosha*s in ayurveda and siddha. But the concept of the vital force and emphasis on what Dr Radha calls 'mind power' is distinctive.

According to Dr Radha, the derangement of the vital force is directly linked to 'mind power'. As she put it, 'if you are able to control the mind, you are healthy. But if your mind power is weakened, your vital force becomes deranged' and you will become sick. She explained the role of mind power in relation to anger:

> In any situation, if two people get angry, one person might be able to handle that situation very easily. That person doesn't take it into the inner level and doesn't think constantly about it like that. So that person doesn't get diseases and all that because she is able to control. But for another person, if she takes a lot of things in her mind and she is always thinking

> about the problem or the issue, then when that mind is disturbed, then the vital force is weakened and then she can very easily get diseases. That is the main thing we are saying.

Controlling the mind does not, however, mean suppressing emotions such as anger. In fact, suppression of emotion is thought to threaten derangement of the vital force and result in illness. Instead, Dr Radha explained that it is best to express emotion. But your mind must be able to effectively control this expression so that it is manageable and does not become an obsession, which would lead to a derangement of the vital force. She explained this in relation to depression and introverted *versus* extroverted personality types:

> Some people have depression. We talk about extroverted and introverted people. There is medicine for introverted people and different medicine for extroverted people. The introversion makes more disease. And we advise people to be extroverted ... We advise them, 'don't keep it inside; don't keep it inside'. Keeping it inside causes disease. If you express your anger in any form, if you just throw something or whatever it may be, your anger will be calmed down. Then you can control yourself. Then no disease will be there. That is the thing.

Here we can see that emotions are symptoms, just as physical experiences are. In both cases, the strength of the vital force, mediated by the power of the mind, affects how one responds to symptoms and how symptoms manifest. The homeopathic doctor must determine the appropriate treatment for the symptoms to address the root cause, but the symptoms themselves should not be suppressed. Suppression of symptoms is detrimental to the health of the patient and also makes diagnosis of the root cause and proper prescription difficult for the doctor.

Homeopathic Treatment

Dr Radha explained that in the theory of homeopathy there is a direct parallel between the dangers of suppressing emotions and the danger of suppressing any physical symptoms, particularly through the use of topical medicines. Homeopathic medicines do not aim to suppress a patient's symptoms. Rather, they aim to restore the deranged vital force that results in the symptoms. This is one of the reasons that medicines are highly individualised because the cause of derangement of the vital force will vary from person to person, even if they exhibit the same symptom. As she said, 'we are only giving medicine to the root cause, not to the symptom', and the root cause is the deranged vital force that is rendered vulnerable by the lack of mind control. Medicines aim, therefore, to redress these underlying psychological and spiritual dynamics. She went on to explain:

> In homeopathy we are giving medicines that affect the inner power more, the subconscious, as we say. For example, how they prepare the medicine in homeopathy is based on the idea of the atom. Even if it is very small, the atom has the power to burst like that. [She gestured with her hands springing upwards and her fingers splayed out.] Take neem,[10] for example. We make that neem minute. That minute particle of neem has the capacity to change things at the subconscious level. The smaller the amount, the more power it has. So in homeopathy, the medicines exist in minute particles like that, not in crude forms.

She contrasts this with siddha medicines, which also use neem but in the form of a paste that will only act externally but not at the level of the subconscious. However, if you break the molecule down to the smallest level to make it more minute, 'it has more power; it will act at the level of the subconscious; it can even act in your mind'. Homeopathic medicines are prepared by breaking down these substances into their dynamic liquid forms, which is then dropped onto tiny white sugar balls that serve as the vehicle for the medicine and are taken like a tablet. She showed us the sugar balls kept in a jar in her clinic alongside vials of the homeopathic liquid medicines that are widely available in pharmacies throughout Tamil Nadu. This concept of the increased power of plants and other substances when reduced to their atomic or sub-atomic level is a core principle of homeopathy and is often mentioned by homeopathic doctors in India in contrast to what they consider the 'crude' form of plants used by practitioners of ayurveda, unani and siddha (Frank and Ecks 2004). In our conversation, Dr Radha makes these contrasts with siddha medicine, because siddha is more widely practised in Tamil Nadu than ayurveda or unani (although there are similarities across these three systems of medicine). Siddha is a system of medicine that is unique to the southern part of India. It is considered an important part of Tamil history, heritage and culture, and is supported by the Tamil Nadu state government. As Hausman (2002) argued, in Tamil Nadu, siddha alone has the status of being a truly indigenous system of medicine.

Using the homeopathic dictum, *similia similibus curantur* (like cures like), known as the law of similars, Dr Radha told us that medicines which produce particular symptoms—both physical symptoms and 'mind symptoms'—when given to a healthy person are given to a sick patient presenting with those same symptoms. For example, she explained, there is a bark called the cinchona bark which, when taken by a healthy person in its 'dynamic atomic form', produces the same symptoms as a patient with jaundice.[11] So when a patient presents with jaundice symptoms, they may be given medicine made with the cinchona bark. But not every patient with the same symptom will be given the same medicine because the doctor must ultimately address the disturbance of the 'mind symptom' to get to the root problem of what has led to the deranged vital force for that particular patient. Although she used the symptoms of jaundice as an example, she emphasised the fact:

> We don't give importance to the name of the disease. We give importance to the symptom. Whatever the symptom may be. That is the thing. We don't give importance to the name of the disease.

This point will be addressed further in the discussion on cancer later.

Another contrast that she made with siddha is that whereas siddha doctors pay special attention to diet as a central part of the therapy, diet plays no role in homeopathic treatment,[12] except for the fact that homeopathic doctors recommend reducing coffee consumption because of the 'antidotal effect' that it has on homeopathic medicines. They also advise against burning camphor[13] because of similar antidotal effects of the camphor smoke. For example, they do not recommend restricting sugar for patients with diabetes. Instead, she explained:

> The main thing we say to all patients is to be relaxed. In every situation if you change your attitude to take everything easy, then in every situation the problem will become easy to you. That vital force will not get deranged, so no disease will occur. That is what we say to all the people. We do not recommend dietary restrictions at all.

Dr Radha's comments about relaxation and controlling the mind reminded me of key aspects of yoga. However, when I asked her if she would recommend yoga to her patients to help them achieve relaxation and mind control in order to strengthen the vital force, she was dismissive of yoga, and simply said, 'No. That is a separate thing.'

Women, cancer and homeopathy in stressful times

Dr Radha has experience treating patients with cancer, particularly women with reproductive cancers (including cervical, uterine and breast cancer), which were the focus of my study and are the most common types of cancer among women in India. She was adamant that all kinds of cancer could be cured with homeopathy. However, she would not treat these patients for cancer *per se*. As she explained, homeopathy does not conceptualise problems according to biomedical disease categories and treat those diseases; rather, it only considers symptoms. As she explained:

> We don't see disease as such. Whether it is breast cancer or TB (tuberculosis) or whatever it may be, we don't give this medicine for TB, that medicine for cancer. We just collect all of the symptoms of what is making the person have cancer. For that we are giving medicine. And when we give medicine for those symptoms, whatever they may be, like pain or whatever else is expressed because of the cancer, it will be reduced.

Here, again, the dangers of suppression come into play. For Dr Radha, standard biomedical treatments for cancer, including surgery, radiation and chemotherapy, are not effective and cause more problems in the long run because they do not address the root cause of the problem, which is the deranged vital force that gives rise to all ailments. I quote her critique of allopathic approaches to cancer treatment here at length:

> If the normal symptom is suppressed, it becomes a more dangerous disease. For example, if a woman has just a small inner growth in her breast, if they are going for allopathic treatment and getting those medicines for a long time, that suppresses the symptom. If they suppress that breast pain or whatever it may be, it may become more pathological. We say that the suppression makes more derangement. Suppression is a very dangerous thing.
>
> ... If you are a person with uterine cancer, if they just do a hysterectomy, if they are only removing the part, the person will not become healthy. The part has been removed but the thing which caused the disease remains there. So if you take that approach, you will have to keep removing parts of the body to get rid of the disease. But if you are removing and removing parts, only the parts are removed but the reason for the problem is not removed. So we advise patients not to do surgery and not to do external things ...
>
> ... One of my patients came to me with a lump in the breast and within one month we completely reduced the lump and pain. But we are treating not just the lump but the whole person.

Most of the cancer patients who had come to her for treatment were women; very rarely had she treated male cancer patients. Most of the women cancer patients who came to see her for treatment lived or worked near the atomic energy plant. She said that in that area, no matter what the symptoms are, people are quick to seek out homeopathic therapies immediately, even before they go to an allopathic practitioner. She attributed this to the fact that people in that area are well-educated and also to the fact that the allopathic doctors working at the atomic energy plant were supportive of homeopathy and would refer patients to her for treatment, so people had become very familiar with homeopathy and appreciated the low cost.

When I asked why she thought most of the patients with cancer who came to see her were women, she said this was not only the case with cancer but that in general, most of the patients who come to her were women. This, she said, was due to the increased levels of stress faced by women as a result of social changes. This added stress was leading to disproportionately increased rates of illness among women, including increases in rates of cancer. She felt that stress accounted for 'more than 50 per cent' of the root cause of the derangement of the vital force of all patients who came to see her. In her view, women's lives have become dramatically more stressful in recent times, leading to increased health problems, including cancers, which she viewed as manifestations of the deranged vital force. According to Dr Radha, women experienced more stress than ever now because of their movement into the workforce, and the fact that they now must juggle the demands of their work outside the house with the continued full responsibility of the household work, including childcare, cooking and cleaning. She explained this to me:

> Dr R.: Nowadays, stress is the main reason for all health problems. Women suffer the most from this. In the past, women didn't have so much stress. But now everything is stressful. They have to do this work within this time; they have to look after their children; they have to look after their husbands; they have to do the cooking and then go to the office; they have to do all these things. So it is a fully stressful life and so the diseases will come.
>
> CVH: So before women didn't have as much stress? Are you saying that it is because now they are trying to manage their job outside of the home and inside of the home? Is that why they have more stress?

Dr R.: Yes, this is the thing that makes more stress. Now it is very competitive, so that makes it more stressful.

CVH: From a homeopathic perspective, would stress be considered one of the causes for cancer?

Dr R: Yes, definitely!

Dr Radha's analysis of social change seems to be based on her perceptions of transformations in the lives of middle-class women, since women from lower-class urban and rural communities in Tamil Nadu have historically been engaged in the labour force while simultaneously also being responsible for much of the domestic labour of their families. However, lower-class women may also be experiencing increased stress in the context of the neoliberal era and an increasingly wide gap between the rich and the poor, forcing people in poverty to take on additional labour or to suffer from increased anxiety associated with under-employment and unemployment.

Given what Dr Radha told me about the ways in which transformations in gendered labour relations and increased competition were negatively impacting women's health, I asked if she considered it part of her job as a homeopathic doctor with training in psychology to provide counselling to patients about the ways in which they might consider working to change the unequal social relationships within their families that were leading to poor health outcomes for women, including increases in reproductive cancers. This, however, was not an approach she advocated. The following excerpt of the conversation with Dr Radha, myself and Shweta Krishnan, in response to our questions about this, conveys her opinion well:

Dr R.: No, we don't give any counselling about family issues. We just say, 'Change your attitude; don't try to change your whole family.' For example, for me, if I had a disease, if ten people are around me, I am not able to correct all those ten people. If I correct myself, then whatever problems are given by those ten people, no derangement will be there if I change myself. So we advise people to change themselves only. We don't give family counselling and all that.

SK: So just as an example: you know how we were talking about how women have to deal with all sorts of different things. So how will you advise them? If I come to you and you feel that my basic problem is that I am doing so many hours of work outside, and then I am coming home and doing so much work inside, and I have so much stress. Then how will you advise them?

> Dr R: You see, the first thing that we will say is, 'don't be introverted. And don't think anything constantly in your mind. Just leave the thing at that time.'
>
> SK: So you would say to just do this and that and let it go?
>
> Dr R: Yes.
>
> CVH: So don't obsess about issues.
>
> Dr R: Yes. And don't take everything as a burden. We also say that. And if one thing is decided, this is a thing that you have to face, so don't take it as a burden. You have to do it, so you have to do this.
>
> SK: Don't fight it.
>
> Dr R: So don't do everything complaining, 'oh, we have to do this; oh we have to do that...' [she said this in a whining voice]. Do everything with happiness and be joyful. That is the thing we say.

Dr Radha also notes that both men and women were at increased risk of disease due to amplified environmental hazards associated with the rising use of pesticides, chemical fertilisers and growing air pollution from cars. She explained that these environmental stressors were weakening people's vital force, but underscored that homeopathic medicines 'will overrule all these effects'. We wondered if she advocated for social movements to combat such environmental hazards, and asked if she recommended getting involved in social movements to change the unequal gender relations and reduce the increasingly competitive environment that were leading to increased stress and disease among women. Again, she was adamant that this was not what she recommended, saying:

> No, no. Whatever social movements may be there, that is one thing. But what we say in homeopathy is that if each of us can overcome all of these situations to make it easier, then no problem will be there. So we are only advising that it is just you who has to change. Whatever the situation and whatever it may be.

Conclusion

Margaret Trawick (1992b) provided a fascinating analysis of a Tamil ayurvedic doctor's theory of cancer, based on her discussions with him in 1975. She interpreted his views of cancer to be a metaphorical critique of the rapacious effects of consumerist capitalism within colonial and a postcolonial India still under assault by foreign companies. She argued that 'his idea that the body itself must acquire the power to carry all the needed materials to all the places within itself, and to gently but firmly expel foreign elements' was a metaphor for an anti-colonial nationalist call for Gandhian local self-government (ibid.: 218). She came to the conclusion that this ayurvedic doctor was expounding his theories to her in the hope that she would convey his critique of imperialistic capitalism to a Western public.

Although Dr Radha also placed blame on social and economic factors (unequal gender relations, increased competition and environmental degradation), this was not conveyed metaphorically through her understanding of the body. It was a very literal diagnosis of social ills. Also, unlike the doctor interviewed by Trawick, Dr Radha's solution to the increased risk of disease in the contemporary era was distinctly apolitical. Like Trawick's ayurvedic doctor, Dr Radha located the solution within the individual, championing the power of both homeopathic medicine and of individual minds. But this remedy did not suggest a call for political self-rule in opposition to systems of exploitation. In fact, she was emphatic that there is no space for political action within homeopathic therapeutics. Although most of the patients who came to her with cancer symptoms were those who lived or worked in the vicinity of an atomic power plant, she did not consider that there might be a connection between exposure to radiation and increased risk of cancer while she extolled the power of homeopathic medicine in its 'atomic form'. This was particularly striking given the fact that controversies have swirled around concerns about higher rates of cancer in communities around this power plant.

This case both diverges from and supports critiques of medicalisation that have been central to critical medical anthropological theory (Scheper-Hughes and Lock 1987). On the one hand, this homeopathic doctor does not locate the cause of health solely in the individual body, but views illness as caused by social and economic factors. On the other hand, she considers the antidote to the problem solely through the lens of homeopathic treatment of the individual, combining targeted medicines to strengthen the vital force and mind control to both prevent and combat stressors that weaken the vital force. This case provides a reminder that biomedicine does not have a monopoly on the phenomenon of medicalisation or pharmaceuticalisation, as other medical anthropologists studying medical pluralism in India have also noted (Ecks 2013; Nichter 1996).

If Dr Radha was eager to share her thoughts with me and saw me as a messenger (in the way that Trawich suggests), I believe it had more to do with her desire to elevate the status and increase the practice of homeopathy than it did with her wish to critique a particular political-economic order. Over the course of our long conversation, she compared homeopathy to allopathy, siddha and yoga to argue that no other approach to health and wellbeing could match that of homeopathy. As multiple systems of medicine and healing compete with one another for patients and for political and economic support from NGOs, state governments and the central government, homeopathic doctors and homeopathic medical schools must struggle to maintain homeopathy's relevance. Although, in a state such as Tamil Nadu, the popularity of homeopathy is evidenced by the fact that there are more registered homeopathic doctors compared with that of any of the other medical systems within the AYUSH umbrella, homeopathy does not carry the mantle of indigeneity in the same way that the other AYUSH therapeutic systems do (particularly siddha in the Tamil context). Since indigeneity is often incorrectly associated with the concept of 'culture', I suspect that this may be one of the reasons for the lack of attention given to homeopathy among medical anthropologists in the past. Just as it took medical anthropologists a long time to recognise biomedicine as a cultural system of knowledge and practice worthy of ethnographic study and analysis, so too medical anthropologists have overlooked homeopathy in India because it has not been viewed as cultural or exotic, or linked to South Asian religious traditions. This chapter represents only the views of one homeopathic doctor, focusing on my analysis of her views on homeopathy in relation to my broader study on women and cancer in India, but it contributes to an emergent medical anthropological interest in homeopathy in South Asia.

Notes

1. This is a pseudonym to protect the anonymity of the doctor. I conducted the interview in English by her choice and recorded it with her consent.

2. 30 July 2015, Kancheepuram District, Tamil Nadu.

3. She referred to the middle class with the term 'literary people', though I believe she meant literate people since she later contrasted this group with people without education.

4. In India, biomedicine is most often referred to as allopathy.

5. 'Yunani' and 'unani' are two spellings of the same system of medicine.

6. These included biomedicine, ayurveda, unani, siddha, naturopathy and yoga.

7. See http://ayush.gov.in/about-the-ministry (accessed 25 January 2017).

8. Ibid.

9. Note that this only represents registered medical practitioners in each system of medicine. We know that in India, people often provide medical services without being registered. Sometimes they will falsify certification and registration. In other instances, a registered practitioner of one system of medicine may also use another system of medicine. For example, a siddha or ayurvedic doctor may sometimes recommend allopathic medicine or homeopathic medicine to patients who can buy most medicines over the counter without a prescription.

10. The leaves from the neem tree are widely used for medicinal and healing purposes in south India and are said to have 'cooling' properties.

11. Cinchona is a tree that is indigenous to South America. It is used for a wide variety of medicinal purposes. It is particularly well-known for the fact that it produces the alkaloid quinine, which is used to treat malaria. See http://www.lib.cam.ac.uk/deptserv/rcs/cinchona.html (accessed 3 February 2017).

12. According to Frank and Ecks (2004), Dr Radha's assertion that diet plays no role in homeopathic treatment reflects a very orthodox approach to homeopathy, which directly follows the ideas laid out by Hahnemann. In their ethnographic study in Bengal, however, Frank and Ecks found that most of homeopathic doctors there blended ayurvedic approaches to diet with their therapies, though in general they too followed Hahnemann's approach quite closely, and did not consider their practice to be a hybrid of homeopathy and ayurveda, contrary to Leslie's (1976a) assertion.

13. Hindus often burn camphor during puja worship.

References

Alter, Joseph (ed.). 2005a. *Asian Medicine and Globalization*. Philadelphia: University of Pennsylvania Press.

———— (ed.). 2005b. 'Ayurvedic Acupuncture—Transnational Nationalism: Ambivalence about the Origin and Authenticity of Medical Knowledge'. In *Asian Medicine and Globalization*, 21–44. Philadelphia: University of Pennsylvania Press.

Arnold, David. 1993. *Colonizing the Body: State Medicine and Epidemic Disease in Nineteenth Century India*. Berkeley: University of California Press.

Bhardwaj, Ruby. 2013. '"No One Medicine is Enough": Accounts of Complementary Therapy Practitioners in Delhi'. In *Multiple Voices and*

Stories: Narratives of Health and Illness, eds Arima Mishra and Suhita Chopra Chatterjee, 46–74. New Delhi: Orient BlackSwan.

Bhardwaj, S. M. 1980. 'Medical Pluralism and Homeopathy: A Geographic Perspective'. *Social Science and Medicine* 14B: 209–16.

Basham, A. L. 1976. 'The Practice of Medicine in Ancient and Medieval India'. In *Asian Medical Systems*, ed. Charles Leslie, 18–43. Berkeley: University of California Press.

Ecks, Stefan. 2013. *Eating Drugs: Psychopharmaceutical Pluralism in India*. New York: NYU Press.

Frank, Robert, and Stephan Ecks. 2004. 'Towards an Ethnography of Indian Homeopathy'. *Anthropology and Medicine* 11(3): 307–26.

Gupta, Brahmananda. 1976. 'Indigenous Medicine in Nineteenth and Twentieth Century Bengal'. In *Asian Medical Systems*, ed. Charles Leslie, 368–78. Berkeley: University of California Press.

Habib, S. Irfan, and Dhruv Raina. 2005. 'Reinventing Traditional Medicine: Method, Institutional Change, and the Manufacture of Drugs and Medication in Late Colonial India'. In *Asian Medicine and Globalization*, ed. Joseph Alter, 67–77. Philadelphia: University of Pennsylvania Press.

Halliburton, Murphy. 2009. *Mudpacks and Prozac: Experiencing Ayurvedic, Biomedical and Religious Healing*. Walnut Creek, CA: Left Coast Press.

Hausman, Gary. 2002. 'Making Medicine Indigenous: Homeopathy in South India'. *Social History of Medicine* 15(2): 303–22.

Jütte, R. 1996. 'Eine Späte Homöopathische Großmacht: Indien'. In *Weltgeschichte der Homöopathie. Länder, Schulen, Heilkundige*, ed. M. Dinges. München: C. H. Beck.

Kumar, Deepak. 2005. 'Health and Medicine in British India and the Dutch Indies: A Comparative Study'. In *Asian Medicine and Globalization*, ed. Joseph Alter, 78–87. Philadelphia: University of Pennsylvania Press.

Langford, Jean. 2002. *Fluent Bodies: Ayurvedic Remedies for Postcolonial Imbalance*. Durham: Duke University Press.

Leslie, Charles. 1976a. 'The Ambiguities of Medical Revivalism in Modern India'. In *Asian Medical Systems*, ed. Charles Leslie, 356–67. Berkeley: University of California Press.

——— (ed.). 1976b. *Asian Medical Systems*. Berkeley: University of California Press.

———. 1992. 'Interpretation of Illness: Syncretism in Modern Ayurveda'. In *Paths to Asian Medical Knowledge*, eds Charles Leslie and Allan Young, 177–208. Berkeley: University of California Press.

Leslie, Charles, and Allan Young (eds). 1992. *Paths to Asian Medical Knowledge*. Berkeley: University of California Press.

Montgomery, Edward. 1976. 'Systems and the Medical Practitioners of a Tamil Town'. In *Asian Medical Systems*, ed. Charles Leslie, 272–84. Berkeley: University of California Press.

Nichter, Mark. 1980. 'The Layperson's Perception of Medicine as Perspective into the Utilization of Multiple Therapy Systems in the Indian Context'. *Social Science and Medicine* 14B: 225–33.

———. 1996. 'Pharmaceuticals, the Commodification of Health and the Health Care: Medicine Use Transition'. In *Anthropology and International Health: Asian Case Studies*, eds Mark Nichter and Mimi Nichter, 265–328. London: Routledge.

Obeyesekere, Gananath. 1976. 'The Impact of Ayurvedic Ideas on the Culture and the Individual in Sri Lanka'. In *Asian Medical Systems*, ed. Charles Leslie, 201–26. Berkeley: University of California Press.

———. 1992. 'Science, Experimentation, and Clinical Practice in Ayurveda'. In *Paths to Asian Medical Knowledge*, eds Charles Leslie and Allan Young, 160–76. Berkeley: University of California Press.

Scheper-Hughes, Nancy and Margaret Lock. 1987. 'The Mindful Body: A Prolegomenon to Future Work in Medical Anthropology'. *Medical Anthropology Quarterly* 1(1): 6–41.

Taylor, Carl. 1976. 'The Place of Indigenous Medical Practitioners in the Modernization of Health Services'. In *Asian Medical Systems*, ed. Charles Leslie, 285–99. Berkeley: University of California Press.

Trawick, Margaret. 1992a. 'Death and Nurturance in Indian Systems of Healing'. In *Paths to Asian Medical Knowledge*, eds Charles Leslie and Allan Young, 129–59. Berkeley: University of California Press.

———. 1992b. 'An Ayurvedic Theory of Cancer'. In *Anthropological Approaches to Ethnomedicine*, ed. Mark Nichter, 207–22. Amsterdam: Gordon and Breach.

Van Hollen, Cecilia. 2005. 'Nationalism, Transnationalism, and the Politics of "Traditional" Indian Medicine for HIV/AIDS'. In *Asian Medicine and Globalization*, ed. Joseph Alter, 88–106. Philadelphia: University of Pennsylvania Press.

WHO. 2007. 'WHO Country Cooperation Strategy 2006–2011'. Supplement, August. WHO Country Office for India, New Delhi. Available at http://apps.who.int/iris/bitstream/10665/161138/1/WHO%20Country%20Cooperation%20Strategy%202006-2011%2c%20India%20Supplement.pdf (accessed 2 February 2017).

Zimmermann, Francis. 1992. 'Gentle Purge: The Flower Power of Ayurveda'. In *Paths to Asian Medical Knowledge*, eds Charles Leslie and Allan Young, 209–23. Berkeley: University of California Press.

Notes on the Contributors

Janet Chawla is Researcher, JEEVA project, and Founder-Director of MATRIKA, a Trust for research and advocacy on traditional midwifery and non-invasive birth methods, Delhi.

Cecilia Coale Van Hollen is Professor and Head of Studies, Anthropology, Yale-NUS College, Singapore.

Maya Annie Elias is a Ph.D. student at the University of Antwerp, Belgium.

Hariramamurthi Govindaswamy is Head, Centre for Local Health Traditions and Policy at the University of Trans Disciplinary Health Sciences and Technology, Bengaluru.

Sarika Kadam is an Independent Health Systems Researcher, Mumbai, Maharashtra.

Renu Khanna is the founder-trustee of SAHAJ-Society for Health Alternatives based in Vadodara, Gujarat.

Praveen Lal is a Research Associate at KRAN Consulting Private Limited, Thiruvanthapuram, Kerala.

Harilal Madhavan is Faculty Member, Humanities, Indian Institute of Science Education and Research (IISER), Thiruvananthapuram, Kerala.

Arima Mishra is Professor, Azim Premji University, Bangalore.

Sultana Mustafa Khanum is Professor, Department of Sociology, University of Rajshahi, Bangladesh.

Moe Nakazora is Associate Professor / Lecturer, Graduate School of International Cooperation and Development, Hiroshima University, Japan.

Devaki Nambiar is Program Head – Health Systems and Equity, George Institute of Global Health, Delhi.

Mark Nichter is Regents Professor Emeritus School of Anthropology, Department of Family Medicine and Mel and Enid Zuckerman College of Public Health, University of Arizona, Tucson, USA.

Unnikrishnan Payyappallimana is Principal Visiting Fellow at the United Nations University-International Institute for Global Health (UNU-IIGH) Kuala Lumpur, Malaysia.

Steffy Dhayalan is Principal Investigator at Rural Development Organisation (RDO Trust), The Nilgiris, Tamil Nadu.

Rajeev B. R. is Program Coordinator, ACCORD, Gudalur, Tamilnadu.

Debjani Roy is Advisor, Quality Council of India, New Delhi.

Sarin Sasikumar is at the Institute of Public Health, Bengaluru.

Brigitte Sebastia is a Medical Anthropologist Researcher, affiliated to the French Institute of Pondicherry and CEIAS (EHESS), Paris.

Shrish N. R. is the Co-Founder, Ideas Unbound, Bangalore.

Pooja Venkatesh is a Ph.D. student in sociology and social anthropology, Central European University, Budapest, Hungary.

Index